FATHERS AND VIOLENCE

Fathers and Violence

A Program to Change Behavior, Improve Parenting, and Heal Relationships

Carla Smith Stover

Foreword by Linda C. Mayes

THE GUILFORD PRESS
New York London

A Division of Guilford Publications, Inc.
370 Seventh Avenue, Suite 1200, New York, NY 10001
www.guilford.com

Printed in the United States of America

This book is printed on acid-free paper.

Last digit is print number: 9 8 7 6 5 4 3 2 1

The author has checked with sources believed to be reliable in her efforts to provide information that is complete and generally in accord with the standards of practice that are accepted at the time of publication. However, in view of the possibility of human error or changes in behavioral, mental health, or medical sciences, neither the author, nor the editors and publisher, nor any other party who has been involved in the preparation or publication of this work warrants that the information contained herein is in every respect accurate or complete, and they are not responsible for any errors or omissions or the results obtained from the use of such information. Readers are encouraged to confirm the information contained in this book with other sources.

Library of Congress Cataloging-in-Publication data

Names: Stover, Carla Smith, author.
Title: Fathers and violence : a program to change behavior, improve parenting, and heal relationships / Carla Smith Stover.
Description: New York : The Guilford Press, [2023] | Includes bibliographical references and index. |
Identifiers: LCCN 2023022991 | ISBN 9781462552986 (paperback) | ISBN 9781462552993 (cloth)
Subjects: LCSH: Family violence. | Abusive men—Psychology. | Abusive men—Behavior modification. | Violence in men. | Father and child. | BISAC: PSYCHOLOGY / Psychotherapy / Couples & Family | PSYCHOLOGY / Psychotherapy / Counseling
Classification: LCC HV6626 .S764 2023 | DDC 362.82/92—dc23/eng/20230626
LC record available at *https://lccn.loc.gov/2023022991*

About the Author

Carla Smith Stover, PhD, is Director of the Fathers for Change Program, Associate Professor at the Yale University School of Medicine Child Study Center, and a licensed clinical psychologist. Dr. Stover received a Career Award from the National Institute on Drug Abuse that initiated her research on interventions for fathers with intimate partner violence (IPV) behaviors. She developed Fathers for Change and has continued to conduct studies of the intervention. She has published widely on the topics of trauma, IPV, and substance misuse; has presented trainings internationally on the topics of family conflict, healthy relationships, family violence, engaging and treating fathers, and interventions for childhood trauma; and is on the editorial board of the journal *Advances in Dual Diagnosis*.

Foreword

In John Steinbeck's novel *The Grapes of Wrath*, after the Joad family has packed up their few possessions and left their dust-buried farm to find work and a way to survive together further west, Ma Joad observes, "All we got is the family unbroke. . . . I ain't scared while we're all here." Stark as the imagery is, this short line captures an enduring wish of many, if not all, families, that they will remain bound together, unbroken, united, and always present for each other, filled with love and caring. Still, just on the other side of that imagery and even for the Joad family themselves, violence and cruelty are often not too far behind. Tragically, domestic violence impacts many families at moments of high stress, is repeated over time, and leaves its mark across generations. Especially tragic is when one parent abuses the other as their children look on or hear from the next room. Not only are children often in danger themselves, they also are left alone psychologically trying to understand the powerful, destructive emotions and behaviors taking over their mother or father. No one in the home or family escapes the negative impact of domestic violence. Families are left broken apart despite the optimistic hopes they had when they came together.

To compound the tragedy, family violence often crosses generations. Adults who abuse children have a higher likelihood of having been abused themselves and/or exposed to domestic violence (Bartlett, 2017; Merrick & Guinn, 2018). Children witnessing or caught in the crossfire of domestic violence are at greater risk of repeating the same behavior when they have their own families. Much work in both human and preclinical models seeks to understand the mechanisms of how family abuse and violence are transmitted across generations. Epigenetic perspectives have added important dimensions to understanding how stress and trauma may alter the regulation of genetic expression, especially in those genes regulating the stress response (Zannas & West, 2014). We understand better how intervening with both children and their parents caught up in family violence may impact not only the immediate generation but generations to come. With the frame of a lasting intergenerational impact, finding effective interventions with a lasting impact becomes an even more urgent imperative. This is the goal of Dr. Stover's work with fathers and families generally caught in the spiral of domestic and intergenerational family violence.

In this volume, three unique features, artful in their presentation and broad in their impact, are worth calling out. The first is an intervention that is specifically geared toward fathers and toward considering the important and unique role fathers play in their children's lives. The second is a steady shifting of how clinicians relate to individuals who are caught up in domestic violence both as perpetrators and as victims. Closely related are Dr. Stover's efforts to have us make every effort to understand, not judge, the motivations, feelings, and beliefs of those who are violent toward their partner (and their children). And third is bringing attachment, mentalization, and lifespan perspectives to understanding the experience of individuals abusing their partners. Dr. Stover has a deep appreciation of the long trail of early childhood adversity reaching well into adulthood and impacting parenting, and how that adult can or cannot sustain intimate, caring relationships. This is one of the core premises of Fathers for Change—that fathers' early adverse experiences in childhood may be expressed in later interpersonal violence.

To the first—focusing on fathers. Historically, interventions with families generally and even normative studies of family functioning have been very maternal-centric and focused on a more traditional model of a two-parent family with a man and woman sharing parenting responsibilities. A few scholars have called attention to the unique role that fathers may play in their children's development (Clarke-Stewart, 1978; Lamb, 1995; Parke, 2002; Paquette et al., 2013). Further, clinical reports suggest that men—for example, in substance use treatment—report they are not asked whether they were fathers now or if they hoped to have children in the future (McMahon & Rounsaville, 2002). Parenting seems to be traditionally associated with mothering and men's experience of parenting often goes unnoticed or is underappreciated for its impact on the man's self-identity. Still, a number of observational studies suggest that when two adults are sharing the responsibility of parenting a child, they may intuitively (or based on their own experience of being parented) "divide" the task (Yaffe, 2020). One may be more focused on conveying ways to manage emotions and needs and interact more verbally while another may be action-oriented, engaging a child in activities and physical play. Of course, there are many other ways to share parenting responsibilities and there is not one model of either a family or parenting. But across studies, co-parenting seems to convey developmental advantages for children (Nunes, 2021) and fathers are key parenting partners. A focus of Dr. Stover's work, stated so eloquently in this volume and elsewhere (Stover et al., 2012), is that fathers have a very important role to play in their children's lives and that this role is also developmentally restorative for them as an adult. She shines a light not primarily on fathers as perpetrators of family violence but on the hope and possibility of restoring fathers' parenting roles in their children's lives and on restoring their coparenting role. In other words, her work puts a strong emphasis on helping men reconnect with their fathering roles and their identities as fathers instead of addressing only their violent behavior and assuming that healthier parenting will follow.

Rather than beginning with the view that fathers involved in domestic violence need remedial help in their parenting, Fathers for Change begins with the premise that fathers seeking help care about their children and want to ultimately feel competent in that role. Further, fathers under scrutiny for their angry, violent behavior may be particularly sensitive and resistant to interventions primarily focusing on the anger and harm they have caused. Instead, finding those moments when a father and his child are positively connected gives fathers the opportunity to see times when they are competent, when their child needs them, and then be naturally incentivized to strive toward more of these moments. Granting that fathers want to do better by their children and to care for and nurture them is a different starting point in considering the impact of domestic violence on children and on an adult's capacity to be a parent. Uniting with fathers around discovering the strengths in their parenting builds a working relationship between clinicians and fathers that potentially more effectively incentivizes fathers to learn more and then bring more of their concerns into the therapeutic space. At the same time, they also begin to understand how their anger and physical violence happens in the context of their relationship with their partner. This shift in emphasis is a key to one of the unique and impactful aspects of Dr. Stover's intervention.

This is difficult work. To bring parenting/fathering to the forefront in work around domestic violence means also confronting head on the strongly held, often unconscious attitudes that both the public and many, if not most, clinicians hold toward those who commit family violence. Especially for those working with children, it is very difficult both to hold the child's experience in mind and, at the same time, maintain an open, curious, and empathic stance toward the adults responsible for—or at least caught in—repeated acts of violence and abuse toward each other. Consciously or unconsciously, clinicians may be repelled, even frightened, by the violence and cruelty they witness in the father's history. They may feel pulled toward defending the partner, protecting the child or children, and judging, shunning, or closing down any effort to empathically connect with the father. Fathers for Change asks clinicians to confront and acknowledge their own biases and attitudes as they engage with families caught up in violence.

The intervention also asks clinicians to balance risk not just for a child but for the family as a whole as they engage the father in work that may be uncomfortable for both, ask him to consider past injuries he has caused or experienced; and, at the same time, offer the hope of being different. Depression with suicidality, posttraumatic stress disorder, crippling anxiety, and personality disorder are among the comorbid conditions commonly associated with those individuals who engage in family violence. These comorbidities make for challenging, sometimes harrowing, work. Clinicians must be comfortable holding in mind the risks for all the children and adults in the family while at the same time be genuinely dedicated to understanding a father's individual needs and wishes as a parent. They must be able to tolerate often considerable aggression or at the least ambivalence toward the father's partner and often child, and, at the same time, see the possibility of a positive outcome for the father. They also need to be comfortable with anger, hate, the possibility of violence, and ongoing breaks in a family that may continue even as the father works hard to change. A difficult balancing act for all involved—holding reality in one hand and hope in the other.

But all too often, the difficulty of working with such dark realities and those deeply held biases about individuals who perpetrate family violence means fathers who have abused their partners are not seen as individuals with unique experiences that shape their response to stress, their parenting, and their responses to their partners. They are seen as volatile, dangerous, and unchangeable. Fathers for Change offers a different, more empathic lens by integrating attachment and mentalization perspectives. In so doing, Dr. Stover encourages clinicians to look beyond the label of "domestic abuser" to better understand the individual's ability to reflect on and understand his own and others' emotions, beliefs, and desires that are driving behaviors. The attachment lens also brings a focus on the father's childhood experiences, including his own childhood adversity. Secure attachments are key to effective stress regulation in adulthood (Nolte, 2011). But early adversity may negatively impact the capacity for developing secure relationships that are stabilizing and present during stressful times.

Understanding that interpersonal violence is often the outcome of multiple adverse childhood experiences impacting adults' capacity to adaptively regulate stress and negative emotions opens up richer and more complex ways of understanding how a father may come to domestic abuse and break what he also loves. This more empathic, attachment-informed view of interpersonal violence and of fathers who abuse their partners puts relationships, past and present, front and center—the father's relationship with his partner and with his children. The power of this individualized, relationship-directed approach is in enhancing the father's understanding of his impact on his child and the salience of his relationship with his child for his own sense of competence and self-worth. Putting the relationship front and center also allows that interpersonal violence—past, present, or both—is not necessarily fate for life. Change is possible. What is broken can be restored. And like the Joad family, unbroken or shattered but restored may be all a family needs to keep going.

Linda C. Mayes, MD
Yale School of Medicine

REFERENCES

Bartlett, J. D., Kotake, C., Fauth, R., & Easterbrooks, M. A. (2017). Intergenerational transmission of child abuse and neglect: Do maltreatment type, perpetrator, and substantiation status matter? *Child Abuse and Neglect, 63,* 84–94.

Clarke-Stewart, K. A. (1978). And daddy makes three: The father's impact on mother and young child. *Child Development, 49*(2), 466–478.

Lamb, M. E. (1995). The changing roles of fathers. In J. L. Shapiro, M. J. Diamond, & M. Greenberg (Eds.), *Becoming a father: Contemporary, social, developmental, and clinical perspectives* (pp. 18–35). Springer.

McMahon, T. J., & Rounsaville, B. J. (2002). Substance abuse and fathering: Adding poppa to the research agenda. *Addiction*, *97*(9), 1109–115.

Merrick, M. T., & Guinn, A. S. (2018). Child abuse and neglect: Breaking the intergenerational link. *American Journal of Public Health, 108*(9), 1117–1118.

Nolte, T., Guiney, J., Fonagy, P., Mayes, L. C., & Luyten, P. (2011). Interpersonal stress regulation and the development of anxiety disorders: an attachment-based developmental framework. *Frontiers in Behavioral Neuroscience, 5,* 55.

Eira Nunes, C., De Roten, Y., El Ghaziri, N., Favez, N., & Darwiche, J. (2021). Co-parenting programs: A systematic review and meta-analysis. *Family Relations, 70*(3), 759–776.

Paquette, D., Coyl-Shepherd, D. D., & Newland, L. A. (2013). Fathers and development: New areas for exploration. *Early Child Development and Care, 183*(6), 735–745.

Parke, R. D. (2002). Fathers and families. In M. H. Bornstein (Ed.), *Handbook of parenting: Being and becoming a parent* (pp. 27–73). Erlbaum.

Stover, C. S., Hall, C., McMahon, T. J., & Easton, C. J. (2012). Fathers entering substance abuse treatment: An examination of substance abuse, trauma symptoms and parenting behaviors. *Journal of Substance Abuse Treatment, 43*(3), 335–343.

Yaffe, Y. (2020). Systematic review of the differences between mothers and fathers in parenting styles and practices. *Current Psychology,* 1–14.

Zannas, A. S., & West, A. E. (2014). Epigenetics and the regulation of stress vulnerability and resilience. *Neuroscience, 264,* 157–170.

Preface

If the consequence for family violence is limited to criminal sanctions or threatened loss of their children and family, fathers who have used violence are put in a position to deny accountability to avoid punishment. They are not given the space to honestly evaluate their behaviors and make meaningful change that will end the cycle of family violence. The system we need to create is one that asks for accountability by offering the support needed to create change.

I did not come to this realization right away. It has been a journey. Developing and advancing work with fathers who have caused harm has been a labor of love. The evolution of my own thinking has culminated in this book. Although it seems like as soon as I feel it's finished, I learn something new that I want to add or share, I want the ideas I've already gathered to be accessible to others as I continue to grow this work throughout the rest of my career. I hope the message of my work will begin to create change in how we approach those who have caused harm to their coparents and children.

I began as a bright-eyed graduate student working with the clinically brilliant Drs. Alicia Lieberman and Patricia Van Horn as they were developing and manualizing child–parent psychotherapy. I worked with mothers and their toddlers who had experienced family violence, and developed my dissertation examining the impact of father–child contact following family separation due to intimate partner violence (IPV). Doing that research was the beginning of my understanding of attachment, including the ways that children are attached to their fathers even when they have caused harm. It became clear that there was a need to find ways to help those fathers have healthy relationships with their children. This understanding grew as I continued my training at the Yale Child Study Center with the Child Development Community Policing Program responding to mothers who had experienced IPV, and to their children. We were providing support to women and children following such violence, and I noticed time and again that fathers were still in the home or would soon return following these incidents. We were there working to engage mothers and children in needed therapeutic supports, and mothers often reported they wanted help for their partners. They wanted a healthy family, and there were not services available to support families that wanted to remain together following an incident of IPV. There were no therapeutic services for their partners who had caused harm. Court-mandated "batterer groups" were the only option. I noticed child protective services often set a treatment plan that required mothers to engage in treatment services due to their experiences of IPV and to get help for their children. They also set expectations that mothers would leave their partners and protect their children. These expectations were not placed on the fathers who had caused harm, and they were also not provided any treatment opportunities. They were expected to leave the home with no supports. These early career experiences started me on the path to the development of Fathers for Change (F4C). I first received a small grant from the Annie E. Casey Foundation to pilot an intervention, and a subsequent Mentored Patient-Oriented Research Career Development Award (K23) from the National Institute on Drug Abuse to further develop the therapy and test it.

Convincing funders that treatment for those who use family violence is important has been much more challenging than I could have predicted. People want to fund and help victims but fail to think about the experiences that cause a person to use violence: What childhood experiences may prompt individuals to use violence as adults? Some have worried that offering individual and family therapy for fathers who have caused harm will put women and children at risk for further violence. My response to this is, what are we doing instead? If we do not offer comprehensive assessment and a treatment plan that we think will address the root causes of that individual's violent behaviors, what are we offering? Criminal justice responses such as "batterer or offender" programs? Jail time? Probation? An expectation that these alone will help people understand themselves and change despite rigorous research indicating the contrary? These approaches can cause feelings of shame, which do not allow people to be in a space to make change. When we use physical punishment with children, they learn to lie and hide their mistakes for fear of punishment. The same is true for adults who have used violence. I have seen it over and over in my work.

Fathers and Violence: A Program to Change Behavior, Improve Parenting, and Heal Relationships presents an alternative way of approaching accountability and treatment for family violence. I believe this individual therapy approach can ultimately keep families safer. To be clear, I am not arguing that there should be no criminal justice or child protection response to fathers' violent behavior toward their coparents or children. I believe the opposite: A coordinated community response must include protection of those who could be harmed, as well as *provision of appropriate treatments and services to help the person who is causing harm to change their behavior.* You will see in this book the ways that practitioners must coordinate with child protection and victim advocates to ensure safety of all family members. I have always approached this work with the safety and healing of those who have experienced violence and harm as a primary goal.

If you are hesitant about approaching fathers in ways that are not punitive or using intervention that is not a group format, I encourage you to read this book anyway. Digest its content and talk to others. I welcome constructive conversation that can move the field forward to benefit families. I have benefited from the tireless work of many amazing researchers and clinicians from a variety of fields (please do read the Acknowledgments section, where I thank the many people who have helped develop this work). In this book you will see therapy techniques drawn from other interventions, and I have acknowledged other treatment modalities that use them. It will take many of us testing different approaches and sharing what we learn to end family violence.

Often the fathers who are causing harm were maltreated or did not feel safe themselves in the past, and sometimes they still feel unsafe in the present. They have maladaptive ways of interacting that must be addressed through understanding and development of new ways of coping, communicating, and relating. This book is for anyone who wants to broaden their thinking about how to intervene with fathers who have caused harm. It is for *clinicians* and *therapists* (terms that are used interchangeably throughout the book) who want to provide this kind of therapy approach, which begins with individual therapy with the father and can flexibly add his coparent in individual collateral sessions, conjoint coparenting sessions, and father–child or family sessions as indicated by the needs of the individual case, family presentation, and safety. F4C focuses on coparenting relationships in all their forms, and any conjoint sessions are *not couple therapy but coparenting communication-building sessions, focused solely on the coparenting relationship to benefit their children.* It is also for individuals working or educating people in the field of family violence broadly (child protection, criminal justice, human services, college professors). It offers a compilation of ideas, some new and some arranged and integrated from other therapeutic approaches, that address the needs of this population.

In this book I describe the rationale for this kind of work, the theory behind it, and what research has told us not only about how family violence impacts children but also what they need and want from their fathers who have caused them harm. We discuss assessment strategies and how those strategies can inform intervention and safety planning with families. We then turn to how to engage a population that has been historically difficult to retain in treatment. We examine why this may be and how to approach engagement differently. The remaining chapters detail different phases of the F4C therapy approach, with case vignettes and examples to provide context for what the intervention looks like.

This book does not provide legal advice. It is imperative that anyone doing work with families who have experienced violence in the home familiarize themselves with local rules, laws, procedures, and reporting requirements that may arise, and, if needed, consult with a legal expert who can provide guidance on these issues. Having a trusted attorney who is familiar with the local laws as a consultant can be very helpful to clinicians working in the field of family violence.

I have not been able to help every father referred to me. This intervention approach is not foolproof, but I have seen it help hundreds of fathers and their families. F4C has been implemented as part of a coordinated community response by the Connecticut Department of Children and Families in their Intimate Partner Violence—Family Assessment Intervention Response (IPVFAIR). We have been training clinicians in the intervention across the state since 2015. There are now clinicians in Florida, Virginia, Rhode Island, and Vermont that are trained in this intervention approach. We have implemented it in substance use treatment programs (both outpatient and residential), community mental health agencies, parent and family mental health clinics, and agencies that provide in-home services, and we soon will start serving veterans in VA health care settings. Information about training and consultation in F4C can be found at the following website: *https://medicine.yale.edu/childstudy/education-and-training/professional-development/fathers-for-change*.

You will notice the use of person-centered language in this book, because I feel each client is a person first, and they are more than their worst behaviors. None of us want to be identified by the worst thing we've ever done. Why would we approach intervention that way? I believe that to provide treatment and create change, we cannot continue to refer to individuals who have caused harm as "batterers," "offenders," or "perpetrators." They are people who have perpetrated, used violence, or caused harm. This is the language you will see used throughout the book. We also use the term *coparent* instead of mothers or partners, because the family constellations and dynamics of relationships are varied, and this intervention can be applied to all different kinds of coparenting relationships. Coparents may be in an intimate relationship, or they may not. We also use *they/them* pronouns throughout the book for the same reason, as the gender identity and sexuality of the coparents should not be assumed.

This book has focused on those who identify as fathers and their use of violence. It does not mean that mothers do not perpetrate violence or need intervention. I felt it essential to focus on fathers, because they have often been marginalized in their importance, and when fathers use violence, the response is often gendered. I hope this book begins to combat preconceived notions about how to intervene and the needs of fathers in therapy.

To The Guilford Press and my editing team, Jim Nageotte and Jane Keislar, your input has been instrumental in developing this book. Without your patience and helpful editing suggestions, I do not think this project would have been finished.

To the fathers with whom I have worked over the last 20 years, thank you for trusting me and allowing me to learn from you. Without you, there would be no book.

Finally, I want to thank my husband, Wes, the father of my two amazing daughters, Madeliene and Charlotte. His support over the last 25-plus years has allowed me to become the best version of myself and to do the work that I do. He is an example of a father who experienced abuse and witnessed family violence, and worked hard to ensure that his own wife and children were loved and supported. Watching him with our daughters and the ways he has influenced their growth and expectations of how to be treated in relationships has been inspiring over the years. Breaking the cycle . . . men like Wes are an inspiration to me and another reason I will fight the rest of my life to ensure that fathers everywhere have an opportunity to receive appropriate, evidence-based treatments to make changes for their health and that of their family.

Contents

Purchasers of this book can download and print enlarged versions of select materials at *www.guilford.com/stover-materials* for personal use or use with clients (see copyright page for details).

CHAPTER 1

Family Violence

Theories and Intervention Approaches for Men

Family violence (FV), which impacts millions of families around the world each year, could be either one partner toward the other, or a parent toward a child. In other contexts, family violence also includes child aggression toward a parent, aggression among siblings, or even elder adult abuse. Interventions are often designed either for those identified as survivors or for those who have used violence. Considerations of family context or how to best conceptualize providing help to an entire family have been lacking, especially when legal systems and child protective services (CPS) are involved with families. Below is an example of a referral a clinician might encounter related to FV with legal and CPS involvement.

George and Susan were referred for assessment and intervention by CPS when a thoughtful social worker was concerned that the case plan was too burdensome for the family and would result in failure to reunify the couple's young children with their parents. George and Susan were homeless and living with Susan's mother when a verbal dispute escalated to yelling and throwing objects. A neighbor called police, resulting in George's arrest. The police notified CPS because the couple's 2- and 3-year-old children were home at the time of the incident. Initially the children remained in their parents' care; however, the parents both tested positive for marijuana and the mother for cocaine upon drug screening. Furthermore, review of CPS records indicated that Susan had been removed from her own mother's care as a child and had aged out of the foster system. Susan's mother's parental rights had been terminated. CPS felt that the home was unsafe for the children, but George and Susan had nowhere else to live. That, coupled with the intimate partner violence (IPV) and positive drug screens, resulted in CPS removing their children and placing them in a foster home about a 30-minute drive away. The initial case plan required both George and Susan to engage in treatment at separate addiction services agencies given their IPV. Susan had to engage in individual therapy and attend a parenting class. As is common, Susan's use of violence was assumed to be reactionary or in self-defense, so no assessment of her use of violence or recommendation for IPV use intervention was included in her case plan. George was required to complete a domestic violence intervention for offenders and attend a parenting class. Both parents were also required to maintain full-time employment, and they were expected to attain their own apartment that was suitable for the children. They were given 1 hour supervised visitation with their two children once per week, but they had to get transportation to the foster home. Neither had a car, and bus service to the foster home was an hour ride each way.

A TYPICAL CASE

This story is not unique. Referrals to multiple agencies/services without consideration of transportation difficulties, financial resources, and time can be frequent occurrences for parents trying to complete case plans to be reunified with their children. The CPS social worker was right to be concerned about the expectations of the department described in the case plan. Upon meeting with this family, the social worker found the parents to be extremely stressed about the requirements they were asked to fulfill, and they were longing to spend more time with their children. The plan was not in keeping with young children's sense of time: To adults, weekly contact seems frequent, but to young children, a week feels like an eternity. The case plan also did not consider the resources of the parents. Safety of the children was highest priority; however, the plan seemed to give no priority to their relationships with their parents and to setting the parents up for success. As this example illustrates, interventions that can meet the many and varied needs of families such as George and Susan's are needed so they are not hindered by the array of different services they are required to attend.

Individual assessments by the clinician with George and Susan indicated two parents in their early 20s who had no models of healthy relationships provided during their own childhoods. Both had experienced significant trauma that included witnessing IPV and their parents' misuse of substances. George admitted that at times he was aggressive and had trouble managing his anger. Susan also reported that she was aggressive toward George, hitting and pushing him when upset. Sometimes this was in self-defense and other times she became physical first. George said, "I just want to be a family. I know I can do better." Susan also wanted to maintain her relationship with George and was not fearful of him. Both wanted help with managing their emotions and communicating with each other. Neither parent was substance dependent, but they did use alcohol, marijuana, and occasionally other drugs to manage stress. George had a full-time job at an auto garage, but he found getting to his job by bus and meeting CPS program requirements difficult. The clinician-administered assessment conducted with both parents, along with a review of criminal and CPS records and an observation of the father with his children and the whole family together indicated young parents who required support and understanding. George needed to feel seen by his service providers as valuable to his children.

Depending on where they live and what service systems are available, interventions may not be available to meet the needs of families like that of George and Susan. Programs have historically focused on mothers and reuniting them with their children, especially when IPV is part of the story. This lack of treatment options has left couples who want to remain together and have a history of IPV behaviors without dyadic or family intervention options. This leads them to hide their ongoing relationship or plans to reunite from providers, especially those connected with CPS agencies. Alternative ways of working with families when family violence is identified is the focus of this book. Fathers for Change (F4C) is a flexible individual therapy program that can include coparent and family sessions as deemed appropriate and safe by the treating clinician. It is designed for fathers with a history of FV, either verbal or physical, in the last 12 months who have at least one child age 12 or younger. Coparents who also used FV (mutual or bidirectional violence is happening within the relationship) or those who are primarily survivors of the violence may participate. The intervention provides a phased and flexible intervention approach to family violence that can be implemented by a range of clinicians, from master's-level social workers in community-based agencies to psychologists in private practice. It is a program that can be offered or suggested by CPS agencies, family courts, domestic violence courts, or community providers. It also is a therapeutic approach that fathers or families can seek out on their own. This treatment comprises 18 "topics" that are organized into four phases, and combines attachment, family systems, and cognitive-behavioral theory (see Table 1.1). What makes it different from most other interventions is the focus on the father–child and the coparenting relationships.

It is important for providers of F4C to have background in both adult and child clinical work. Understanding child development and the impact

TABLE 1.1. Phases of F4C and Corresponding Topics and Session Types

Phase	Topic	Participants	Session type
Assessment	Father assessment	Father	Individual
	Coparent assessment	Coparent	Individual
	Child assessment	Child	Individual
	Family	Father, child (coparent optional)	Conjoint
1. Engagement and Motivational Enhancement	1. Introduction to Fathers for Change	Father Coparent	Individual Parallel individual
	2. Fathers' Roles and the Importance of Fathers to Child Development	Father Coparent (optional)	Individual Parallel individual
	3. Reflecting on Father–Child Interactions	Father Coparent (optional)	Individual Parallel individual
	4. Reflecting on the Family of Origin	Father Coparent	Individual Parallel Individual
2. Reflective Functioning and Skills Building	5. Exploring Triggers for FV, Need for Control, and Use of Substances	Father Coparent (optional)	Individual Parallel individual
	6. Understanding Emotional Arousal and the Body's Stress Response	Father Coparent (optional)	Individual Parallel individual
	7. Physiological Reactivity and Management Skills	Father Coparent (optional)	Individual Parallel individual
	8. How Thinking Impacts Behavior	Father Coparent	Individual Parallel individual

3. **Coparenting Communication**	9. Increasing Coparent Positive Interactions	Father Coparent	Individual in parallel OR conjoint
	10. Positive Communication Skills	Father Coparent	Individual in parallel OR conjoint
	11. Coparent Problem Solving, Part I	Father Coparent	Individual in parallel OR conjoint
	12. Coparent Problem Solving, Part II	Father Coparent	Individual in parallel OR conjoint
4. Restorative Parenting	13. Parenting Skills	Father Coparent	Individual in parallel OR conjoint
	14. Preparing to Make Amends	Father	Individual
	15. Taking Responsibility	Father Child	Conjoint
	16. Father–Child Play	Father Child	Conjoint
	17. Father–Child Feelings Identification and Expression	Father Child	Conjoint
Final Session	18. Ending Treatment	Father Coparent	Individual Individual in parallel

on children of witnessing violence is crucial to being able to help fathers develop better reflective functioning related to their children. Without this background, therapists may focus too heavily on the father's individual skills and not enough on helping him hold his children's experiences and needs in mind (which are key features of F4C). Importantly, the intervention addresses reflective functioning, emotion regulation, communication, and relationship difficulties, all while holding the safety and well-being of the children and their mothers as paramount.

CLARIFYING THE TERMINOLOGY

The terms *intimate partner violence* (IPV), *domestic violence* (DV), and *family violence* (FV) are often used interchangeably despite some notable differences between them. In this book I differentiate and will be as specific as possible when referring to forms of violence as defined below. The Centers for Disease Control and Prevention (2015) defines IPV as physical violence, sexual violence, stalking, or psychological harm by a current or former partner or spouse, occurring between heterosexual or same-sex couples, that does not require sexual intimacy. IPV differs from DV, which was originally introduced to define violence between married partners who were living together; DV has since expanded to include violence broadly among family members, such as an aunt toward a niece, between two adult brothers, and so forth. In this book, I most frequently use the term FV to indicate violence within the nuclear family, which may be either one partner toward the other, or a parent toward a child. In other contexts, FV also includes child aggression toward a parent, aggression among siblings, or elder adult abuse, but for purposes of this book, FV focuses on partner and parental use of violence toward each other or their children. Like IPV, FV occurs in multiple forms, including stalking, physical, sexual, and psychological violence. All forms have harmful consequences for family members. I use the term FV because F4C is an intervention approach designed to address violence between both current or former intimate partners, as well as parental violence toward children. When I use IPV or DV instead of FV, it is because the specific study, sample, or case is describing that form of violence in particular. I want to be consistent with how the research authors defined their sample and findings, or how a case is specific to IPV without other forms of family violence included.

Aside from these definitions, further distinctions have been made between different forms of FV in the literature. IPV, in particular, is often characterized by two frequently used categories: *situational couple violence* and *intimate terrorism* (Johnson, 2010). The first involves violent outbursts in the context of an escalating argument with an intimate partner. It is not planned and is usually the result of overwhelming emotion. This form of IPV can be used by both partners in the relationship and escalate bidirectionally. In contrast, intimate terrorism involves continuous coercive behavior used to progressively build and maintain power and control over the partner (Nielsen, Hardesty, & Raffaelli, 2016). The violence is manipulative, more frequently planned, and is used more often by men than by women. Sometimes patterns and different FV episodes do not fall neatly into these two categories. However, assessment of the level of power and control dynamics in a relationship and whether violence is reactive or planned are issues to which we return later, as they are important to assessment and intervention planning.

You will also notice the use of person-first language in this book to describe individuals who have inflicted violence. This is a purposeful choice, in that use of words like *abuser, offender,* or *perpetrator* have a negative connotation that sets the frame not for treatment, but instead for punishment. This book focuses on describing a treatment approach and therefore use of those words is minimized to focus on the individual process of changing behaviors that are harmful.

Last, I most frequently use the term *coparent* rather than spouse, wife, partner, husband, or mother throughout the book. Coparent is intended to encompass all the possible coparenting relationships that exist regardless of marital or relationship status, gender, and so forth. If a specific case example includes a mother and father, I may use those terms specifically in the case, but otherwise use the encompassing term *coparent.*

THEORETICAL EXPLANATIONS AND TYPOLOGIES OF FV USED BY MEN

There are multiple theoretical models of FV described in the literature. Some of these models have included feminist/power theory, social learning theory, trauma theory, and personality theory. The feminist or power theory emerged in the 1970s as the first intervention approaches were developed to hold men accountable for violence against women. This theory focuses on patriarchal gender roles and men's use of power and control over women (Burelomova, Gulina, & Tikhomandritskaya, 2018; Dobash & Dobash, 1979). Social learning theory posits that individuals learn violent ways of responding from figures in the home or community environment and fail to learn alternative ways of responding to conflict (O'Leary, Van Hasselt, Morrison, Bellack, & Hersen, 1988). This results in individuals repeating patterns learned in their family of origin related to use of FV. Trauma theory (Taft, Vogt, Marshall, Panuzio, & Niles, 2007) suggests that exposure to traumatic events across the lifespan leads to activation of neural structures that are related to the body's threat (fight-or-flight) response (Baldwin, 2013), which results in the brain and body being in persistent survival mode (Silove, 1998). Living in this mode can then result in the use of intimidation, threats, and rejection in response to distorted perceptions of threat in interactions with others (Chemtob, Novaco, Hamada, Gross, & Smith, 1997). Finally, personality theory focuses on the development of personality types via formative early experiences and relationships including borderline, antisocial, and narcissistic traits that are present in those who have used FV (Burelomova et al., 2018). Most research on these traits is associated with different typologies or categories of men who use violence. Some studies have also examined how different personality profiles respond to intervention. There is an indication that those with antisocial personality traits are less likely to complete interventions (White & Gondolf, 2000) and that different treatments may be needed depending on the personality characteristics of an individual who causes harm. For example, those with antisocial personality traits may respond better to cognitive-behavioral therapy (CBT), while those with dependent personality traits may do better in a more psychodynamic process-oriented treatment (Saunders, 1996).

Interventions have been designed based on these theoretical models of why men use violence against their partners or children. Power theorists argue that interventions should aim to shift the dominant discourse around which society is structured, whereby females are consistently perceived as subordinate to their male counterparts (Connell & Messerschmidt, 2005; Rothenberg, 2003). Social learning theory points to learning skills to manage emotions and conflict in nonviolent ways as the best course of intervention given that individuals did not previously learn these skills in their developmental environments (Beck & Fernandez, 1998). Trauma theory interventionists target social information processing related to perceived threat (Taft et al., 2013), while personality theorists assess personality styles and target interventions to specific traits such as narcissism. Generally, the power/feminist theory has had the most traction in intervention development and dissemination, but studies of broad implementation of group interventions based on this theory have not produced consistently effective findings (Arias, Arce, & Vilariñ, 2013; Babcock, Greene, & Robie, 2004; Cheng, Davis, Jonson-Reid, & Yaeger, 2021).

Aside from specific theories of FV, attempts have been made to categorize those who use violence into battering typologies. Gottman and colleagues (1995; Jacobson, Gottman, & Shortt, 1995) defined two: *Type 1 batterers,* who showed cardiac slowing (hypoarousal), and *Type 2 batterers,* who showed cardiac speeding (hyperarousal), each in response to a marital conflict discussion presented in a laboratory setting. Type

1 had more psychopathic traits and were thought to become calm and calculated in their use of violence, whereas Type 2 had greater substance misuse and psychopathology, and were considered reactive in their use of violence. Replication studies have not fully supported the broad distinction of these two types (Babcock, Green, Webb, & Graham, 2004; Meehan, Holtzworth-Munroe, & Herron, 2001). Holtzworth-Munroe, Meehan, Herron, Rehman, and Stuart (2000) proposed that rather than typologies per se, the focus should be on dimensions that fall on a continuum to help with understanding the etiology and nature of violence that may point to intervention. These dimensions include factors such as severity of violence (frequency and intensity), generality of violence (intimate partner only, others in the family, outside the family), psychopathology, and personality characteristics. The use of FV is not a psychiatric diagnosis but a behavior, and there is evidence for varying origins of the use of violence, differing characteristics and dimensions of importance for various individuals (Holtzworth-Munroe et al., 2000), and potential utility to examining individual motivations for the use of FV (Wride, 2020). Therefore, individual assessment that leads to the development of an intervention plan to meet the needs of each person who uses FV is needed, especially for those parenting children who may be impacted directly or indirectly by court-based decisions around custody and visitation.

INTERVENTION APPROACHES FOR MEN WHO HAVE CAUSED HARM

Intervention for FV by men has been addressed most frequently by what are referred to in the field as *batterer intervention programs* (BIPs). Currently, many BIPs comprise men's groups focused on the nature of power, control, and abuse in relationships, and in many states and jurisdictions are the standard response to FV following arrest and court involvement (Karakurt, Koç, Çetinsaya, Ayluçtarhan, & Bolen, 2019). This is not universally true, but is the most typical approach. Broadly and universally applied to all men appearing in court who use violence, without considering traits and typologies, BIPs have not been shown to be effective in randomized controlled trials (Cheng et al., 2021). The restriction and laws requiring use of men's groups as a response to FV is not identical across states, but it is common (Stover & Lent, 2014; Voith, Logan-Greene, Strodthoff, & Bender, 2020). There has been increased focus more recently on development of alternative interventions recognizing heterogeneity of needs of those who cause harm. Below are descriptions of some of the most commonly implemented and known interventions in the field at present.

Gendered Group Interventions

The Duluth model (Pence & Paymar, 1993) is the best known and is considered the most widely implemented BIP. Despite this, there is frequent confusion in the field about what the Duluth model entails, and evaluations of the program have focused on its psychoeducational group aspect. However, the group is intended to be embedded within a coordinated community response that encompasses arrests for IPV, sanctions for noncompliance with court orders, support and safety planning for survivors, and referrals to other agencies. The group component is characterized by its developers as a gender-based cognitive-behavioral approach to counseling and educating men arrested and mandated by the court to attend an IPV program. The group is focused on the *power and control wheel,* which outlines a variety of behaviors that constitute the constellation of possible abusive behaviors. This model also focuses on teaching and developing alternative skills for avoiding abuse and violence (Paymar & Barnes, 2007). Aside from the Duluth model, there are many gender-specific group BIPs. CBT groups focus on teaching ways of recognizing and managing anger. Others are a combination of both the gender-based model and CBT. Most of these models have not been rigorously tested in research trials.

Several other group-based approaches have been developed to target FV, including Achieving Change Through Value-Based Behavior (ACTV; Lawrence, Langer Zarling, Orengo, & Aguayo, 2014), Substance Abuse and Domestic Violence (SADV; Easton, Crane, & Mandel, 2018), and Strength at Home (SAH; Taft et al., 2013). All have shown promising evidence for the specific populations for which they were designed. Development of ACTV was based on acceptance and commitment therapy (ACT) principles. ACT builds on CBT and emphasizes using psychological flexibility, focusing on what is most effective rather than acting based on emotions or psychological responses (Hayes, Strosahl, & Wilson, 2009). Destructive behavior patterns are targeted through developing skills such as present-moment awareness, acceptance of difficult emotions or thoughts, decreasing believability of thoughts, perspective taking, identification of values, and committed action in service of values. The ACTV model does not involve teaching or requiring that participants change the *content* of their thoughts but instead involves change in the way they *respond* to their thoughts in order to change their behavior (Zarling, Bannon, & Berta, 2019). ACTV has been shown to reduce IPV recidivism in randomized trials compared to the Duluth model, but it has higher dropout rates (Zarling et al., 2019).

Strength at Home (SAH) is a CBT group model developed using trauma theory. It was implemented initially with veterans or active-duty service members returning from deployment. This model focuses on information processing deficits that may interfere with partner interactions. The 12-session group includes psychoeducation on IPV and trauma reactions, conflict management skills, identifying and correcting negative thought patterns, and communication skills (Taft et al., 2013). SAH participants had significantly greater reductions in IPV than those in enhanced standard services within the VA setting (Taft et al., 2013).

Delivered in both group and individual formats, SADV targets the intersection of substances misuse and violence in each session (Easton et al., 2007, 2018) and development of coping skills for both violence and substance misuse. Both the group and individual format of SADV showed significantly less use of IPV on days of substance use than either group or individual drug counselling (Easton et al., 2007, 2018).

All these group approaches consider some of the possible factors that can contribute to a person's use of violence (e.g., gendered views on women's roles, distorted cognitions, trauma reactivity, and substance use) and each has strengths. What is lacking in these approaches is an individually tailored focus on family interactions and dynamics, as none of these provide one-on-one sessions with fathers to address the impact of violence on their children. Completion of any one of these programs alone would not address the coparenting and restorative parenting required to make amends with children and develop healthy father–child relationships (see Chapters 8 and 9), or how to safely consider father–child relationships following FV. Coparenting includes the shared responsibilities of raising a child, whether in an intimate relationship or not. Restorative parenting is an approach that focuses on repair rather than punishment. It allows those who have caused harm to take accountability and make amends for their mistakes to those they have hurt. In this case, fathers take accountability for the harms they have caused to their children through use of FV and make amends.

Couple Interventions

Although often controversial (and, in the United States, not acceptable in some states as a court-ordered intervention for IPV offenders), couple interventions have been developed and a few tested in research studies. The intervention with the most clinical and research writing is domestic-violence-focused couple therapy (Stith, McCollum, & Rosen, 2011). It is a solution-focused, brief therapy intended for couples who are experiencing mild to moderate situational couple violence and want to stay together and end the violence in their relationship. It has two possible formats: a multicouple group approach or an individual couple treatment approach (Stith et al., 2011). The 18-week model utilizes two cotherapists who first work separately with the male partner and the female partner (typically for about 6 weeks), bringing them together only after the individual components are completed and the therapists believe that working with the couple together is clinically appropriate and safe. The intervention continually emphasizes use of violence as a choice. This therapy addresses the interactional nature of relationships and provides treatment for both members of the couple that may support ongoing assessment of safety and change. This could be especially helpful to survivors of violence as they determine whether a healthy relationship is possible with the person who harmed them. This treatment does not address family dynamics and father–child relationships specifically; however, it provides a great framework for how to initiate intervention with each member of a couple when there has been FV and consider how to safely facilitate conjoint sessions. This strategy of parallel sessions with each member of the couple and coming together only when deemed safe and appropriate by the treating clinicians is the same strategy used in F4C. Parallel sessions with coparents are done in the early stages of treatment, with the possibility of conjoint coparenting sessions later in treatment.

Father-Specific Interventions

There are several well-known interventions in the field which have been used with fathers who caused harm that focus on their roles as fathers. These include: the Caring Dads program (Scott, Francis, Crooks, & Kelly, 2006); Child–Parent Psychotherapy (CPP; Lieberman, Ippen, & Van Horn, 2015), and Alternative for Families—Cognitive-Behavioral Therapy (AF-CBT; Kolko, Herschell, Baumann, Hart, & Wisniewswki, 2018).

Caring Dads is a group parenting intervention for fathers who have used violence toward either their partners or children. It includes contact with children's mothers and coordinated case management to mitigate the risk fathers may pose to their partners and children. The intervention has shown promising reductions in FV (Scott & Crooks, 2007; Scott & Lishak, 2012), and focuses on fathers' behaviors and understanding their children's needs but offers no direct treatment of the children together with their fathers. Completion rates in a large implementation study in Australia were 63% of fathers who started the program. The program increased the amount of time fathers spent with their children; however, it did not appear to impact use of violence or mothers' fear of fathers based on the small number of coparenting mothers who provided pre–post data in the evaluation (Diemer et al., 2020).

CPP is a treatment for trauma-exposed children ages 0–5. Typically, children are seen with their primary caregiver, and that dyad is the unit of treatment. The CPP model aims to examine how trauma and the caregiver's relational history affect the caregiver–child relationship and the child's developmental trajectory. A central goal is to support and strengthen the caregiver–child relationship as a vehicle for restoring and protecting the child's mental health (Lieberman et al., 2015). CPP has been shown to improve posttraumatic stress symptoms for both young children and their mothers who experienced IPV (Lieberman, Ippen, & Van Horn, 2006). CPP was not designed specifically for dyadic work with fathers who have caused harm. It was first developed and tested with survivors of FV and their young children, but it has since been provided to fathers and their young children with anecdotal success (Iwaoka-Scott & Lieberman, 2015; Lieberman & Van Horn, 2011). CPP has been adapted to provide a coparenting model whereby a single therapist provides therapy to both mother–child and father–child dyads in parallel, allowing the therapist to understand the dynamics children are experiencing in their triadic relationship with each of their parents. This approach has not yet been tested in a randomized trial.

AF-CBT is a trauma-informed CBT-based treatment designed for parents who have caused harm and their children. It is intended to reduce the effects of exposure to child or family anger, aggression, and child physical abuse. AF-CBT teaches parents and children (ages 5–17) skills to enhance self-control, promote positive family relations, and reduce violent behavior. Other goals of AF-CBT include promoting nonaggressive discipline and interactions, reducing child physical abuse risk or recidivism, and improving the level of child safety and family functioning (Kolko et al., 2012). The intervention includes both individual sessions with the caregiver and child, and conjoint parent–child sessions. A randomized trial revealed that children who received AF-CBT had lower posttraumatic stress disorder (PTSD) symptoms compared to treatment as usual at 6-month follow-up but not at 18-month follow-up. There was also a greater reduction in family dysfunction, conflict, and reports of child physical abuse for the AF-CBT group (Kolko et al., 2018).

What Is Missing?

Overall, there is now a range of interventions to address FV. Many are group-based, with a few individual or dyadic options that address both the individual and family needs. Few provide guidance on work with coparents together or how to intervene with fathers and their children. Furthermore, the current system of care for FV is often siloed, with those who cause harm and their families being treated separately, without coordination among providers or across systems. This is quite concerning because, in most cases, children from homes where there has been violence continue to see the fathers who have caused harm, either because the family has reunified, the father has shared custody, or the court has ordered visitation. Thus, not only does intervention for children exposed to FV need to target traumatic stress symptoms and the relationship with the nonoffending parent, but it also needs to consider ensuring an end to children's exposure to violence. This may be achieved in some cases through effective treatment for the parent who caused harm, and reparative intervention for the children to restore a safe and healthy relationship with that parent. There is ample justified concern for how to implement such work, and what is needed for fathers who cause harm to be ready to participate in treatment safely with their children.

The field has developed many interventions that focus on maltreating mothers and repairing the mother–child attachment and relationship. The field has not advanced as quickly in work with fathers who have used FV. Clinical treatment for FV largely comprises services aiding survivors. Far fewer treatment providers (individuals and agencies) offer services to those who have caused harm, who are more typically men and often fathers. There is ample need for treatment approaches to work with fathers safely, so they can develop healthier relationships with their children. Adapting those interventions that were designed for survivors and their children (e.g., CPP) must be done carefully with fathers who have caused harm, with deliberate attention to assessment and fathers' readiness to engage in a fully dyadic model. AF-CBT was designed specifically to work with offending parents and their children, but it is not intended for infants, toddlers, or preschool-age children.

In most states, following an incident of FV reported to the police, CPS is notified if children are in the home. In CPS-involved families, mothers and children often receive intensive in-home safety planning and counseling that is focused on their needs. Fathers are often ordered to leave the home and are frequently court-ordered to a batterer intervention group because it is the only treatment option available. This may be because the state where they live requires a gender-based group BIP, or because alternative interventions are not offered in their community. There is limited ability to tailor the topics of this type of group to the specific needs of fathers, or to focus substantial time on parenting and fatherhood, since fathers make up only a proportion of participants, limiting group cohesion around this topic. Services are often not offered to fathers that would address their roles as father or coparents. Instead, they are labeled as batterers, offenders, or perpetrators, putting them in a defensive position that may limit their willingness to engage and minimizes their importance as fathers. This gap also means the burden of protecting the children and addressing their mental health needs is placed on mothers.

F4C was developed to fill these gaps in evidence-based interventions for fathers who use FV and to provide an alternative or adjunctive treatment when appropriate. F4C was originally developed through funding by the National Institute on Drug Abuse (NIDA) through a K23 career award, with an initial focus on fathers with co-occurring IPV and substance misuse, and was broadened to encompass fathers, with a dual focus on IPV and child maltreatment as the intervention was implemented within the community. This intervention provides services to fathers to benefit their children, an area of significant need in the field (Gordon, Oliveros, Hawes, Iwamoto, & Rayford, 2012; Labarre, Bourassa, Holden, Turcotte, & Letourneau, 2016; Maxwell, Scourfield, Featherstone, Holland, & Tolman, 2012), and is in keeping with calls for interventions that will work with families impacted by FV in different ways to address the needs and wishes of survivors (Arroyo, Lundahl, Butters, Vanderloo, & Wood, 2017).

As stated earlier, F4C was designed to provide detailed guidance on individualized assessment of families and a phased approach toward coparenting and father–child intervention that maps onto individual family needs safely. With F4C, a clinician can assess and understand a father and his family and provide interventions to help him individually (based on what is driving his violent behavior) and in his relationships with his coparent and children. It brings in components of other evidence-based interventions such as motivational interviewing (Miller & Rollnick, 2023), CBT (Beck & Fernandez, 1998), dialectical behavior therapy (DBT; Linehan, 2020), behavioral couples therapy (O'Farrell & Fals Stewart, 2012), CPP (Lieberman et al., 2015), and parent–child interaction therapy (PCIT; McNeil & Hembree-Kigin, 2011). The unique features of F4C are (1) a phased approach to addressing the needs of fathers who use FV that moves from assessment through individual focused work and ends with coparenting and family components, (2) flexible inclusion of coparents and children, and (3) a continual focus on reflective functioning related to self, partner, and children. Chapter 4 provides both a description of the intervention and the theoretical framework.

In the coming chapters I present the theoretical underpinnings of the F4C approach. First, in Chapters 2 and 3, we consider the importance of fathers in the lives of their children, the parenting behaviors of fathers who have caused harm, and what children will need from their fathers following FV, as well as the research supporting F4C. Chapter 5 gives details on how to assess and select appropriate cases, Chapters 6 through 9 provide step-by-step guides for conducting the work—covering 18 topics—in sessions with fathers, their coparents, and children. Chapter 10 gives details on ending treatment and referrals.

CHAPTER 2

Parenting by Men Who Have Caused Harm

There is now ample evidence to support the positive role fathers play in children's development. Meta-analytic findings indicate that fathers' involvement is associated with their children's improved cognitive, academic, and social functioning (Amodia-Bidakowska, Laverty, & Ramchandani, 2020; Rolle et al., 2019). Increased father involvement and positive father–child play are associated with better school performance (improved measures of learning, including reading and math), especially if fathers are involved with their children's academics (Cano, Perales, & Baxter, 2019; Rolle et al., 2019). This association has been found to be particularly strong among children who are disadvantaged, including those in low-income communities and attending subpar educational systems (Mathwasa & Okeke, 2016). Fathers' and mothers' parenting styles and relationships with their children can individually and uniquely influence child academic performance (Waterman & Lefkowtiz, 2017). Although not universally true for all fathers or mothers, studies indicate generally that fathers tend to focus on preparing their children for the future through modeling and problem solving, providing structure, discipline, and responsibility (Henry, Julion, Bounds, & Sumo, 2020), which benefits children's overall functioning across domains. Specific to emotional expression and regulation, a study of 3- and 4-year-old children indicated that children with more positively expressive fathers also showed more positive emotional expression. Fathers' emotion coaching, but not mothers', was predictive of children's increased positive expression in laboratory observations 1 year later.

This outcome indicates fathers' unique contributions to the development of their young children's emotional socialization (Gerhart et al., 2020).

Conversely, children exposed to suboptimal father involvement may experience social–emotional, developmental, and educational challenges that can extend into adolescence and adulthood (Gillette & Gudmunson, 2014), including increased likelihood of substance misuse, involvement with the criminal justice system, and teen pregnancy (Harper & McLanahan, 2004). Father involvement is often dichotomized into fathers' presence or absence in their children's lives. In reality, this demarcation is rarely clear and simple, and can be influenced by many factors, including marital and residency status, race, and coparenting relationships (Cabrera, Hofferth, & Chae, 2011; McLanahan, Tach, & Schneider, 2013). What constitutes enough contact to be considered present versus absent is difficult to distinguish, especially since children of different developmental ages experience time differently. For example, is one full weekend a month the same as one night a week? Are overnight visits necessary? It is likely not simply the quantity of contact with the father that is most important, but the quality of the time spent and the range of parenting activities the father engages in during his time with his children.

Although greater positive father involvement has significant benefits to children, when there has been family violence, there may be negative impacts, such as ongoing stress, chaos, fear, or trauma. The impact of that violence and ongoing safety concerns must be considered, and determinations are needed about how children can reap the benefits of a positive father–child relationship, while mitigating the negative impacts that exposure to FV have on children's development (Jouriles & McDonald, 2014). Furthermore, there is evidence that harsh parenting by fathers has a greater association with adolescent delinquency than does father absence (Simmons, Steinberg, Frick, & Cauffman, 2018), indicating that time with fathers on its own in the absence of supportive parenting may not be better for the child. Therefore, interventions that can help fathers have supportive and healthy relationships with their children are needed to combat these potentially negative outcomes. F4C aims to have fathers maintain contact with their children while working to reduce conflict in both the father–child relationship and the coparental relationship.

RESEARCH ON FATHERS WITH HISTORIES OF FV

Depending on the nature of FV, children may be experiencing violence between their parents, be direct targets of violence themselves, or both. When thinking about parenting in this context, it is necessary to disentangle IPV from abuse directed toward the child (e.g., physical or psychological abuse of the child). Approximately half of children who live in homes with IPV also experience child maltreatment in the form of physical abuse, psychological abuse, or neglect (Ahmadabadi et al., 2018; Hamby, Finkelhor, Turner, & Ormrod, 2010) by one or both parents. Children who experience multiple forms of child maltreatment and witness IPV are more likely to experience the poorest outcomes (Osofsky, 2003; Stover, Ippen, Liang, Briggs, & Berkowitz, 2019). Whether fathers directly maltreat their children or expose them to IPV, there are some characteristics of fathers who use FV that are important to understand when considering intervention and how they may engage with service providers.

Studies of men with histories of IPV indicate that they display more gender-stereotyped beliefs and behaviors, and use more authoritarian and abusive parenting methods compared to fathers with no history of IPV (Fox & Benson, 2004; Maliken, Fainsilber, & Katz, 2013). Community-recruited samples of fathers with histories of IPV self-report more hostile, aggressive parenting toward their children (i.e., "I yell at my children when they do not deserve it," "I hit my children when they don't deserve it") and taking part in fewer stimulating activities with their children (e.g., reading books, playing games, telling stories; Adhia & Jeong, 2019; Stover, Easton, & McMahon, 2013). However, these fathers report no differences in use of spanking for discipline compared with men without histories of IPV (Adhia & Jeong, 2019). Also of concern is that some fathers who use IPV are unaware of the consequences of this behavior on their children (Mohaupt & Duckert, 2016; Rothman, Mandel, & Silverman, 2007; Salisbury, Henning, & Holdford, 2009). They focus on not using physical abuse toward their children while failing to understand the detrimental impact of the treatment of their children's mothers (Stover & Spink, 2012).

Beyond physical violence toward their children, fathers who use IPV may be more likely to use an authoritarian parenting style, view their children as possessions, and disregard their thoughts and feelings (Bancroft, Silverman, & Ritchie, 2012), which have harmful impacts on child development. These characteristics may also play out in the way they engage in a therapeutic intervention that includes restorative parenting. They may attempt to use participation in the intervention in order to look good to the court or prove they are interested and involved fathers but have limited interest in fully engaging in the therapeutic process. These issues are explored further in Chapters 5 and 9.

Some studies have indicated that fathers who have used IPV express a strong desire to have close and warm father–child relationships (Fox, Sayers, & Bruce, 2002; Perel & Peled, 2008; Rothman et al., 2007). This finding is important, because paternal sensitive caregiving has been found to interrupt the path that leads from children's IPV exposure to poor representations of their father–child relationships (Zvara & Mills-Koonce, 2021). When fathers who have used IPV behaviors can provide sensitive caregiving to their children, this can be protective to the father–child relationship. Some fathers who are violent and abusive toward their intimate partners can contrastingly be sensitive and warm with their children, particularly their very young children (Stover, 2015b). However, this is not global, so one should not make assumptions about a particular father–child relationship without careful assessment.

Mohaupt, Duckert, and Askeland (2021) found that one of the key issues preventing sensitive caregiving by fathers who had used FV was that they seldom explored their children's experiences. They failed to make efforts to understand their children's inner lives, an indication of impaired *reflective functioning,* the inability to imagine feelings and thoughts of themselves and others. Instead, their fathering was influenced by their own past relationships and negative expectations for the future. They defined their success as fathers through their children's well-controlled behavior, and they often felt their good parenting was not recognized by others. Another key finding was that fathers who had used FV found their emotional arousal (in the form of physiological or bodily responses) difficult to control and understand. These types of reactions indicate fathers' poor emotional understanding and reflective functioning, and how they impact their behaviors and parenting. Intervention that both focuses on a father's life experience and context and how it is influencing his parenting and helps him consider the emotions and experiences of his children, may increase positive connection in the father–child relationship.

Coparenting

The few studies on coparenting in IPV have found greater coparenting conflict and less feelings of support reported by couples with a history of IPV (Fainsilber & Low, 2004; Stover et al., 2013); however, different types of IPV behaviors are associated with greater coparenting conflict. Men who used *situational couple violence* (violence that occurs in the context of an argument and lacks coercion and control) exhibited less conflictual coparenting than those who used coercive controlling behaviors (Hardesty, Khaw, Chung, & Martin, 2008). In a recently divorced sample, fathers with coercive controlling behaviors had lower coparenting quality, higher levels of conflict, and less interest in fostering positive father–children relationships than those with situational couple violence (Hardesty, Crossman, Khaw, & Raffaelli, 2016; Hardesty et al., 2017).

A study of the narratives of fathers who have used FV revealed overwhelmingly negative evaluations of ex-partners, predominant patterns of blaming mothers for difficulties, and lack of insight into the impact of coparenting conflict on children (Thompson-Walsh, Scott, Dyson, & Lishak, 2018). Of significant concern, some men may try to control or terrorize their ex-partners by refusing to return children after visits or threatening to harm, abduct, or keep the children from the mother (Greif & Hegar, 1993; Johnston & Girdner, 2001). Ongoing conflict over visits and concerns about safety make coparenting in families with FV challenging and sometimes impossible, and can put mothers and their children at ongoing risk for poor physical and mental health outcomes. However, if coparenting can be improved, it can significantly benefit children, as healthy coparenting can buffer the impact of past conflict and IPV (Fainsilber & Low, 2004) making it a key consideration for assessment and intervention.

Risks to Children by Fathers Who Use Violence

Children exposed to ongoing FV are at risk for a host of psychosocial difficulties and symptoms. Stopping exposure to violence is crucially important to optimal child development. As mentioned earlier, father involvement and healthy father–child relationships are also associated with improved child developmental trajectories. Balancing these two factors is key in making decisions about children's ongoing contact with fathers who have caused harm. There are other risks to children from these fathers that must be assessed and considered: their potential use of the children to control their partners, or to gather information about the mother and purposefully lying to the children about the mother or otherwise trying to alienate them from her. This ongoing stress to children is harmful and must be considered in making custody and placement decisions, and it must be evaluated as part of any treatment program that will work with fathers who have been violent and their children. Details about assessment and suggested instruments are provided in Chapter 5.

Safety and Legal Considerations

When approaching this population to provide treatment, there are safety and legal issues that need to be considered at the forefront. Safety of all members of the family and the clinician, as well as legal requirements for mandated reporting, court orders related to contact of family members or treatment requirements must be assessed and understood to develop plans for parenting focused intervention. The following two sections address some of these important issues.

Safety Considerations

Fathers in general are often ignored or minimized in their roles as parents by service providers from all areas of health and education. Clinics, health care centers, and schools have historically not prioritized contact with fathers or father engagement, although there have been recent efforts to change this (Cox, Smith, Brown, & Fitzpatrick, 2007; Lawrence, Watson, & Stepteau-Watson, 2013; Maxwell et al., 2012). Add FV into the equation and children's services have often avoided contact or prohibited involvement of fathers who have caused harm in services, in the name of ensuring safety of the mother and children. Safety is paramount, and providing safe spaces for survivors is necessary, but universal exclusion or lack of contact is not the best policy, since father absence even following IPV can have negative impacts on children, such as increased depressive and anxious symptoms (Stover, Van Horn, & Lieberman, 2006; Stover, Van Horn, Turner, Cooper, & Lieberman, 2003). Treatments for child trauma and PTSD are designed specifically for the nonoffending parent and child, and little guidance is provided about how a provider might include or engage the parent who caused harm in a therapeutic way. CPS agencies have traditionally put service requirements on mothers (including keeping the father away from the children) and failed to provide access or opportunity for appropriate therapeutic services to a maltreating father that would be provided to a maltreating mother. The following vignette provides an example of how including a father who has caused harm in treatment following FV can have significant benefits to their children's recovery.

CASE EXAMPLE: SUSAN AND PETER

Five-year-old Jimmy and his mother, Susan, were in treatment at a community-based mental health clinic following an incident of IPV in which Jimmy's father, Peter, broke into their house and attempted to strangle Jimmy's mother. Jimmy and his older sister fled the house to a neighbor's and called the police, who arrived and arrested their father. Peter and Susan had recently separated and were going through a divorce. Peter was diagnosed with bipolar disorder and was not taking his medications. When Jimmy and Susan began CPP, Peter had completed his domestic violence diversion program and was in individual treatment for his bipolar disorder. There was a no contact order pertaining to Susan, but the order allowed for Peter to have several hours of visitation with his children each week. The agency where the therapist worked normally did not contact or engage fathers who had used IPV, and its treatment services focused on survivor mothers and their children. During dyadic CPP sessions, the topic of Jimmy's visits with his father came up. There were themes in his play about characters visiting their fathers and wanting to be in control of the timing of their visits and for how long. Jimmy was nervous talking about visits with his father in front of his mother, so the therapist used the play to attempt to understand Jimmy's wishes and translate them for his mother. The character in Jimmy's play did not like visiting his father on a given day, because he wanted to play that day with his friends. He also did not like the way that sometimes the visit dates changed and came up unexpectedly. The therapist reflected back, "The boy doesn't like it that his dad changes the visits sometimes. It makes him feel worried. He wants to know when the visits will happen in advance. He also doesn't like to miss time with his friends. I wonder if talking to his parents would help?" At this point, Jimmy looked up at the therapist, then looked quickly at his mother. The mother, bewildered, looked at the therapist, who then said, "I'm wondering if sometimes you get worried when visits are changed with your dad?" Jimmy nodded. "Jimmy, do you think it would be OK if I contacted your dad? I could talk with him about the visits and see if we can find a schedule that works better?" Jimmy nodded and looked at his mother. She smiled and responded, "That would be OK." The therapist and Susan discussed this plan together after the dyadic session to ensure that Susan felt comfortable with Peter having contact with the therapist and knowing where their therapy was conducted. She felt that as long as he did not know the days/times of their sessions, this would be OK. The therapist contacted Peter, explained her role, and invited him to meet with her. She was unsure what to expect from this father given his prior violence. When he arrived, he was dressed professionally and appeared very anxious. He wanted to be sure the therapist knew he cared about his son. She used his stated motivation to do what was best for his son to talk with him about his son's symptoms related to the IPV incident, and his need for a consistent routine with visits and to have some control over contact with his father. Peter understood and agreed to modify the visiting schedule to make it less stressful for Jimmy. When Jimmy arrived at session the next week, he began playing with the toys and said he had had a good visit with his dad, and they went fishing. He looked at his mom carefully to ensure that she was OK with this disclosure. The therapist asked him follow-up questions and said she was glad he had a good visit.

In this example, the therapist's willingness to reach out to the father and have contact with him made a big difference to her client. She did not engage him in the CPP but began to include him in collateral sessions when she deemed it would advance the treatment. Assumptions could have been made that this father would be unreasonable or unwilling to change his behavior or visitation plan, or that contacting him would put his ex-wife or children in danger without talking about the issue of safety directly with the mother. Not including the father in the treatment process would also have deprived him of the opportunity to know how his behaviors were impacting his son. If Jimmy's father had responded differently to her outreach or been unwilling to make accommodations for his son's needs, the therapist would have understood the reality of the tension that would remain related to visits and the father's inflexibility. She would then be able to work with Jimmy and Susan in CPP to help Jimmy cope with the uncertainty of visits. Either way, she learned salient information to inform and enhance the treatment.

Another consideration is that sometimes safety concerns can be misused to prevent fathers from having contact with their children. Even when visitation is granted, mothers can gatekeep or prevent children from seeing their fathers. There are multiple reasons this can happen: (1) Mothers may be truly fearful of fathers' involvement with their children; (2) mothers' own posttraumatic symptoms are triggered by their children's contact with their father, who caused the mother harm; (3) mothers are using access to the children to get something that they want (e.g., money, to control the father's other relationships). No matter the reason, assessment of whether lack of contact is truly in the child's best interest is valuable.

CASE EXAMPLE: MOIRA AND MALCOLM

A domestic incident between Moira and Malcolm resulted in a full no-contact protective order. Malcolm moved out of the house and Moira filed for divorce. Malcolm followed the protective order and did not contact the family. When the protective order ended and Malcolm tried to arrange visits with their 6-year-old son, Zahid, Moira indicated she was not comfortable with Malcolm visiting with Zahid because she thought Zahid was afraid of him. She said he did not want to be alone with his father. Malcolm was enrolled in F4C, and his therapist contacted Moira regarding setting up therapeutic contact with Zahid in which the therapist could be present to help reintroduce Zahid to his dad in a safe and therapeutic way. Moira agreed to starting with a phone call between Malcolm and Zahid, facilitated by the therapist. At the time of the phone call, Moira was listening in and interrupted the conversation to ask Malcolm when he would sign documents for Zahid to attend an expensive summer camp. Malcolm reported that he wanted to learn more about the camp first. Moira responded, "You haven't changed. This call is over!" She hung up.

In this example, Moira's response was reactive likely due to her past experiences of Malcolm trying to control her, but it was not in line with the goal of the phone call. She used the call to ask for something she wanted from Malcolm, then reacted in an inappropriate way in front of Zahid. Her gatekeeping of Zahid's contact with his father was likely causing confusion for Zahid. The therapist in this case reached out to Moira to try to discuss what happened, but she was unresponsive. Instead, she filed a restraining order for herself and Zahid, asking the judge to grant a 10-year restraining order and full custody to her. We return to this case again in the next section.

Legal Considerations

The handling of FV cases in criminal courts is extremely varied from state to state and country to country. Whether protective orders are issued and the nature of these orders have a substantial impact on not only family safety, but also the father–child relationship. When a full no-contact order is issued, there should be substantial concern that mother and children will be harmed if the father has contact with his children. There are cases where a no-contact order is absolutely needed and other cases where supervised visitation with children could and should be allowed but is prohibited, sometimes for many months or years at a time, following an incident of IPV between the parents. Having available assessment and intervention approaches to determine if supervised visiting is safe and in the child's best interest would be an asset to the courts in making their decisions. The following vignette provides an example of ways that therapeutic intervention that included the father who caused harm, may have been beneficial to his children after a FV incident.

CASE EXAMPLE: LATOYA

Six-year-old Latoya had not seen her father in nearly 2 years. There had been an ongoing restraining order in place following an incident of IPV between her parents in which the father was yelling, and pushed and hit the mother. Latoya, then age 4, tried to intervene by getting in the middle and was knocked down. The father swore he did not mean to hurt Latoya. During divorce proceedings, the mother filed for a restraining order for her and Latoya, and a 2-year order was issued. Now, 2 years after her last contact with her father in her first clinical visit, the therapist asked her about her father. Latoya responded, "Do you know where my dad is? Where has he been? I want to see him!" The therapist asked what she had been told about why she wasn't seeing her dad, and Latoya responded, "He and my mom had a big fight and he had to stay away, but that was a loooong time ago. I don't know where he is now, and I miss him. I've been making drawings for him. Do you know how to find him?"

This scenario highlights the ongoing confusion that children can experience and the longing they have for their absent parent even in the face of FV. Latoya's mother had explained the situation to her in the beginning, when she was 4, but was having a hard time helping Latoya understand where her father was and why he still could not visit her. Latoya's mother was concerned about this and wondered how to help reintroduce the father safely to her daughter while maintaining her own distance. The long-term nature of this restraining order did not consider the children's relationship or development, and no one had assessed whether supervised or therapeutic visits could be beneficial to the child even while maintaining no contact between the parents.

Crucially important to the provision of interventions to fathers who have caused harm is the consideration that these individuals, especially those who have used systematic power and control tactics with their partners, often utilize the court systems to continue to control and abuse their partners. This control can take the form of never-ending motions in family court related to custody and visitation. Providing intervention for fathers who have caused harm can result in fathers using a clinician or program to benefit their court case without really engaging in the needed therapeutic work. Providers who engage fathers with a history of FV must be aware of this distinct and likely possibility in their work. Developing clear guidelines about who to see in the F4C treatment, and parameters around engagement and successful treatment outcomes, are important. (These issues are discussed in more detail starting in Chapter 5.)

Saliently, though, *how* we engage with fathers who have caused harm is crucial to their commitment to behavior change. When fathers feel minimized and think everyone views them as criminals or monsters, they are more likely to shut down and not follow through with suggested intervention programs, and if they have the financial means to hire lawyers, they will instead try to prove their innocence in court.

CASE EXAMPLE: THERESA AND JULIO

Julio was involved in a domestic dispute with his wife, Theresa. She reported that he was screaming at her and he pushed her while she was holding their 2-year-old daughter Lily. She dropped the child as a result. Lily was not physically injured. Julio then left the house, and Theresa filed a police report. CPS was also notified. Julio was arrested and a full no-contact protective order was put in place for both Theresa and Lily. Julio was required to complete a group Family Violence Diversion program. He completed this requirement, and his case was dismissed. During this time, his wife filed for divorce and applied for a restraining order. The judge granted a 3-year restraining order for both Theresa and Lily, and indicated that Julio needed to participate in reunification therapy with his daughter as part of the divorce order. He initiated reunification services as the 3-year restraining order was coming to an end. In his first meeting, on the verge of tears, he stated to the therapist,

"Everyone thinks I'm a monster. I'm not a monster. I just want to have a relationship with my daughter. I've followed the order. I haven't contacted them, and now my daughter is 5 years old, and she probably doesn't even know me!" Julio felt significant shame that made it hard for him to seek help or agree to F4C and ongoing supervised visits. He initially stated that he was going to "get a lawyer and go to court to fight this. I don't need anyone to help me reconnect with my daughter. I'm a good father!"

The therapist gently asked Julio, "How does it make you feel when you think about having someone supervise your visits with your daughter?"

"I feel ashamed," he responded, and hung his head.

"I hope that shame doesn't get in the way of your seeing your daughter again. I can see how painful it has been that you haven't seen her for so long and how much you want to be an active father again. Fathers are really important to their children. Let's talk about how we can make that happen. The fastest way for you to be able to see her is to follow what the court is asking. I know it's hard, but a legal battle will only prolong your separation. You are right that your daughter is much older now and it will take time to rebuild a relationship with her. I can help you plan an initial meeting with her and work with her mother to help Lily be prepared to see you, and we can do that here in my office together when everyone is ready. We can start working on those goals today."

Julio responded, "If I can see my daughter soon, I'll do it. Thank you."

This example shows two important things: (1) Shame can get in the way of fathers' ability to take responsibility and to participate in treatment; and (2) when fathers feel that they can be important to their children and that you, as the provider, want to help them with that goal, they are able to move forward with the treatment.

Fathers often come to programs and services with the expectation of bias and feel they need to convince the provider that they are "not a monster." They see the therapist in a position of power that can prevent them from seeing their children if they do not convince them that they are a good parent. Keeping these concerns in mind is a tenet of the F4C program. Showing that you are approaching your work with them with an open mind is paramount, while also not allowing them to minimize or downplay their own behavior and the impact on their family. Methods of engagement and the importance of motivation will be further outlined in Chapter 6.

Returning to the case of Moira, Malcolm, and Zahid, the legal issues in this example are also about Malcolm's access to the child, but contact with his son was used as a control tactic by Moira in response to Malcolm's request to know more about the summer camp. The therapist tried to intervene directly with Moira without success. She therefore wrote a letter for Malcolm detailing the work he had been doing in F4C and his wish to reconnect with his son through a therapeutic reunification process. She detailed the efforts that had been made to begin that and Moira's unwillingness to allow Zahid to participate. She detailed the steps that could be taken to support safe and healthy contact between Malcolm and Zahid. The letter was helpful to Malcolm in court. The judge ordered the restraining order for Moira but did not include Zahid, so that Malcolm could legally begin reunification therapy with his son.

When we consider legal issues in families with FV, we are often most focused on protection of mothers and children from harm, but work with families with FV may also need to include advocacy for safe, restorative parenting work for fathers and their children. With children's needs in mind, Chapter 3 focuses on what fathers can do to help their children following FV.

CHAPTER 3

Needs of Children Following Violence and Research on Fathers for Change

A large body of literature has shown that exposure to FV has a deleterious impact on children's emotional and behavioral development (Graham-Bermann, Castor, Miller, & Howell, 2012; Kitzman, Gaylor, Holt, & Kenny, 2003; Wood & Sommers, 2011). This chapter is not intended to review that entire body of literature, but instead to give a broad overview of how FV impacts children's development and functioning to inform what is helpful to their recovery. The focus is specific to fathers who have caused harm and how they may promote recovery of their children. Following the review of what children need from their fathers following violence, this chapter presents a review of the research conducted so far on F4C and needed future directions of investigation.

RESEARCH ON CHILDREN'S EXPOSURE TO VIOLENCE AND DEVELOPMENTAL IMPACT

Data have demonstrated that exposure to violence in childhood is associated with concurrent and prospective indices of child behavioral problems including aggression, conduct problems, and juvenile delinquency, as well as psychiatric diagnoses including depression, anxiety, PTSD, and attachment disorders (e.g., Evans, Davies, & DiLillo, 2008; Jouriles & McDonald, 2014; Kitzmann, Gaylord, Holt, & Kenny, 2003). Witnessing IPV can be a significant traumatic experience for children and may have a long-lasting impact on their well-being and future development (Siegel, 2013). This recognition has led to the classification of exposure to IPV as a form of child maltreatment evidenced by its inclusion in worldwide mandatory reporting legislation (Dubowitz, 2014; Mathews & Kenny, 2008). Exposure to IPV in early life is also associated with polyvictimization and greater psychosocial difficulties (Stover, Ippen, et al., 2019). The association with polyvictimization such as concurrent child physical or sexual abuse or neglect increase the likelihood of poor outcomes, including increased psychiatric diagnoses. As reported in Chapter 2, the overlap of IPV and child maltreatment is high (Hamby et al., 2010) and children who experience both are at highest risk for poor developmental outcomes (Osofsky, 2003). Polyvictimization has been shown to be more highly related to posttraumatic stress symptoms than repeated exposures to a single type of violence (Turner, Finkelhor, & Ormrod, 2010).

There is now a wealth of data indicating that children who have experienced FV are at increased risk for a host of health concerns. They are more likely to experience physical health conditions such as asthma and other nonsexually transmitted diseases that require hospital treatment (Lanier, Jonson-Reid, Stahlschmidt, Drake, & Constantino, 2010). Meta-analytic findings from 37 studies of FV (including exposure to IPV and physical and psychological abuse of children) found moderate associations between FV and child internalizing, such as anxiety, and externalizing symptoms, such as verbal and physical aggression (Chan & Yeung, 2009). Compared to participants not exposed to FV in childhood, those exposed have been shown to be at higher risk of engaging in early sex, dropping out of high school, entering early into full-time employment, marrying early, and becoming parents early (Maneta, White, & Mezzacappa, 2017; McTavish, MacGregor, Wathen, & MacMillan, 2016). Studies have revealed FV may also be associated with physical changes in the brain (Teicher et al., 2004, 2018; Choi, Jeong, Polcari, Rohan, & Teicher, 2012). The auditory and visual cortex and the hypothalamic–pituitary–adrenal (HPA) axis are particularly affected (Mueller & Tronick, 2019). These brain changes may be related to cognitive and other health outcomes experienced by these children and adolescents. For example, Kiesel, Piescher, and Edleson (2016) found that children exposed to child maltreatment and IPV, individually or in combination, underperform at school, with children exposed to IPV having the poorest outcomes.

Important to the impact of exposure to IPV is children's level of involvement. When variation in children's involvement is assessed, more involvement resulted in increased risk for poor mental health outcomes (Bayarri Fernandez, Ezpeleta, Granero, de la Osa, & Domènech, 2011; Jarvis, Gordon, & Novaco, 2005). Although both mother and child reports of children's increased involvement are significantly associated with negative outcomes for children, child reports may more accurately predict outcome variables. This may be due to the impact of children's perceptions of IPV, which are more closely related to outcomes than the descriptions of the violent incidents (Spilsbury et al., 2008). Children's *perceived* threat and blame related to IPV were more associated with child behavioral outcomes than the actual frequency and intensity of IPV (Grych, Jouriles, Swank, McDonald, & Norwood, 2000). Furthermore, children who reported fear during IPV episodes were more likely to meet diagnostic criteria for PTSD and depression (Zinzow et al., 2009) and reported reduced connectedness and attachment to their family (Owen, Thompson, Shaffer, Jackson, & Kaslow, 2009). These studies indicate that inclusion of children's reports of FV and their perceptions of the violence are important to understanding how the FV will impact their mental and behavioral health functioning. Children who report ongoing fear of their fathers' violence (that he will physically injure them or their mothers) need careful assessment to determine whether father–child sessions will be helpful. Clinicians using F4C when working with fathers who have caused harm must assess fathers' commitment to change, their understanding of the impact of the violence on their children (Howell, Barnes, Miller, & Graham-Bermann, 2016), and the benefit to their children of father–child treatment when making determinations about conducting joint sessions with children. These issues are further explored in Chapter 5 related to assessment and case selection and Chapter 6, which pertains to motivational engagement.

Developmental Considerations of FV at Various Ages

Exposure to FV can have differential impacts on children depending on their ages. Generally, earlier exposure, especially when prolonged, has the most detrimental impact on children's developing brains and nervous systems as described previously. Infants do not have the capacity to process fearful stimuli the way older children and adolescents do, and their brains are developing rapidly, which makes the impact of experiences and adversities potentially more potent. Although infants and very young children do not have language to express their experiences, they are deeply affected by the moods, sounds, and actions of their primary caregivers. Infants and toddlers do not have well developed nervous systems. They depend on co-regulation with their primary caregivers. When caregivers are unable to help children regulate and actually stimulate dysregulation through loud and scary experiences, infants and toddlers do not develop the regulation skills needed, resulting in poor emotion regulation and inability to soothe themselves in healthy ways as they get older (Mueller & Tronick, 2019). Furthermore, young children are very egocentric and assume everything that happens around them is something they caused, which can impact their developing sense of self. They are prone to self-blame, and this inclination can continue into adolescence.

Exposure to violence in early childhood can impact cognitive development and functioning. When children reach school age, those exposed to FV are at higher risk for learning and behavior problems in school. Adolescents exposed to FV are at increased risk for substance misuse (Halpern et al., 2018), antisocial behaviors (Braga, Gonçalves, Basto-Pereira, & Maia, 2017; Wilson, Stover, & Berkowitz, 2009), and sexual risk taking (Kugler et al., 2019; Thibodeau, Lavoie, Hébert, & Blais, 2017). The developmental tasks of children's age/stage impact the kind of symptoms they can exhibit and how they will respond to FV. This chapter is not intended to review the vast literature on this topic. For further reading to understand the impact of FV on child development, see suggested resources in Appendix B.

Addressing Children's Needs Following FV

Children need safety and security first and foremost following FV. They need to feel that they are safe, and that their physical and emotional needs will be met. They may experience significant symptoms and difficulties following FV that need to be addressed through treatment as indicated earlier. Aside from meeting these primary needs, there are things that can help children recover. A study of children whose fathers had been violent reported results of interviews about what these children wanted from their fathers following violence. They identified wanting (1) the violence to be acknowledged, (2) an apology for the violence, and (3) the behavior to change (Lamb, Humphreys, & Hegarty, 2018). Each of these areas is described below in relation to the person who has caused the child harm.

Acknowledgment

FV is often minimized, ignored, and not discussed in families in which it is occurring. There is either a spoken or unspoken rule that the violence is not talked about or acknowledged. Parents who have caused harm, as well as coparent recipients of harm, often assume that talking about the violence will "retraumatize" their children or cause them further undue distress. In fact, acting as if violence either did not occur or does not deserve to be talked about can be very confusing to children, who have no means of processing these events on their own. This lack of acknowledgment also colludes with a primary symptom of PTSD: avoidance. The longer the violence is not talked about or processed, the harder it can become to talk about it. It feels wrong and can cause the child to be uncomfortable and dysregulated. That does not mean talking about it is harmful especially within a therapeutic setting that can provide appropriate support. Acknowledgement of what children have experienced is crucial to allow them to begin to heal. This does not mean that children need lengthy discussions with acknowledgement of every detail of the violence they witnessed or experienced, but a general admission that FV occurred is a place to begin—with timing of more detailed discussions done at the child's pace and with the help of a therapist.

Apology

Following the acknowledgment of FV, a heartfelt apology without the expectation of forgiveness is the next step. Healing takes time; it's not helpful for parents to say they are sorry with the express purpose of expecting forgiveness or to close further discussion. The apology must be genuine and given with a mindset of repair that may take significant time. Something akin to "I'm sorry for what happened, OK!? Do you forgive me?" is delivered not for the benefit of the child but for the parent. This kind of apology is made by a parent who caused harm and is seeking to ease their conscience of any guilt or shame, with forgiveness signaling to all the ability to move on and not speak of it again. This kind of discussion is not in the best interests of their children. Opening discussion about what happened, acknowledging that it was wrong, and signaling that work is being done to make change are all needed to repair the relationship. An apology followed by continued FV either toward the child or mother is frustrating and harmful, as children will distrust the apology and shut down from further discussions about the topic (Lamb et al., 2018).

Change Behavior

In order to heal from FV, children need their fathers to change their behaviors and show them consistently that they are working hard to interact differently. Children also flourish when their fathers are communicative, cooperative, and consistent coparents. Parents who repeatedly change their parenting time, do not show up for scheduled planned time together, or make parental exchanges conflictual and difficult are only causing further stress and harm to their children. Clear communication about coparenting, shared time, and children's needs in this regard is an essential part of intervention with fathers following FV. Fathers must keep their children's developmental needs in mind as they plan their parenting time and communication. Young children, in particular, need to see their coparents on a consistent schedule that is predictable to them and in keeping with their sense of time (Kelly & Lamb, 2000). A week is a long time to a 2-year-old, so visits should be more frequent and for shorter amounts of time, when possible, rather than longer visits spread out over the month. Consistency helps children feel a sense of control over what will happen. They know when they will see each parent and for how long. This consistency reduces their stress.

BENEFITS OF REPAIR IN FATHER–CHILD RELATIONSHIPS

We know that men who have caused harm continue to have a role in their children's lives. Women take an average of 8 years to leave a violent relationship, and 68% of women exiting domestic violence shelters return to live with the perpetrating partner (Lerner & Kennedy, 2000; Martin et al., 2000). Specific to children exiting domestic violence shelters with their mothers, one study found postshelter contact between children ages 4–9 years and their mother's violent partner was positively associated with child conduct problems (Jouriles et al., 2018). It was not clear how many of these partners were biological or psychological fathers to the children in the study. In nonshelter, community samples in which fathers used IPV, high percentages of children lived with or had contact with offending fathers following arrest for IPV, with rates in the range just over 70% in three different studies (Hunter & Graham-Bermann, 2013; Israel & Stover, 2009; Stover et al., 2003); fathers with a history of IPV also frequently had joint custody of their children following divorce (Forssell & Cater, 2015), and mothers often reported their children were attached to their fathers who had used violence (Israel & Stover, 2009).

Few studies have examined how contact with fathers may impact community samples of children following family dissolution due to IPV. In one study, preschool-age children who had limited or no contact with their previously violent fathers had higher levels of depression and anxiety than children who had frequent (at least weekly) visits 6 months or more following family separation. The associations with father contact were consistent even when researchers controlled for the severity of violence exposure (Stover et al., 2003). In addition, preschool-age children, especially boys, who saw their fathers more regularly had fewer negative representations of their mothers in play (Stover et al., 2006). In a sample of 6- to 12-year-old children, Hunter and Graham-Bermann (2013) found that frequency of father contact was not associated with child internalizing and externalizing scores overall. However, frequency of contact did moderate the association between IPV and child behavior problems, suggesting that contact with certain fathers who engaged in less frequent violent behavior may protect children against higher levels of behavior problems. The authors indicated that if fathers were able to model appropriate emotion regulation strategies and help their children effectively work through feelings about the violence they witnessed, children might be less likely to resort to using aggressive and problematic behaviors to convey their feelings. Together these findings support consideration of therapeutic interventions with fathers who have caused harm that focus on helping fathers make amends for their violence and change their behavior for the benefit of their children. F4C was designed to meet this need.

DEVELOPMENT AND OUTCOMES OF F4C

F4C has been studied in two small, randomized trials and an open trial (Stover, 2015a; Stover, McMahon, & Moore, 2019; Stover et al., 2022). F4C was developed and first implemented within a substance misuse treatment clinic in a department of psychiatry. Ten clients received F4C to test out components and assess initial feasibility (Stover, 2013). This was followed by studies in an outpatient clinic, a residential substance use treatment facility, and within six community agencies as part of a statewide implementation by the Connecticut DCF. Each of these studies provides important information about how F4C may benefit families.

Do Participants Find F4C Acceptable?

Ten fathers of children ages 1–6 years who had co-occurring FV and substance misuse (and their coparents) participated in an open trial of initial feasibility of F4C. They had high completion rates at 80%. This 20% dropout rate was significantly lower than other studies of IPV and substance misuse interventions, which see dropout rates ranging from 40 to 60% (Stover, Meadows, & Kaufman, 2009). Additionally, all fathers who completed the program remained nonviolent during treatment and reduced their substance misuse, with 80% being abstinent during treatment. There were very high rates of satisfaction from participants. All men reported liking all three components of the model (individual, coparent, and child-focused sessions) and stated they thought the program was either just right in length or too short. These data indicated good potential for the intervention's acceptability by fathers.

Subsequently, a small, randomized pilot study was conducted with 18 fathers of children ages 1 to 6 years who were randomized to F4C or individual drug counseling (IDC). These fathers were recruited from the same substance misuse clinic as the initial 10 participants. They all had substance misuse problems and had reported IPV behaviors in the last 12 months. Fathers were 52% African American, 19% Hispanic/

Latinx, 14% White, 10% multiethnic, and 5% identified as another ethnic group. The primary substance of choice in the sample was alcohol, with a smaller number of participants using marijuana or opioids. About half the fathers were unemployed. Those randomized to F4C were more likely to complete treatment (67 vs. 33%, p = .10). They also reported greater satisfaction with the treatment, feeling that it better helped them with their problems (Stover, 2015a).

Acceptability in the Community

Clinicians from six community mental health agencies were trained to offer F4C to CPS-involved families through a statewide initiative in the state of Connecticut. In this initiative, F4C was implemented as part of a larger Intimate Partner Violence–Family Assessment Intervention Response (IPV-FAIR) funded by the Connecticut Department of Children and Families. IPV-FAIR included assessment of all members of the family (father, mother, and children), safety planning, treatment for mothers and fathers, and case management services. Each family was assigned a clinician and family navigator team. The clinician provided F4C or other clinical treatment needed by the mother and father, and the family navigator assisted with case management, connection with other services, and advocacy. Based on a program evaluation by the Injury Prevention Center at Connecticut Children's Medical Center, 204 fathers and their coparents were referred for F4C and attended at least one session of the program, with a 73% completion rate. There were no differences in completion due to fathers' age, severity of IPV, employment, education, or ethnicity, indicating broad acceptability of the program when implemented in community settings. The sample was 37% non-Hispanic White, 30% Hispanic/Latinx, 22% non-Hispanic African American/Black, and 10% multiracial or other identified race/ethnicity. Fifty-five percent of fathers were married or cohabitating, 36% were single, and 9% were divorced or separated. Fifty-six percent of fathers were employed, and 30% had less than a high school diploma, 37% graduated high school, and 33% had some postsecondary education (Stover et al., 2022).

Acceptability within Residential Substance Misuse Treatment Settings

The intervention was modified and implemented within a residential treatment program for substance-dependent men. Forty-four fathers participated in the pilot program provided once per week over 16 weeks while they were living in the residential treatment facility. Participants had completed 6 months of a 12-month residential program when they started the intervention. Interviews were conducted prior to beginning F4C and posttreatment to assess the impact of the intervention on anger, hostile thinking, and emotion regulation problems. Focus groups were also conducted with the participants to gain further insight into their needs as fathers and their recommendations for intervention that they would find helpful. Impressively, 84.1% of participants completed the program in its entirety and were highly satisfied with the content (Stover, Carlson, & Patel, 2017).

The feedback from these participants in the focus groups was used to further enhance materials related to talking to children about substance misuse and to alter the program to be provided using 12 sessions in residence and four aftercare sessions following discharge to assist with reintegration into family life in the community. This revised residential application was pre-piloted within a 6-month residential facility with 10 participants (Stover, Carlson, Patel, & Manalich, 2018) to assess feasibility and acceptability. Eight of the 10 participants completed the full intervention and booster sessions. Next, 60 fathers were randomly assigned to F4C or a parenting education (PE) comparison program. PE was selected because it represents the kind of psychoeducational parenting program that might typically be offered in substance use treatment settings and met the expectation of study participants to receive an intervention focused on their roles as fathers. Fathers in the study were primarily in residential treatment due to opioid or alcohol addiction. They were provided 12 sessions of F4C or PE during the last 3 months of their 6-month residential treatment and four aftercare sessions following discharge. Fathers were assessed for IPV, substance use, emotion regulation, and anger pretreatment, postresidential treatment, postbooster sessions, and at 3-month posttreatment follow-up. Completion rates were higher for the PE group than F4C (F4C = 76.2% and PE = 95.8%) (Stover, McMahon, et al., 2019). Importantly, the F4C group had more participants discharged from the facility for breaking rules. Several of these were before F4C even started. None of the participants in either group dropped out of F4C or PE only. If they discontinued, it was because they chose to leave the residential facility and therefore could not continue in the study. Still, the PE group was focused only on parenting guidance and not IPV. It may be that this was more acceptable to fathers in the context of their residential treatment. Further study is needed to understand these completion differences.

Does F4C Reduce FV and Substance Misuse?

Several studies have found significant reductions in IPV behaviors and substance misuse by men during and after F4C. In the initial randomized trial (Stover, 2015a) F4C fathers showed a trend toward greater self-reported reduction in violence that continued following treatment compared to IDC fathers. Not only did men report reductions in their violence, but they also reported less use of violence by their partners as well on the Conflict Tactics Scale—Revised. There were comparable reductions in substance misuse for the F4C and IDC groups (Stover, 2015a). IDC is an evidence-based intervention for substance misuse, so showing comparable reductions in substance misuse while improving IPV indicates multiple benefits for F4C. The addition of F4C within the residential substance-use-treatment setting revealed significantly less substance use during the 3 months following residential discharge for the F4C group than for those that received the PE add-on intervention, suggesting that F4C better supported fathers' abstinence from substances and may have additive benefit for those in residential treatment for substance use (Stover, Moore, & McMahon, 2019).

In the community implementation study of F4C (Stover et al., 2022), pre- to posttreatment assessments revealed significant reductions in IPV and children's exposure to conflict based on mothers' reports using the Abusive Behavior Inventory (Shepard & Campbell, 1992) and the Children's Exposure to Conflict Scale on the Coparenting Relationship Scale (Feinberg, 2003). Further, a propensity score match study by the Injury Prevention Center at Connecticut Children's Medical Center assessed the impact of F4C on repeat maltreatment reports to the DCF. Fathers who had completed F4C were matched using propensity score matching to comparable fathers who received other treatments as usual in the community following CPS involvement due to IPV. Two hundred ninety-seven F4C fathers were matched with 297 control fathers on variables such as severity of IPV, prior CPS involvement, father age, father race, and gender of child. Fathers who received F4C were half as likely to have a repeat maltreatment report for any FV made to CPS in the 6 months following the treatment period than the control group (Beebe, Clough, Bernstein, Grasso, & Stover, submitted for publication).

Does F4C Improve Father–Child Interactions and Child Symptoms?

Men in F4C showed gains in their videotaped interactions with their children from pre- to posttreatment compared to fathers randomized to IDC (Stover, 2015a). Fathers' interactions were coded using the Child Interactive Behavior Rating Scales (Feldman, 1998). These were coded by masked, reliable coders. Men who received F4C showed less intrusiveness during free-play interactions and more consistency of style postintervention than did men who received IDC. Fathers who received the intervention allowed more child-led activities by less frequently disrupting or redirecting the child's activities or attention, and the fathers' interaction styles were consistent and predictable (i.e., lacking abrupt changes in affect, tone of voice, level of activity, or parent's interest in the child activity) to the children following the intervention. Fathers in the IDC condition did not improve in these areas and actually seemed to get worse. It is possible that fathers in the IDC group showed worse interactions posttreatment because they were no longer using substances, but they did not gain any father–child-focused intervention as part of their treatment to improve their relationships with their children.

In the community study, coparents of F4C-enrolled fathers completed pre–post F4C caregiver reports of their children's PTSD and other mental health symptoms using the Structured Trauma-Related Experiences and Symptoms Screener (STRESS; Grasso, Felton, & Reid-Quinoñes, 2015) and Strengths and Difficulties Questionnaires (SDQ; Goodman, 2002). Mothers reported improved PTSD and other mental health symptoms in their children post-F4C (DiVietro, Beebe, Geisler, & Stover, 2017) in a sample of 74 children whose fathers received F4C. These findings need to be tested next in a larger randomized trial of F4C.

Does F4C Improve Intervention Targets of Emotion Regulation and Reflective Functioning?

Two studies indicated F4C improved intervention targets of emotion regulation and reflective functioning. The residential treatment implementation study found that those who received F4C had significantly greater improvements in emotion regulation difficulties than the PE group (Stover, McMahon, et al., 2019). In the open community trial, fathers reported significant improvements in emotion regulation, hostility, and prementalizing as measured by the Difficulties with Emotion Regulation Scale, Multidimensional Anger Inventory, and Parental Reflective Functioning Questionnaire.

ONGOING STUDIES AND WHAT WE STILL NEED TO KNOW

There is an ongoing study of F4C to provide further support for its efficacy. There is a current randomized trial of the intervention compared to a Duluth model batterer intervention program (BIP) being conducted at the Yale School of Medicine within their Parent and Family Development Clinic. Fathers are referred for the program by CPS due to concerns related to FV. They are randomly assigned to one of three treatment groups—F4C, Duluth individual, or Duluth group intervention—and participate in 18 sessions of their assigned intervention. The findings from this study will provide evidence for the efficacy of F4C in reducing FV compared to treatment as usual for IPV (Duluth model). Results of this study should be available in 2023. There are also plans for a multisite randomized trial. These studies are needed to replicate efficacy followed by further tests of real-world effectiveness. F4C has been used with a diverse sample of fathers to date, including monolingual Spanish speakers, but further testing modifications for specific cultural and language groups are needed to provide evidence with other groups.

Providing intervention for fathers that keeps their children's needs in focus while helping them change their harmful behaviors can improve outcomes for children. Chapter 4 details the theoretical underpinnings of how to implement the F4C work and describes the intervention targets.

CHAPTER 4

Theoretical Rationale for the Fathers for Change Intervention

F4C was developed by integrating research and theories about the most common causes of FV. This chapter outlines the strategies F4C uses to motivate fathers in the early sessions and the rational for the targets or focus of the intervention. Several main issues commonly seen in fathers who use FV are highlighted before describing the theoretical underpinnings of the F4C model: (1) a history of childhood adversity, such as maltreatment or witnessing IPV in their own families of origin; and (2) co-occurring substance misuse. These features are not universally seen in fathers who use FV, but they occur frequently enough that they must be assessed and understood as they impact case formulation and provision of appropriate intervention. Intergenerational transmission of FV is a well-known phenomenon (Franklin & Kercher, 2012; Madigan et al., 2019; Stith et al., 2000) and histories of childhood trauma and maltreatment are associated with adult use of substances and substance use disorders (Halpern et al., 2018). Overlap of substance misuse, especially alcohol, and FV is substantial, with moderate associations between alcohol, cocaine, marijuana, and FV (Choenni, Hammink, & van de Mheen, 2017; Crane, Godleski, Przybyla, Schlauch, & Testa, 2016).

Important to the associations of FV with intergenerational patterns of childhood experiences of maltreatment and substance use is the impact of chronic childhood adversity on brain development. As discussed in Chapter 3, early adversity in the form of neglect and exposure to IPV or other forms of violence or maltreatment have been shown to have significant impact on the developing brain. This is particularly true for the prefrontal cortex and amygdala. Chronic childhood adversity is associated with reduced prefrontal cortex functional connectivity and attention control in adults (Liston, McEwen, & Casey, 2009). The prefrontal cortex is associated with attention, concentration, and impulse control. Another study has linked increased amygdala volume in adolescents (Lupien et al., 2011; Whittle et al., 2013) with chronic childhood adversity. The amygdala interprets external stimuli such as sights and sounds as potentially dangerous and sends that information to the hippocampus. This process activates a release of energy so people can respond to and protect themselves from external threats. These data corroborate the idea that childhood adversities, like maltreatment or witnessing IPV, impair higher prefrontal cortex cognitive functions and strengthens amygdala–striatal affective responding that may be oversensitive to threat (Arnsten, 2015). Disruption of higher-order prefrontal-cortex-mediated functions during and following adversities may manifest psychologically and behaviorally as heightened emotional reactivity (e.g., hypervigilance to threat), emotion dysregulation (inability to manage intense emotions), and weaker understanding of one's own mental states or reflective functioning (inability to understand one's own thoughts and feelings and how they impact behaviors) (Arnsten, 2015; Duffy, McLaughlin, & Green, 2018; Germine, Dunn, McLaughlin, & Smoller, 2015; Hein & Monk, 2017). As detailed below, these deficits are associated with increased risk for use of both FV and substances. Figure 4.1 illustrates these associations and proposed intervention targets for F4C.

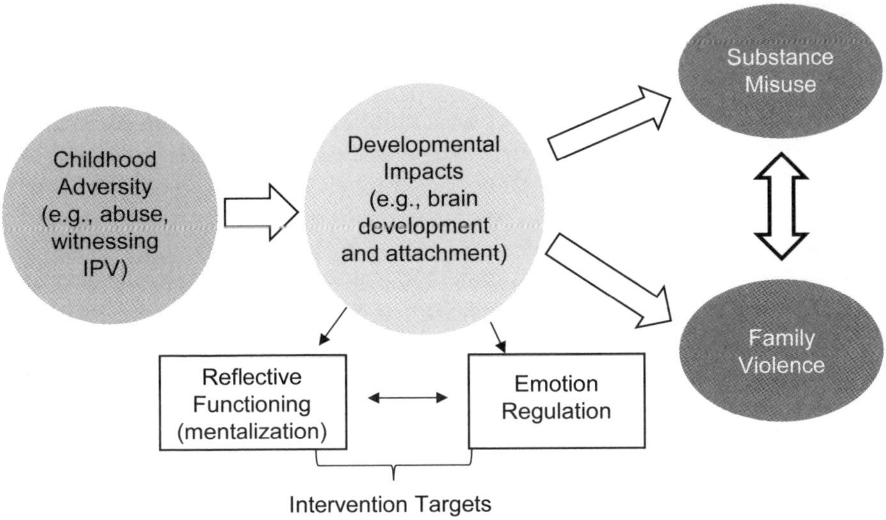

FIGURE 4.1. Theoretical underpinnings of F4C targets.

What all this means is that many of the fathers who are referred for intervention due to use of FV and/or substance misuse were in the same position during childhood that their children are in now; through helping these fathers, we help their children with this intervention. These men experienced significant early life adversities and did not develop the mentalization (see below for more on mentalization and reflective functioning) and emotion regulation abilities needed to have healthy relationships or manage stress. Holding this phenomenon in mind helps the clinician to have empathy for the father and work to understand his difficulties and provide him with support to build skills he never learned as a child.

FATHERHOOD AS A MOTIVATOR FOR CHANGE

Low motivation to change and treatment noncompliance are serious problems that can affect the success of intervention programs for FV (Daniels & Murphy, 1997; Eckhardt, Holtzworth-Munroe, Norlander, Sibley, & Cahill, 2008; Scott & Wolfe, 2003). Those who cause harm often deny their use of or blame others for their violence, making it difficult to engage in a self-reflective therapeutic process of behavior change (Birkley & Eckhardt, 2015; Eckhardt, Samper, & Murphy, 2008; Kistenmacher & Weiss, 2008). This nonacceptance has led to a focus on motivational enhancement for those referred to FV programs. Motivation for change has been associated with treatment engagement and completion; however in FV cases, many individuals are ordered to treatments by the courts or referred by CPS agencies. Both sources of referral provide external pressure with potentially significant consequences for failure to comply (jail time, loss of contact with children). In fact, Maldonado and Murphy (2021) found that court referral status was a greater predictor of treatment completion than self-reported motivation to change, but that a focus on motivation may be particularly important for those referred by the court, since this population tends to be less motivated at the start of treatment, and there is some evidence that increased motivation for change is associated with better treatment outcomes (Semiatin, Murphy, & Elliott, 2013). So although external pressure to engage and complete intervention may increase completion rates, individual motivation is associated with how much a father may get out of the program offered.

One motivational strategy that has shown promise is a focus on fatherhood. Fathers may be more likely to complete court-mandated treatment and have higher self-reported rates of behavioral and cognitive change following treatment for FV than their counterparts who are not fathers (Poole & Murphy, 2019). Therefore, the central premise of

F4C is that focus on men as fathers and increasing their feelings of competence and meaning within their parenting role can provide motivation to change maladaptive patterns that have led to use of aggression and substances to control negative or inefficacious feelings. When clinicians approach men as parents (rather than as perpetrators or offenders) and stress the important role they play with their children, they may have more success in motivating them to engage in treatment. This individual father approach is unique in the IPV batterer intervention world, which often treats individuals who caused harm as "offenders" and works with them in groups using a standard approach. There has been a lack of individual assessment and treatment planning to address the needs of fathers who have used FV, which is why F4C was developed. The specific strategies used for engagement of fathers is described in detail with case examples in Chapter 6.

FOCUS ON REFLECTIVE FUNCTIONING

Mentalizing or *reflective functioning* (RF), terms that are often used interchangeably, is the capacity to imagine and think explicitly about mental states, namely thoughts, feelings, intentions, beliefs, motives, emotions, desires and needs. It is the ability to imagine mental states in the self and in others. A key aspect of F4C is working toward helping fathers have better reflective capacities related to their own experiences, as well as those of their partners and children. Through reflective capacities, we develop the ability to understand our own behavioral responses and the responses of others as a meaningful attempt to communicate those inner mental states (Fonagy, Steele, Steele, Moran, & Higgitt, 1991). Parental RF refers to the parent's capacity to hold the child's mental states in mind (Slade, 2005). Individuals with high levels of RF are better able to recognize their own and others' thoughts, emotions, intentions, and desires (Fonagy et al., 1991). Poor RF is associated with emotional dysregulation and increased violent and aggressive behavior (Fonagy, 2003; Fossati et al., 2009; Taubner, White, Zimmermann, Fonagy, & Nolte, 2013).

There are limited studies on the RF of fathers, especially those who have used FV. Those that exist indicate that such fathers have very poor self and parental RF (Mohaupt et al., 2021; Mohaupt & Duckert, 2016; Stover & Kahn, 2013; Stover & Kiselica, 2014; Stover & Spink, 2012). Studies of mothers indicate a significant association between poor RF related to their children and maltreatment (Edwards, Shipman, & Brown, 2005; Shipman & Zeman, 1999). While there is less research on the relationship between paternal RF and child maltreatment, poor RF is a potential core element driving men's FV (Asen & Fonagy, 2017). Reading of the larger literature suggests a common and potentially modifiable pathway to FV through RF. Men at risk for FV often misperceive threat (acute threat sensitivity), especially from their partners (Holtzworth-Munroe & Hutchinson, 1993), and instead respond to innocuous or ambiguous stimuli with emotion dysregulation and violence (Babcock, Green, Webb, & Graham, 2004; Costa & Babcock, 2008; Dankoski et al., 2006; Finkel, DeWall, Slotter, Oaten, & Foshee, 2009). Poor RF can result in (1) misperceptions of partners and children's intentions or behaviors; (2) lack of understanding of one's own emotions, triggers, thoughts, and behaviors; and (3) poor regulation of emotion that can result in violence. In F4C, the clinician must continually think about the reflective abilities of the father and how to help move him toward better self-reflective, coparent- and parent-reflective functioning to impact this chain.

EMOTION REGULATION

Emotion regulation is the ability to understand one's emotions and mental states, and then apply strategies to manage overwhelming feelings. Poor emotion regulation has been associated with violent behavior generally, as well as FV specifically. Fathers in a pilot study to develop F4C who had used FV in the last 12 months exhibited poor emotion regulation skills compared to matched community control fathers (Stover et al., 2013). Consistent with the literature, poor emotion regulation was associated with aggressive parenting and IPV (Dankoski et al., 2006; Finkel, 2007; Finkel et al., 2009) and substance misuse (Heatherton & Wagner, 2011; Winters, Botzet, Fahnhorst, Baumel, & Lee, 2008; Witkiewitz & Villarroel, 2009). Meta-analytic findings indicate that maladaptive emotion regulation strategies such as suppression and rumination were moderately associated with substance misuse and violence (Aldao, Nolen-Hoeksema, & Schweizer, 2010), and rumination about hostile thoughts predicted violence over time (Caprara, Paciello, Gergino, & Cugini, 2007). Experimental studies have indicated that improving emotion regulation reduces violence (Denson, Capper, Oaten, Friese, & Schofield, 2011; Finkel et al., 2009), and providing emotion regulation training in addition to standard CBT has been shown to improve a range of psychiatric symptoms (Berking et al., 2008) and to reduce violence. Other evidence-based treatments, such as Dialectical Behavior Therapy (DBT) for borderline personality disorder, focus heavily on developing skills to manage overwhelming emotions and distress (Linehan, 2020). Although not tested specifically with men who have used FV, a recent meta-analysis indicates that DBT reduces anger and aggression transdiagnostically (Ciesinski, Sorgi-Wilson, Cheung, Chen, & McCloskey, 2022). Given these findings related to RF and emotion regulation, a focus on both RF and emotion regulation would impact FV behaviors and thus make them the primary intervention targets in F4C (see Figure 4.2).

FAMILY SYSTEMS AND FAMILY VIOLENCE

Family systems approaches to FV, especially IPV, have been controversial in the field for several reasons. Feminist theory about IPV purports that IPV is caused by men's societal views and desire to dominate women. If an offender wants control over his partner, then focusing on family interactions and communication during dyadic or family therapy sessions may increase risk of violence. These are important concerns, and safety of partners and children are a prominent feature of any intervention. There are, however, dynamics that exist for some families in which FV is occurring that can benefit from systems thinking and working on healthy communication skills. If one partner is attempting to use a new skill to manage emotions or to communicate and the other partner is not supportive or is even hostile or negative in response, it can shut down the possibility of the person using that skill again. For example, if Jorge is in therapy for FV and learns a new way of communicating using "I statements" and his partner Cora laughs at him and says, "I don't care how you feel," when he tries to use them, he is not likely to use them again. Interactive communication patterns sometimes need both

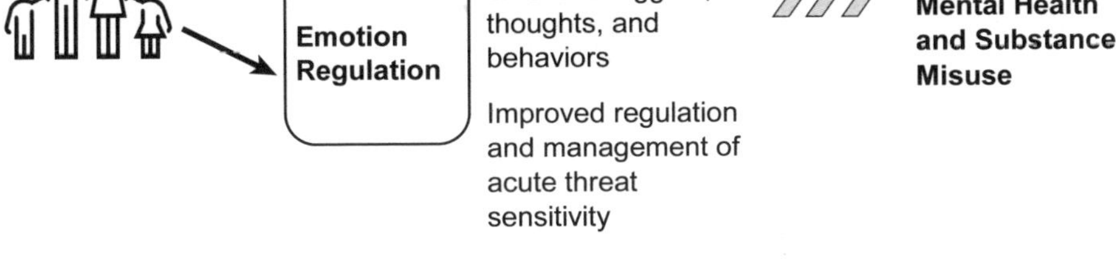

FIGURE 4.2. Intervention targets in F4C.

partners involved in treatment to address the issue more effectively. This can only work if all members of the family feel free and safe to comment during sessions and do not feel at risk of harm by participating. How to assess these issues will be further addressed in Chapters 5 and 8.

Important to the consideration of family systems approaches is the high number of families in which there is reciprocal or bidirectional violence, with both partners using violence with each other. Surveys indicate this occurs in 50–60% of U.S. couples reporting IPV (Langhinrichsen-Rohling, Misra, Selwyn, & Rohling, 2012; Whitaker, Haileyesus, Swahn, & Saltzman, 2007). In these cases, interventions that address couple interactions and communication may be appropriate. Armenti and Babcock (2016) in their review of couple-based approaches for IPV such as domestic-violence-focused couple therapy (DVFCT; Stith et al., 2011), recommend that these approaches are only for those with strong evidence of situational violence, or violence that is not largely motivated by a desire to control and dominate one's partner, with little risk of physical injury, where there are no substance or mental health issues that could compromise safety, and where some accountability for violence is taken, and violence results from maladaptive responses to situational conflicts (Antunes-Alves & Stefano, 2014). They further recommend that concerns such as substance misuse, an intense desire for control over one's partner, and refusal to accept accountability for violence would likely need to be addressed in individual treatment before entering into couple sessions (Antunes-Alves & Stefano, 2014). If these issues are addressed, the focus can shift to conjoint work to address dyadic communication and problem-solving deficits that may be contributing to FV. With these recommendations in mind, along with the acknowledgment that communication and relationship dynamics contribute to difficulties for many fathers referred following FV, F4C works in a phased approach to assess the family, address individual needs of the father (and the mother if she chooses), followed by a coparental phase, and finally a family focus.

INTERVENTION AND THEORETICAL RATIONALE

F4C is designed to be offered to fathers who have young children (under 12 years) with a *history of FV*, defined as threatened or actual physical or psychological violence against an intimate partner and/or child (F4C is not designed to address child sexual abuse by a father). Fathers may have co-occurring substance misuse problems, since the co-occurrence of FV and substance misuse is high and the factors contributing to substance misuse are often the same as those for use of FV (e.g., a history of childhood adversity/trauma, poor RF, and poor emotion regulation, as described earlier; Brady & Backs, 2012; Cunradi, Todd, Mair, & Remer, 2013; Fonagy & Bateman, 2016; Fuller-Thomson, Roane, & Brennenstuhl, 2016), which are addressed in the F4C program. The goals of the intervention are to (1) decrease FV, (2) decrease substance misuse when indicated, (3) improve coparenting communication, (4) decrease negative parenting behaviors, and (5) increase positive father–child relationships.

Following a comprehensive assessment, F4C addresses nine individually focused core topics, four coparent-focused topics, and five father–child-focused topics in 60-minute individual or family therapy sessions over 16–24 weeks (see Table 1.1 in Chapter 1). In the context of a strong working alliance developed through a focus on fatherhood (Brown & O'Leary, 2000; Taft, Murphy, King, Musser, & DeDeyn, 2003), an F4C therapist motivates the father to change by continually recognizing his desire to be a better parent (Maiuro & Murphy, 2009; Scott & Wolfe, 2003) and facilitating his ability to reflect on his own experiences and those of his coparent and children, and to learn new skills to manage his emotions and thinking to improve outcomes for his family. F4C improves RF and emotion regulation through awareness of thoughts, emotions, and antecedents (body sensations), and teaching skills for self-soothing in stressful situations. These skills are reinforced by homework practice to reduce shame responding (shutting down, becoming defensive, or appeasing the other person), rumination on hostile thinking, and impulsivity.

The program progresses through four distinct phases following assessment (covered in Chapter 5): (1) Engagement and Motivational Enhancement (Chapter 6), (2) Reflective Functioning and Skills Building (Chapter 7), (3) Coparenting Communication (Chapter 8), and (4) Father–Child Restorative Parenting (Chapter 9) (see Figure 4.3).

As shown in Figure 4.4, each phase of F4C works to increase RF first toward a father's own mental states, then toward his coparent and child. Each of the phases of F4C covers specific content, for example, the genogram in Phase 1, physiological arousal and coping in Phase 2, showing appreciation in Phase 3, and co-regulation/emotion coaching in Phase 4.

Following assessment, individual work begins with the goals of (1) putting fathers' behaviors within a context both in terms of their own experiences of being parented and their wishes for their own child and the likely disconnect between the two, and (2) building RF and coping skills to aid in emotion regulation. Coparents are invited to participate in assessment and parallel individual sessions from the start of treatment to allow the clinician to better assess the dynamics and risks within the family and to provide the coparent the opportunity to reflect on her wishes about the father's role in the family going forward and to learn the same skills he is learning in his individual sessions. Inclusion of the coparent is particularly important if the family is struggling with mutual violence. In this instance, individual sessions with coparents focus on their own use of violence in the family and dynamics with the father that result in violent episodes. How and when to incorporate coparents are discussed in Chapters 5 through 9.

Coparenting work can proceed individually with each parent in parallel or in conjoint sessions with the goals of (1) increasing understanding of the importance of coparenting, (2) defining coparenting and common coparenting pitfalls, and (3) learning communication skills to strengthen the coparenting relationship in the best interest of their children. Positive coparenting, even in the context of a conflicted intimate relationship, can be protective and result in better child adjustment (Camara & Resnick, 1989). Additionally, coparenting has a much stronger influence on parenting and child adjustment than other aspects of the couple relationship (Abidin & Brunner, 1995; Bearss & Eyberg, 1998; Feinberg, 2003; Snyder, Klein, Gdowski, Faulstich, & LaCombe, 1988). If it is possible to improve coparenting interactions, this will serve to benefit the children in the family (Teubert & Pinquart, 2010).

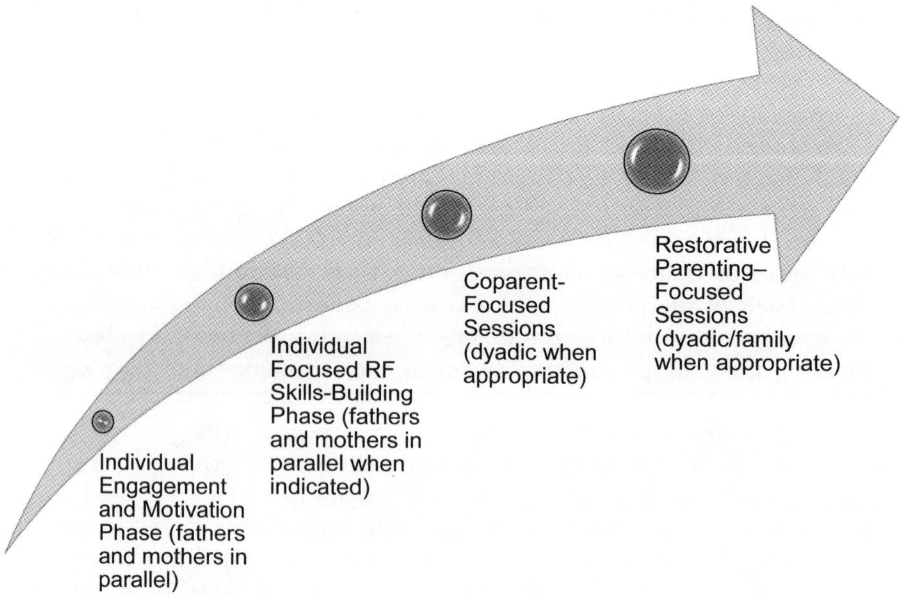

FIGURE 4.3. F4C intervention phase progression following assessment.

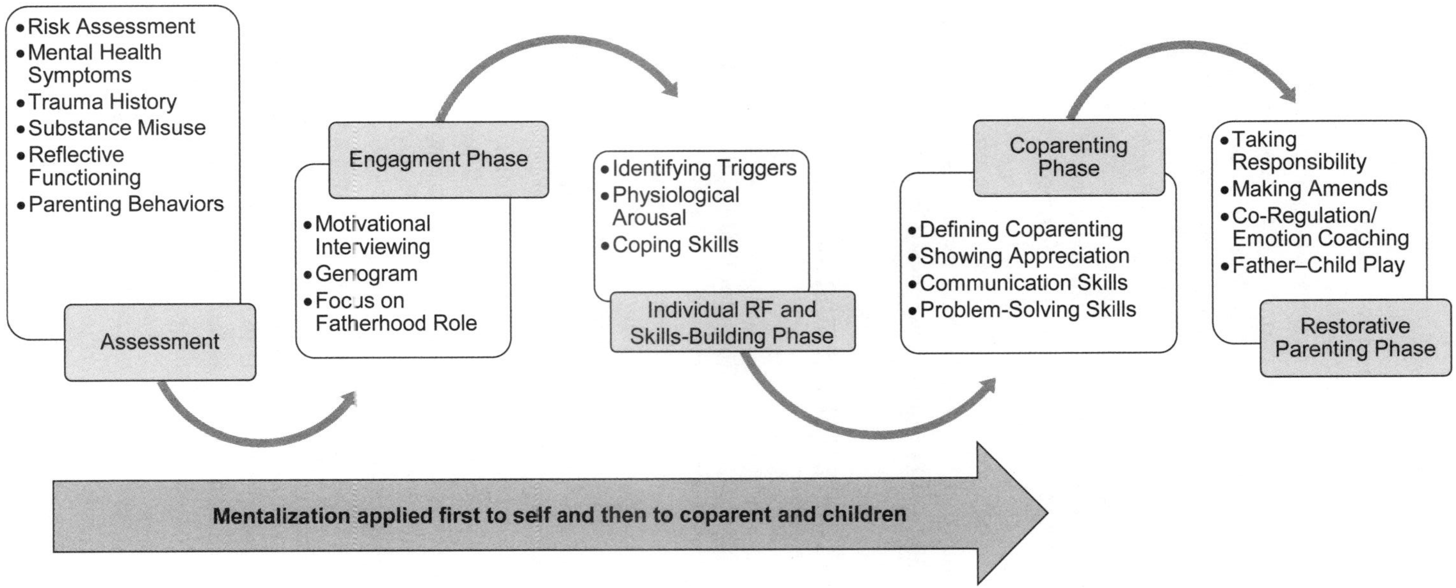

FIGURE 4.4. Phases of F4C.

The last phase of the intervention focuses on restorative parenting and may include dyadic sessions with the father's children. The goal of these sessions is to help fathers take responsibility for their past actions relative to their children and enhance the father–child relationship through improved communication and emotion coaching. Fathers work with the therapist to talk to their children using age-appropriate language to take responsibility for their past behaviors and begin to heal their relationship through activities such as co-regulation and father–child play (see Chapter 9). Dyadic treatments with mothers and young children have a positive impact on the parent–child relationship and decrease posttraumatic stress symptoms for both mothers and young children (Lieberman, Van Horn, & Ghosh Ippen, 2005; Toth, Maughan, Manly, Spagnola, & Cicchetti, 2002). These approaches have been used with both mothers and fathers who have used family violence and young children safely and with positive outcomes (Lieberman et al., 2015).

TRAINING AND COMPETENCY REQUIREMENTS TO DO THIS WORK

F4C is a unique intervention program for families impacted by FV and/or substance misuse that offers participation to mothers, fathers, and children. Therefore, it is intended for master's- or doctoral-level clinicians who have prior training in both adult and child psychopathology and intervention. The treatment combines individual, coparent, and family treatment. A therapist implementing the treatment must feel comfortable and have adequate skill in individual, couple, and family therapy. Prior training in motivational interviewing (Miller & Rollnick, 2023), CBT, and parent–child treatments such as child–parent psychotherapy (CPP; Lieberman et al., 2015) or parent–child interaction therapy (PCIT; McNeil & Hembree-Kigin, 2011) are very helpful to implementation of this therapy approach; however, certification in these therapies is not needed to deliver F4C. Additionally, significant understanding of early child development and the impact of trauma on development (physical, emotional, and social) for both children and adults is needed to be an effective F4C clinician. It is vital that clinicians possess clear training and understanding about the dynamics involved in FV, including power and control and psychological abuse. Clinicians must be interested in the health and well-being of both survivors of FV and those who have caused harm, and be able to have empathy and understanding for all members of the family. They need to be open to working with families from diverse backgrounds and to have cultural awareness and curiosity. The impact of racism for Black, Indigenous, and people of color (BIPOC) clients and their experiences with previous therapists, providers, and systems must be held in mind when working with families. White therapists must have had training in cultural humility, systemic racism, microaggressions, and the impact of colorism on families. An openness to learning about and understanding differing views of gender based on religion and culture is also important. Roles of men and women differ across cultures and religions. Working with families to stop violence while being considerate and conscious of religious beliefs, cultural context, and the impact of racism can require ongoing learning and consultation about how to apply F4C.

AVAILABLE TRAINING AND CONSULTATION IN F4C

To be a fully trained in F4C, clinicians must attend a 2½-day basic training with an F4C Master Trainer and participate in twice-monthly consultation calls for 12 months following training while implementing their first cases. These requirements ensure full understanding in the context of real cases and fidelity to the model. Information about training and consultation can be attained at *https://medicine.yale.edu/childstudy/education/practitioner/fathers*. Training includes didactic and experiential exercises to build skills described in this book. Consultation is done by video conference, and participants present cases for consultation. It is expected that participants will see three cases during the consultation year and do two case presentations to further learning. The consultation is intended to be supportive and is reflective in nature helping new F4C therapists think wholistically about families they are serving, the systems with which they interface, and the complexity and rewards of this work.

ONGOING SUPERVISION AND CONSULTATION

It is recommended that practitioners using the F4C model participate in ongoing consultation or reflective peer supervision following training. Working with families impacted by FV is challenging, and each case is unique. Even with years of experience, clinicians can benefit from support, reflective supervision about their own responses and biases toward families, frustration when progress is not made, or when systems intervene in unhelpful ways with families. Finding joy in small successes is important. Changing long-learned reactive and aggressive responses is hard, and relapse to use of FV behaviors is common. Clinicians should be prepared for this likelihood and be open to hearing from clients even after treatment ends. Sometimes clients who finish F4C will contact their therapist months or years later, when they find they are struggling again. This is a sign of growth, as clients recognize they need help and can reach out. This behavior is often a significant change for clients from their prior ways of thinking and should be celebrated and praised by therapists who have made a difference in their client's lives.

Developing a peer supervision group in your community or staying connected with those who are in your original training group can be helpful and support best practice. Reflective supervision is needed, because clinicians can become jaded in this field, and unexplored biases may impact the work. Therapists with training in individual adult and family therapy, as well as FV, know that the starting point for safe and effective intervention is comprehensive assessment. In Chapter 5, we turn to how to conduct assessments that inform your case conceptualization and treatment implementation, and how to select appropriate cases for F4C work.

CHAPTER 5

Assessment for Case Selection and Treatment Planning

Assessment and case conceptualization are important to implementation of F4C and determining the best interventions for families impacted by FV. Using an individual intervention allows for more tailored case conceptualization and is something that makes F4C different than other interventions for individuals who cause harm. This chapter outlines components of a comprehensive assessment and how these measures and tools can be used to inform F4C practice and case selection.

CLINICAL ASSESSMENT

Prior to commencement of F4C, fathers are assessed to determine appropriateness for this type of therapy. Areas of assessment include severity, nature, and context of FV; risk and safety of all family members; psychopathology, psychopathy, emotional dysregulation/anger, reflective functioning; and coparenting and father–child relationship/parenting. Prior to involvement of the child in treatment, mothers must consent to their child's participation (unless fathers have sole legal custody), and some assessment of the children must be completed to determine that dyadic treatment with the father is appropriate and not contraindicated at the present time (e.g., when a child is extremely symptomatic and treatment with their father could exacerbate present symptoms). F4C is designed to allow for coparent participation, if the coparent wishes to participate. This can be through individual parallel sessions throughout treatment or begin as parallel individual sessions, then move to conjoint sessions during the coparenting phase (see Table 1.1 in Chapter 1). If parents are living together and/or both want to participate in the treatment, the appropriateness of this should be determined during the assessment and continually as treatment progresses toward conjoint sessions. Furthermore, if both parents are using violence, inclusion of both partners in F4C is ideal.

Initial Contact with the Father

Cases can be referred to F4C through a variety of mechanisms, including courts, CPS, other agencies, or the fathers themselves. Fathers who have been referred by courts or CPS may not fully understand the nature of the program and what will be required. It is also not clear at this phase whether a father or family is right for this treatment approach. An initial phone call with a father following their outreach with you or your agency, or another agency referral to F4C, to describe the program and its components is the first step, with an introduction such as the following:

> "Hello, Mr. Fields. This is Dr. Stover calling from the Fathers for Change program at your local community agency. I received a referral from your social worker, Ms. Kimble, to our program. I wanted to tell you a bit about it and schedule your intake appointment. Fathers for Change is a program where you will meet one-on-one with a therapist/counselor. We focus on your role as a father and coparent to improve your relationships. It has some optional joint sessions with your coparent and your children if we decide together that it's a good match for you."

If fathers are not interested in having their child participate in treatment with them, they are usually not appropriate for this intervention. However, some fathers may be interested, yet hesitant to participate at first or have concerns about how their child will be involved, or there may be limitations to the father's contact with his child initially that are likely to change. For example, CPS or the courts may have put an order of protection or stay away order in place that prohibits the father going to the home or having any contact with his coparent and/or children at the present time. Getting a clear understanding of the current orders of protection is an important part of the assessment. Clinicians will need to develop strategies to gain this information from referring agencies in their area, such as CPS or the court. This can be done by requesting that agencies or other providers complete a referral form that provides this information (see Form 5.1 in Appendix A). It is also important to develop relationships with individuals at the referring agencies, whom you can contact when a new referral is received, to request information about whether there are current orders of protection if the information was not provided on the referral form. For example, in Connecticut, each CPS regional office has an IPV specialist who can be a point of contact on cases that are referred from CPS. Similarly, within the judicial branch, the Victim's Advocate Office or Family Relations Office can usually provide information about active orders of protection.

A clinician can opt to proceed with the intervention and further assess these legalities with the father as they begin to develop a rapport. It is important to discuss confidentiality up front, so that clients are clear about when and whether clinicians would need to break confidentiality. This is important for any therapeutic relationship but especially when CPS or legal systems are involved. An example of a general clinician statement follows:

> "Everything we talk about together is confidential, which means I will not share it with anyone, unless I learn that you or someone else is in danger. I am a mandated reporter, so I am required by law to contact help if you are a danger to yourself or someone else, or if I hear about child or elder adult abuse. I will ask you to sign releases of information for previous treatment providers and child protection. These are so that I can gather information to make the program as helpful to you as possible. I will not provide information back to those agencies (except for those required, as I stated before) unless you would like me to. This means I will not be sharing what we talk about week to week related to things you share about your family history or interactions with your coparent or children. Often clients want me to report their progress to their child protection social worker or to notify the courts that they have participated. We can discuss exactly what you might like me to provide or not as we go along. Usually, child protection and the courts will want to know the dates of attendance and receive documentation that you completed the program and that the treatment goals were met. Do you have any questions about any of this? I want to be sure you understand that what we talk about is between us unless you say otherwise, and to make you feel comfortable."

Fathers should be informed that their child's coparent will be contacted to gather information about the child and their coparenting relationship, and to consent for child participation. If a father refuses this, he is not appropriate for the intervention.

An individual assessment is held with the father prior to contacting the coparent to ensure he arrives and completes his appointment and consents for treatment. During the initial assessment sessions with the father, it is important to clarify that contact with the coparent will not involve sharing information about the father with the coparent; the clinician will only discuss the program itself and how she and their children might participate. The father should not be told when the clinician will have contact with the coparent or be given any indication that their consent or information they provide will impact his involvement.

At the end of the clinical assessment, say something like the following:

> "In this program we contact the coparent of your children. This is to explain to them how your child will be involved in the program and to outline what the program provides overall. It is important for both parents to be informed. I will not share any information you and I have talked about. Our conversations are confidential. Do you have any questions or worries about that?"

Detailed information about plans for assessment with the coparent or their involvement should not be provided to the father at this time, so that coparents are not coerced or intimidated from participation by the father. Additionally, let the father know the following:

> "I will review your assessment information and attain the court and treatment records we discussed. Once I have reviewed all the information, I will contact you about starting the program, if we feel it is the right fit for you. At that time, you will either be scheduled for your first program appointment, or we will offer referrals to other services we think are a better fit."

Contacting the Coparent

There are several ways to gain the coparent's contact information. If you (or your agency) implement the F4C program, use Form 5.1. Incoming Referral Form. Courts (family relations counselors, attorneys, etc.), CPS, or other community providers can complete this referral form to provide contact information for the family. The form includes the coparent's name and contact information. It is also helpful if the referral source, such as CPS, asks the coparent's permission for F4C to contact them. This request for contact (Form 5.2. Request for Coparent Contact Form) can be sent to victim's advocates offices, family relations, and so forth,. if they did not include the coparent information on the referral or if the father referred himself. It offers you (the clinician) the coparent's information, so that you do not have to get it from the father directly and gives the coparent the option to tell the referral source or their victim's advocate that they do not wish to be contacted by an F4C clinician.

If the father is self-referred, it is important to proceed with caution related to coparent contact. The clinician can try to locate the mother's contact information with the contact request form (Form 5.2) sent to the victim's advocate or other court/state agency to see if they can assist with providing the number. If this is not possible, the clinician should indicate to the father that in this program we typically have contact with coparents and inquire whether he can provide their phone number. If the father does not want the coparent contacted, then he is likely not appropriate for F4C. If contact is made with the coparent of a self-referred father, the same safety guidelines detailed earlier should be followed. Fathers should not know when coparents will be contacted or notified that information they provided was used to determine whether he was appropriate for the program.

When you have the contact information for the coparent, it is essential to phone and speak with them independently of the father. Do not leave detailed voicemails that might not be confidential or safe for coparents to receive. A simple "This is JoAnn and I'm calling to tell you about a new program at our agency. Please call me back at this number . . . " will suffice.

When you are able to speak directly to the coparent, describe the treatment program to them and set up an intake appointment to meet with them and the child on a different day than the father is scheduled for assessment. This appointment should be *after* the father has completed his initial appointment. As a safety precaution, let them know that if they do not want the child to participate, or if it is determined that the father is not appropriate due to dangerousness or safety risks (see below), the clinician will take responsibility for telling the father that he does not meet program requirements.

Note: As mentioned earlier, the father should at *no time* be informed that the meeting with the coparent or information they provided impacted his eligibility. The father should then be provided with alternatives for treatment either within the same clinical setting or in the community. As noted earlier, participation of coparents in the program is recommended, but their participation is voluntary unless they were also violent and were referred together with their coparent. Coparents should be invited to participate by explaining the goals of F4C and how they can participate. You might say, for example:

> "Fathers for Change is an individual and family treatment for fathers that focuses on reducing conflict and aggression, improving coparenting communication, and improving parenting through teaching skills. We find that it is helpful to have coparents partner with us in this program. We would like to invite you to come in to help us understand from your perspective what is happening in your family and what might be helpful."

Assessment Structure

A comprehensive assessment with both parents and the children will take approximately 4.0–5.5 hours in total (see Figure 5.1). Individual father and coparent sessions *must* be scheduled on separate days to ensure that coparents are not coerced into treatment by the father. Children should not attend the initial assessment sessions with the coparent or father. This should be made explicit on the phone with each parent prior to their appointment. The flow of the assessment should be as follows:

1. Individual assessment meeting with the father (up to 2 hours), along with having him sign releases to collect criminal, court, mental health, and CPS records.
2. Individual assessment with the coparent that includes their interest in participating and parent reports about their children (1.5 hours).
3. Child self-report assessments (30 minutes), father–child play assessment (30 minutes), and if appropriate, family play assessment (30 minutes).

After his intake/assessment appointment, the father should be told that the clinician will review his assessment materials, gather records from the court, criminal justice system, and CPS, and be back in touch with him for next steps.

Note: When making alternative referrals, the clinician should be careful to provide clear reasons for referring to an alternative provider (see Chapter 10); be clear that the court or referring agency will be notified that the father completed the intake but was not accepted into the F4C program based on the program requirements. As stated earlier, at no time should information provided by the coparent be revealed as a reason for nonenrollment. This will help protect coparents from retribution.

Areas of Assessment during Individual Meetings with the Father and Coparent

There are several factors to consider during assessment; these and suggested instruments of evaluation prior to enrollment in F4C are described below. After reviewing their results, if the clinician deems the father appropriate for treatment, the father and family can move on to the next stage of assessment, which include father–child and family play assessments (see the list of disqualifying circumstances below).

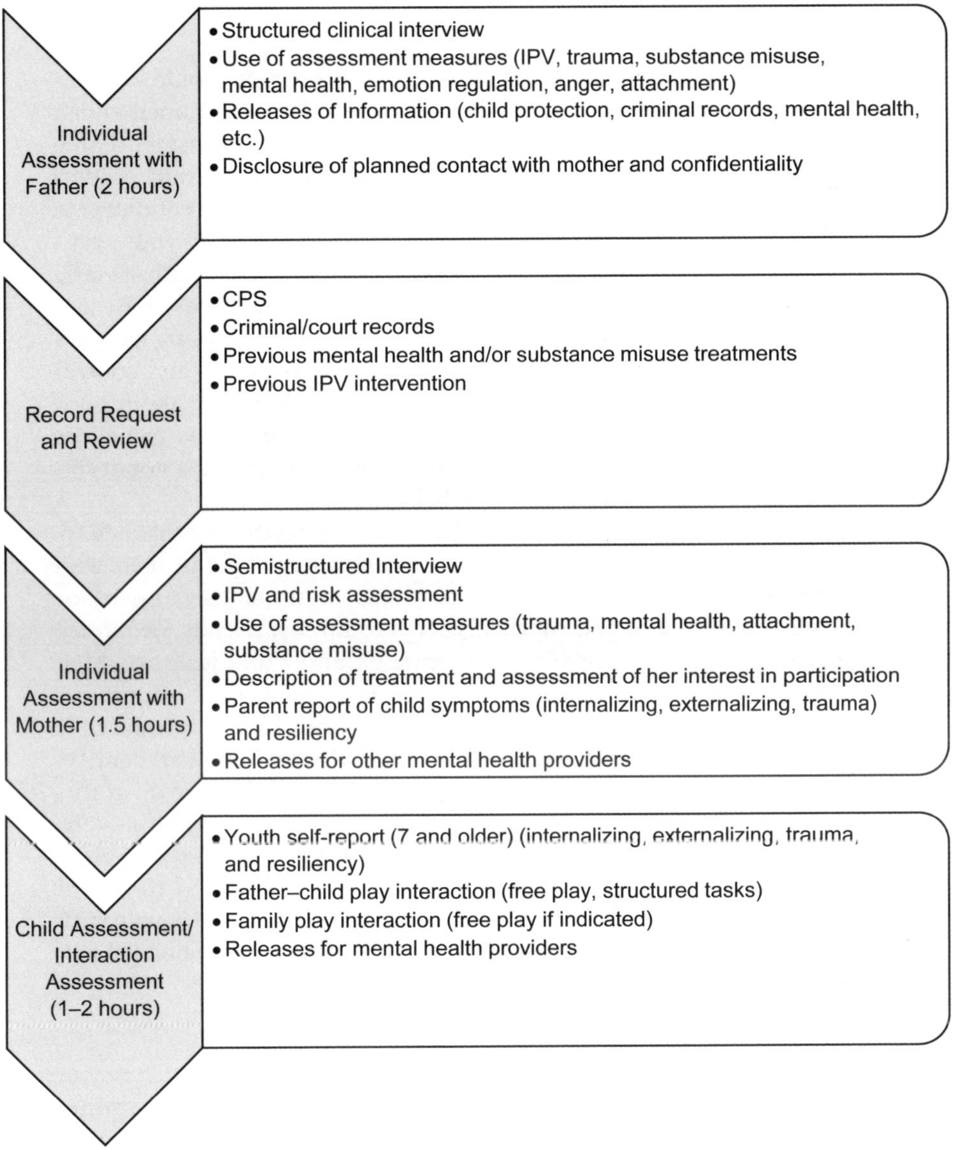

FIGURE 5.1. Assessment components.

Severity of IPV

Direct individual interviews with the father and coparent should be completed to assess severity of IPV and dangerousness. Start with open-ended questions about how they resolve conflict in their relationship. Three examples of such questions include "All couples disagree from time to time. What are the kinds of topics that you and your co-parent disagree about?"; "What happens when you disagree?"; and "How do your arguments end?" This can be followed by a structured interview with specific questions about IPV behaviors. One such measure is the Abusive Behavior Inventory (ABI; Shepard & Campbell, 1992). This measure assesses both physical and psychological violence, as well as power and control tactics. It is helpful to modify this measure to include asking about both fathers' behaviors toward their coparents and the coparents behaviors toward them. This can reduce fathers' defensiveness, and it is not atypical for both partners to use some IPV behaviors.

F4C was not designed for men who exhibit intimate terrorist behaviors. The following are likely not a match for this program: men who stalk their partner frequently; check up on them continuously at work or when they are out; and control their access to family, friends, or money in order to control them or out of extreme paranoia and jealousy. Men who use significant power and control tactics would not be appropriate for inclusion of coparents in conjoint sessions. Take the coparent's assessment of risk seriously. Survivors are typically very good at identifying their level of risk. They know their partners better than we do at this stage. As clinicians, we can advise and make suggestions but, ultimately, we want survivors of FV to be in control of safety planning and their involvement in this program. Responses on the ABI related to use of weapons or significant injuries experienced, as well as assessment with the coparent using the Danger Assessment Scale (DAS; described below), are helpful in determining risk severity.

Dangerousness/Risk of Recidivism

Coparents should complete the DAS (Campbell, Webster, & Glass, 2009) or other similar risk assessment scale. Clinicians should use this scale to assess the level of risk of the coparent and engage in safety planning discussions with the coparent as indicated. A very useful tool for safety planning is the Victim Inventory of Goals, Options, and Risk (VIGOR; Hamby, 2013; Hamby & Clark, 2012). Typically, safety decisions are in the hands of the survivor coparent; however, there are instances when clinicians may need to take action if severe risk is uncovered. A score of 9 or higher (as indicating by summing the number of Yes items) on the

DAS suggests severe risk of domestic homicide, and clinicians need to discuss the level of risk and concern with the coparent immediately by saying something like "I'm concerned about the things you are telling me and whether you and your children are safe. Where are you staying and how safe do you feel?" Clinicians may need to call CPS (domestic violence specialist, if available) and assist the coparent in calling the Domestic Violence Services hotline in their area to determine if emergency shelter is available or to assess a safe place for the coparent and children to stay. (Clinicians should always know the contact number for their local domestic violence services.) If the coparent is not interested in shelter, do they have family members or friends in the area with whom they can stay and will be safe? Scores below 9 may also be of concern, depending on the items endorsed (e.g., a combination of threats to kill, owning a gun, and threatened suicide are very high risk for dangerousness) and may necessitate the need for more safety systems, as suggested earlier.

During their assessment, fathers need to sign releases for clinicians to review police/criminal histories and CPS records. If the father refuses to sign releases, then he should not be enrolled in the program. Clinicians should review records for seriousness of risk. If the father has threatened the coparent with a gun (and he owns a gun), caused severe injuries resulting in a need for hospitalization, or caused injuries to the children requiring medical attention, he should not be enrolled, and other interventions should be considered. See Chapter 10 for alternative treatment options.

Severity of Alcohol/Substance Misuse

Assessment of the severity of the father's substance use helps to determine whether outpatient treatment is appropriate for him. Comparable reductions in substance misuse have been found with F4C compared to individual drug counseling in a small randomized trial (Stover, 2015a), and those in residential treatment have had less use of substances in the 3 months following discharge if they received F4C while in their residential program (Stover, McMahon, et al., 2019). The skills fathers are taught and their increased motivation to become better parents is thought to result in reduced substance misuse and increased abstinence, and studies of F4C support this. Still, there are instances in which F4C will not be a sufficient level of intervention and either substance use treatment is needed first or adjunctive substance use treatment is indicated. A structured substance use screening such as the Addiction Severity Index (ASI; McLellan et al., 1992), the Drug Abuse Screening Test (DAST-10; Skinner, 1982), or the Alcohol Use Disorders Identification Test (AUDIT; Saunders & Babor, 1993) and a urinalysis screening should be done at the initial assessment appointment. This can be implemented weekly during treatment to assess ongoing substance misuse if it is a concern. It is very common for fathers to have a substance misuse problem or addiction, and this alone does not rule out suitability for F4C. The severity and level of care needed to address the addiction will dictate whether a father can participate in the program. Fathers who report daily use of a substance that is interfering with their daily functioning in such a way that outpatient therapy is not a sufficient level of care means F4C is not appropriate, and referral to an intensive outpatient, residential, or inpatient detox should be made. Additionally, fathers who are using phencyclidine (PCP) are not appropriate for F4C, as PCP is an unpredictable drug that can cause severe violence. Fathers using PCP should be referred for intensive substance use treatment (e.g., intensive outpatient).

Breathalyzer and urine screenings should be given regularly during treatment to assess level of substance misuse and confirm fathers' reports of their use. An increase in substance misuse during F4C over several weeks can indicate that additional substance misuse treatment is needed (or even a higher level of substance misuse care through intensive outpatient or residential treatment) and discontinuing the F4C treatment may be necessary.

Assessment of substance misuse by the coparent is also recommended. This provides the clinician with an understanding of the severity of substance misuse in the family and what support the father will have for his abstinence at home. It also provides a context for dynamics happening within the home and child safety.

Trauma History

Assessment of childhood history of abuse and other significant traumas for both parents using a trauma history screening measure such as the Trauma History Questionnaire (Hooper, Stockton, Krupnick, & Green, 2011), the Traumatic Events Screening Inventory (Scher, Stein, Asmundson, McCreary, & Forde, 2001), or some other comprehensive trauma history or adverse childhood experiences (ACEs) tool is necessary. It is important that clinicians also assess parents' experiences of systemic racism or other forms of discrimination. The results will provide them with an understanding of the kinds of traumas and adversity each parent is bringing to their roles as coparents and partners, and indicate whether posttraumatic stress symptoms or consequences of complex trauma may be contributing to the difficulties in the family. Although helpful for case conceptualization and treatment planning, trauma history or ACEs do not impact appropriateness for F4C. In fact, approximately 90% of F4C fathers have significant histories of childhood trauma.

Psychopathology/Psychiatric Symptoms

Coparents and fathers should be assessed for psychiatric difficulties, as these may impact F4C treatment. It may be that significant depression, anxiety, or PTSD symptoms need to be addressed and considered as part of the treatment plan. These would not preclude participation in F4C, but it can be integrated into the treatment, and it may be that additional therapeutic supports or medication treatment also are indicated. A structured clinical interview that covers the range of psychiatric and personality symptoms is suggested. Some common measures to assess these areas are the Brief Symptom Inventory (Derogatis & Melisaratos, 1983), Beck Depression Inventory (Beck, Steer, & Brown, 1987), Psychopathy Checklist—Revised (Hare, 2003), and the Posttraumatic Checklist (Weathers, Litz, Herman, Huska, & Keane, 1993). Instead, clinicians may choose to administer a measure such as the Structured Clinical Interview for DSM-5 (First, Williams, Karg, & Spitzer, 2016) to assess all areas of psychological functioning. The goal is to understand the client's symptom picture, as well as any concerns about borderline, narcissistic, or psychopathic/antisocial behaviors. Clients (fathers or coparents) with untreated psychotic disorders, bipolar I, or narcissistic personality disorder are not a good fit for F4C. Many F4C clients have some borderline, narcissistic, or antisocial traits, and this is to be expected when serving this population. Coparents with significant mental health symptoms who are not already in treatment, should be offered referrals for appropriate services. For example, if a coparent has PTSD or major depression, making suggestions for possible therapy options is helpful.

Attachment in Romantic Relationships

Assess both the father's and the coparent's general approach to intimate relationships. Insecure attachment has been shown to be associated with IPV (Velotti, Rogier, Beomonte Zobel, Chirumbolo, & Zavattini, 2022). Associations are stronger for anxious attachment style, but associations have been noted for all forms of insecure attachment. Is the father generally avoidant (he does not like to be close to others or likes to be on his own) or anxious in his style (worries that he will lose his partner or he loves the partner more than they love him)? This information can inform how the clinician works with the father, especially as related to coparenting. There are also attachment dynamics between partners that can be particularly volatile. Two partners with different insecure attachment styles (one avoidant and one anxious) have been found to experience the highest levels of IPV. The Experiences in Close Relationships—Short

Form (ECR-SF; Wei, Russell, Mallinckrodt, & Vogel, 2007) may be used to assess each coparent's attachment styles. This information can be helpful in case conceptualization and development of treatment goals. An insecure attachment (anxious or avoidant) would not preclude inclusion in treatment but it would inform strategies during Phase 2 of treatment in particular.

Problems with Emotion Regulation

Although this may be obvious given a father's referral for F4C, it is important to get a sense of how he approaches his emotions. A structured assessment of these constructs is helpful. Some freely available measures that can be used are the Difficulties in Emotion Regulation—Short Form (DERS-SF; Kaufman et al., 2016) and the Multidimensional Anger Inventory (MAI; Seigel, 1986). In general, it is valuable to understand how the father describes his understanding of his emotions and how he regulates/copes with strong feelings. Is he overwhelmed by emotions? Does he avoid them? Does he seem to have a poor understanding of his own feelings? Does he deny having any problems with emotions? Again, his responses would not rule him out for F4C treatment, but they would be very informative for case conceptualization and planning for how to approach Phase 2 of treatment.

Reflective Functioning

Given the focus on RF in the intervention, getting a baseline of both self-RF and parental-RF can be helpful. The Reflective Functioning Questionnaire (RFQ) and the Parental Reflective Functioning Questionnaire (PRFQ; Fonagy & Bateman, 2016; Luyten, Mayes, Nijssens, & Fonagy, 2017) are relatively brief measures that assess these constructs. A semistructured interview such as the Parent Development Interview (PDI; Slade, Aber, Bresgi, Berger, & Kaplan, 2004) can provide clinicians with a wealth of information about how the father thinks about his children, himself as a father, and his reflections on the parenting he received as a child. This semistructured interview approach also does not allow for "faking good," as can happen with Likert scale items when fathers think they know the answers that will make them appear in the best light. The PDI, a lengthy interview of 30–60 minutes, will add time to assessment; however, fathers' RF skills will be relevant to all aspects of F4C. Clinicians understanding of his RF skills will inform treatment planning and the intensity of intervention needed in this area during F4C sessions throughout treatment, but would not preclude participation in F4C.

Coparenting Relationship

Assess the level of cooperation between parents. Is there a general sense that parents respect each other's parenting, and they can communicate about the child? Is the relationship completely contentious, and they never agree on how to parent? Is the child put in the middle of arguments between the parents? Is the child used by one parent to make the other parent angry? The Parenting Alliance Inventory (Abidin & Brunner, 1995) and the Coparenting Relationship Scale (Feinberg, 2003) are possible tools that could be used to assess coparenting. Each parent should be asked questions about coparenting support and conflict. Overall, do they think their coparent is a good parent to their child? Do they feel supported by their coparent? What kind of coparenting relationship do they want? This information is needed to help determine whether it is likely that parents will engage in conjoint coparenting sessions during F4C and what kinds of coparenting communication goals might be appropriate for F4C treatment with each family.

Parenting Beliefs and Behaviors

Structured interviews with fathers and coparents (as collateral informants about the fathers' parenting) help to assess fathers' parenting styles and approaches to discipline and father–child activities. For structured valid tools, the Adult–Adolescent Parenting Inventory (AAPI; Bavolek, 1984) or Parental Acceptance–Rejection Questionnaire (PARQ; Rohner, Khaleque, & Cournoyer, 2005) are two options. It is also possible to assess the father's approach to parenting and his understanding of how children should be treated without using these structured measures with them. This could be done in a semistructured interview by asking questions such as "Tell me about how you respond as a parent when your child misbehaves?"; "What kinds of discipline strategies do you or will you use with your child?"; "How do you see your role as a father in shaping your children's behavior?"; "Tell me about your relationship with your children"; and "What kinds of activities do you do with your children?"

As with other areas of assessment, this information is used to develop treatment goals related to the restorative parenting focus in F4C. If the father reports poor parental RF and strong beliefs about corporal punishment, this will inform the clinician's focus on these issues in treatment. Unless concerns arise related to child safety from fathers' responses (e.g., the clinician hears that the father blames the child for his issues with child protection or criminal justice system), then he would be appropriate for F4C even if he has used physical abuse or other maltreatment in the past. The clinician continually assesses safety of coparent and children during treatment and can discontinue child or coparent involvement in treatment at any time if safety concerns arise.

Child Development and Symptoms

Parent-report measures of child symptoms (internalizing, externalizing, posttraumatic responses, resilience) provide needed information about the current symptom picture of the child or children in the family. If the child is old enough (age 7 and older), clinicians should meet with the child directly to assess their symptoms and get a gauge of their comfort level with the father. Asking simple questions (e.g., "Tell me about your dad; what is your relationship with your dad like?"; "What kinds of things do you do with your dad?"; "What is your parents' relationship like? How do they get along?") can help assess the relationship and what they have observed about their parents that they are willing to share.

Note: If a child is in their own therapy, prior to meeting with them, get a release from the parents to talk with their therapist. This will provide information about the child's current symptoms and functioning, and assist in determining whether it will be therapeutic and helpful for the child to participate in F4C assessment and later conjoint sessions with their father.

There are many validated measures of child symptoms that could be used to assess symptoms across a variety of domains. The Child Behavior Checklist (CBCL; Achenbach & Rescorla, 2001) and the Behavior Assessment Symptom Checklist (BASC; Reynolds & Kamphaus, 2002) both have parent, youth, and teacher report versions that can be utilized. Keep in mind that these do not assess PTSD specifically; therefore, it is also suggested that a PTSD symptom measure such as the Child Posttraumatic Symptom Scale (CPSS-5; Foa, Asnaani, Zang, Capaldi, & Yeh, 2018) be used. If the child is very young, assessment of development and functioning using the Infant–Toddler Social and Emotional Assessment (ITSEA; Carter & Briggs-Gowan, 2006) or Ages and Stages Questionnaire (Singh, Yeh, & Blanchard, 2017) might be helpful. The Young Child PTSD Screen (YCPS; Scheeringa, 2019) is also useful to assess trauma-related symptoms specifically. If a child is experiencing significant symptoms, it is important that clinicians talk with the parents about the child's need for treatment and facilitate referrals. If the child has untreated PTSD that is related to violence by the father, it may not be appropriate for the child to participate in F4C prior to having some treatment of their own. If the child indicates they are afraid of their father or do not want to see him, then they should not be included in F4C sessions without treatment of their own and coordination with their individual therapist. There are many evidence-based trauma treatments available for children, and clinicians offering F4C should be knowledgeable of appropriate referrals for treatments such as Trauma-Focused CBT (TF-CBT), CPP, or other evidence-based trauma treatments available in their communities.

Eligibility Criteria to Determine Moving Forward with Child and Play Assessments

Play assessments would not be needed if ineligibility is determined following individual father or coparent assessment meetings or record review. A father would not be appropriate for F4C under the following circumstances and should be referred to other services:

1. He has a history of severe physical violence (e.g., significant injuries causing hospitalization) or risk of violent recidivism is high based on danger assessment. A DAS score of 9 or higher would disqualify a father, and safety planning should commence with the coparent immediately.

2. He has an active *no-contact* protective order pertaining to his child (unless this can be modified during the treatment to allow fathers to have sessions with their children). Sometimes a full no-contact order is in place initially but is modified right away. In this instance, F4C can be appropriate. If a father has a no-contact order, the clinician can ask the father when his next court date is scheduled and have contact with the court (via family relations or the victim's advocate) to determine if the protective order will be modified. If it is likely to be modified, then F4C could proceed.

3. He is currently in withdrawal from substances or in need of detoxification or residential substance misuse treatment based on the substance use assessment conducted (AUDIT, DAST, and urine toxicology). He should be referred for these services first, and F4C could be offered after his residential treatment stay has ended successfully. If F4C is initiated with a father who has a substance use problem, monitoring of his ongoing use during treatment will be needed, and if a significant increase in substance use occurs, he should be referred to additional substance use specific treatment.

4. He has cognitive impairment such as an intellectual disability or neuropsychological impairments that would prevent him from benefiting from the material that could not be mitigated by adaptation or simplification.

5. He has a lifetime history of any psychotic or bipolar disorder that is not currently treated and managed, or he is currently in an episode of major depression with suicidal thinking. If this is the case, he should first be referred for treatment for his primary mental health disorder and could be reconsidered once those symptoms are managed.

6. He has narcissistic personality disorder.

7. He is currently suicidal or homicidal. He should then be referred for inpatient treatment or a primary mental health program commensurate with the level of care needed.

8. He refuses to sign release of information forms for criminal records or CPS. This can be an exclusion, especially if there are other safety or program fit concerns. Note that some fathers may initially be hesitant to sign releases or admit to their use of violence or substances at the time of assessment. For CPS referrals and those mandated by the courts, fathers may feel concerned about how information shared will be used. They may fear that disclosure will result in further CPS involvement, removal of their children, or further action by the courts. They may also be advised by their attorneys not to disclose or admit to any criminal behavior. We have seen that some fathers are more forthcoming and take more responsibility following the initial individual sessions of the F4C model. If after completing the motivational engagement phase a father is still not able to acknowledge that there are aspects of his behavior that could be improved and does not agree to a review of case records going forward, then he will not be able to successfully complete the program, and certainly conjoint coparenting sessions with the coparent should not take place.

Observational Assessments

The father's relationship with his child(ren) and symptoms of the child(ren) should be observed during a structured play assessment. Following individual assessments with the father and coparent, schedule a play assessment session for the father with his children. The clinician will have a sense from these individual assessments about the functioning of the family and a father's relationship with his children. If there are clinical/safety concerns (e.g., his child has indicated a fear of the father or has significant PTSD symptoms as a result of father's violence that has not yet been addressed in any treatment) that suggest the child(ren) should not participate in an assessment with the father, then clinicians can determine that the father is not appropriate for F4C at this time. As mentioned earlier, if there are concerns about holding the play assessment and the child is in their own treatment, it would be helpful to get a release to talk with their therapist, describe the plan for the assessment, and learn whether the therapist would have any concerns about the child participating. This scenario would be atypical if the family members are living together or the child is seeing the father regularly for visits. The play assessment is nonthreatening and should not be stressful for the child(ren) or family.

Setting Up the Play Assessment

When you schedule the play assessment, let the father know that you want to get a sense of the father–child relationship and to meet the child(ren). Fathers need to know the clinician is supportive of them as a parent and enthusiastic to meet their children. You can say something like the following:

> "In this program, it is important for me to get a sense of you as a father and how you play with your children. I'd like to have you come in and play with some toys and games with your children. I'll be recording the play so that we can talk about it together. I like to share the positive things I notice between fathers and their children when they come for the visit. Usually, dads and their kids enjoy the playtime, and although I know the recording part can cause anxiety, I'm not trying to catch you doing something wrong. In fact, I'm looking for everything you already do right or ways you are important to your child. I just want you to come in and have fun playing. Do you have any questions?"

Video Recording All Play Assessments Listed Below for Use during Phase 1

If possible, the clinician should *not* be in the room. If a one-way mirror or video viewed on a monitor in another room is not possible, the clinician should sit in one corner of the room out of view of the camera or record the session and view it later. The clinician should not be involved in the play at all; their role is as quiet observer only. If possible, the camera should be set up and ready to go prior to the father and child's arrival to reduce focus on the recording aspect of the observation.

Free Play

Set up the room where the play assessment will occur with pretend toys appropriate to the children's ages. Toy food, dishes, dolls, baby bottles, cars, trucks, animals, dinosaurs, plain blocks, or Lincoln Logs are all good choices. If children are older school age (ages 10 to 12) a deck of cards, Jenga, or other game can be included. Leave educational and electronic toys out of the room. (Fathers are likely to go into teaching mode if educational items, such as alphabet blocks or books, are available.) Invite the father and child into the playroom and simply say, "I've put out some toys for you to play with together. Play together as you normally would."

Cleanup

After 15 minutes, the clinician should instruct the father to have the child "clean up the toys." This allows the clinician to observe how the father handles giving directives that may not be pleasing to the child. Observe: Does the father clean up the toys himself? Does he scold the child or become hostile/angry? If the child is an infant, then this cleanup step can be omitted.

Structured Tasks

Following the cleanup of toys, the clinician may opt to ask the father to complete several structured tasks with the child to see how the interaction changes under these circumstances. Remove the pretend toys and provide the father with a puzzle or shape sorter, or ask him to build a tower with the child. Make the tasks challenging for the child based on their developmental age, requiring the father support the child in completing them. Clinicians are assessing the following:

- How the father handles this situation
- The father's strategies for supporting or encouraging his child

Family Play Assessment

If the family members are living together now or planning to live together again, it is appropriate to have the coparent join the father and child(ren) for a family play assessment. Remove the structured task items and put the pretend toys back into the room. Tell the family members to play together as they would at home for 15 minutes. This will allow the clinician to observe the dynamics with both parents in the same room with the child and assess the following:

- How the child interacts with each parent
- How the parents interact with each other and with the child collaboratively

- The level of tension or discomfort in the room
- The way the parents support or hinder each other as parents or in their relationship with the child (e.g., does one parent take over and exclude the other parent?).
- Whether the child's behavior changes (e.g., there was no aggression with the father alone, but a 3-year-old boy is aggressive toward his mother when she joins the session).

How to Think about the Play Assessment

The play assessment is a chance to observe the connection between the father and his child(ren) and how he interacts with them. Fathers are often nervous and are trying to showcase their skills. Some level of anxiety is normal. The clinician who observes the play assessment should take note of the following areas to help inform their work with the father later in the program:

1. Overriding/intrusive behaviors (parent not following child's lead in play, making demands of how the child will play)
2. Parent negative affect (hostility/aggression)
3. Parental positive affect (smiles, warmth)
4. Affectionate touch (hugs, sitting on lap, child touching parent's face)
5. Dyadic reciprocity (Was there a nice back and forth between parent and child that allowed for a consistent flow of play? Was the parent not overriding or intrusive with the child? Did the child allow their parent to support and help them? Did the parent and children interact consistently without tension or constriction of emotions?) The clinician should view the play assessment as an example of how the father and children or family can interact. Parents are usually trying to showcase their strengths. The observation is a place to begin the discussion about the father–child and family interactions as the treatment moves ahead.

HOW THE CLINICIAN DETERMINES CASE APPROPRIATENESS AND THE NEED FOR ADDITIONAL REFERRALS

Recall that F4C was designed for fathers with a history of either verbal or physical FV in the last 12 months. This history can include contact with police and coparent- or self-reported violence. Fathers can have co-occurring concerns with substance misuse if their use does not require inpatient detox. F4C can be provided in residential substance-misuse treatment settings or outpatient substance-use settings in collaboration with those treatment providers (see further details in Chapter 10). As mentioned earlier, if fathers are using substances daily and their use impacts their functioning, whereby reduction of substances would require intensive outpatient or residential treatment, referring fathers for engagement in those programs first is needed with later consideration of F4C. Fathers or coparents who have significant symptoms of depression, anxiety, or PTSD that would benefit from a referral for psychiatric evaluation and medication management should be referred as soon as these are uncovered. Typically, one would not refer a father to multiple other treatments simultaneously. Referral to other parenting programs, individual, or family therapies would not be done until the father is further along in F4C and it is clear those services are needed, and the father wants to engage in them. Importantly, many fathers and their families are in need of case management and connection with resources. *Stress related to financial difficulties, unemployment, and food insecurity all contribute to FV. Be aware of available agencies and resources in your community; connect fathers to vocational, educational, and resource referrals as soon as those needs are uncovered.* If anyone in the family (father, coparent, or children) is receiving other treatments, getting a release of information for these providers will help with coordination of care and making decisions about conjoint sessions for coparenting or fathers and children going forward.

If a father is not appropriate for F4C, a discussion with him about the treatment recommendations is needed. Clinicians can set up a meeting with the father in person to discuss the assessment feedback and recommendations or talk with him on the phone. The clinician can report something like the following:

> "After reviewing your assessment results and reviewing your records, we think that Fathers for Change is not the right fit for you right now. We think that your use of opioids is really the most important thing to focus on first. Your urine toxicology screen was positive for fentanyl, and you reported very regular use with an inability to stop. We think it would be most appropriate for you to enroll in a residential program to help you detox from the opioids. We have a program in mind that I can talk with you about. We will be letting your case worker who referred you know that you completed the assessment and were cooperative with everything we asked of you. We will let her know our recommendation as well. Do you have questions?"

If the reason the program is not offered is due to safety/risk concerns, the clinician would be less specific and say something like the following:

> "We reviewed your assessment results and records and we do not think you are a fit for this program right now. We will be in touch with your caseworker who referred you to think about some other possible programs that will meet your needs. We think that an individual therapy may be best. We have a provider in mind and we can help you connect with them. Do you have any questions about what I've said?"

If a father presses the issue of why he is not a fit and there is evidence received from CPS or criminal records that meet exclusion criteria, those can be shared. The clinician might say, "We saw in your criminal record that you have previously threatened your partner with a gun and she was hospitalized due to injuries from your last domestic dispute. That makes you ineligible for this therapy program, but we can find you another appropriate program."

If the information came from the coparent's report only (e.g., she reported that he threatened her with a gun, had threatened to kill her, was using PCP), then the clinician may need to be more vague: "The focus of this program is not a match for your needs. You did not report the kind of behaviors that we usually work with here." This response relates back to the assessment, but instead of identifying behaviors that make him ineligible, it frames it as the father does not have the kind of problems that this program addresses. This strategy is particularly helpful if the father minimized his violence and you want to ensure that he does not think you are excluding him because you know about his violence from his coparent's report.

The following examples provide insight into the types of clients referred to F4C, how they're assessed, and selected, or not, for this program. Realize that each case is different, yet they all include the evaluating criteria discussed earlier.

CASE EXAMPLES

ZANE

Zane, a 27-year-old Puerto Rican father, was referred following two arrests for IPV in rapid succession. In the first incident, he was arrested when employees at a fast-food restaurant called police after hearing a couple yelling in the parking lot and observed his partner with a red mark on her face. The second arrest was several weeks later, when an altercation in the home turned physical. His live-in partner, Emily, threw keys at him following a shouting match. He pushed her up against a wall and punched the wall beside her head, breaking his hand. Zane was referred by DCF. Zane and Emily were living together with their 2½-year-old son, Jaime. During assessment, Zane was open about the difficulties he was having. He admitted to frequently swearing and yelling, as well as some use of physical violence (pushing, shoving, and breaking objects in the home). He was concerned about the impact these things had on his son. He had a great deal of anger toward Emily, who had an opioid addiction in early remission. She had abandoned the family for several months when Jaime was just over 1 year old. She had been abstinent for the last 6 months and was taking an active role in parenting Jaime, who stayed with her while Zane worked full time. Zane often compared Emily to his own mother and felt she was not measuring up as a coparent or partner. Zane admitted to significant difficulty managing his feelings and ruminating on negative thoughts about his partner frequently. He experienced joy in being a father and wanted very much for his son to have both parents in his life. Zane felt that he and Emily were sometimes supportive of each other, but that they had frequent conflict in front of Jaime. His attachment style was disorganized in that he felt suffocated by Emily's desire for closeness and avoided it, but he also was anxious that she would relapse and abandon the family again. Zane endorsed a significant history of trauma, including witnessing IPV between his parents, abandonment by his father, and community violence in his housing project. He indicated that he constantly worried about his mother and stepfather's fighting when he was a child and whether they would become homeless. He met partial criteria for PTSD and endorsed symptoms of depression and anxiety. He reported recreational use of alcohol and marijuana but no other substance use. He had previously completed an IPV intervention group mandated by the courts. He stated that he did not like groups and talking in front of other guys about his problems.

Emily, Jaime's 22-year-old, White mother, was early in recovery and was invested in remaining abstinent and parenting her son. She felt that Zane did not understand her addiction and thought she was weak for using drugs. She reported that she was quite verbally abusive with Zane at times, but at others was loving and supportive. She endorsed name-calling, swearing, and some physical violence, similar to Zane's report. She registered a low score (1) on the DAS (violence had increased). She was not concerned about his use of substances. She had a diagnosis of PTSD and had experienced physical and sexual abuse as a child. She felt that Zane was a dedicated and generally good father: "He treats Jaime really well. He just doesn't treat me that well sometimes." She reported that she generally was not afraid of Zane and that she sometimes started the fights with him: "The last time he got arrested, I started it. I was mad he got home late, and I threw his keys at him."

The play assessment with Zane and Jaime was filled with pretend play. They built block towers and used the pretend phone to make phone calls to family members. Jaime copied Zane's statements and smiled up at him. Zane was warm and showed some affectionate touching. Jaime was clearly comfortable with his father, and they exhibited nice dyadic reciprocity. During the family play assessment, the dynamic was different. Jaime had been settled and calm with his father alone, but now seemed to have trouble settling to play with his mother there. He immediately kicked the blocks and was swinging them around recklessly. Emily became nervous, as if he were trying to strike her with the blocks. Jaime fell over the pile of blocks and yelled, "Ow!" The parents both became active then in trying to settle him and play together, but the play was not fluid.

After the interview with Zane, an interview with Emily, as well as the play assessment, results reveal a family that could benefit from F4C. The father and mother report similar levels of violence, and the risk level for severe violence is considered low. The father is invested in parenting and appears to be struggling with emotion regulation and RF due to his own history of trauma. The emotion regulation and RF focus of the F4C intervention, along with coparent and child involvement, are motivating for Zane, and he is eager to participate in treatment.

ERIC

Eric was a 32-year-old African American father of three daughters ages 3, 9 and 11. He was referred by a family relations counselor from the criminal court for assessment for F4C following an arrest for IPV. During the referring incident, Eric was yelling at his wife and punching her in the face while driving on the highway. He and his wife had been married for 9 years. Eric reported that it was his wife's fault that he was in trouble and being referred for treatment. He was sure she was having an affair and that was why he was angry at her. He admitted to some use of verbal and physical violence (threatening, hitting, yelling and swearing). He worked night shifts and took care of his daughters during the day while his wife worked. He reported getting only 2–3 hours of sleep per night. He worked in a factory but had grandiose ideas about his abilities and intelligence. He reported symptoms of mania and command hallucinations.

His wife had reported a significant increase in violence and stalking behaviors in recent weeks. Her DAS score was a 10, and she was very afraid he would harm her and their daughters. She said his behavior had become erratic. She reported symptoms of depression and anxiety but no history of trauma prior to the IPV she was experiencing at present.

Given the severity of the symptoms reported, a play assessment was not scheduled, and safety planning was initiated with the mother. The clinician helped the mother plan where she could stay with the children and what to bring with her. She was also provided instructions for contacting the police immediately if she felt unsafe. Eric was scheduled for an immediate session to discuss his case (he had significant concerns about his arrest and was motivated to finish the assessment). He was assessed again for danger to self and others and admitted for involuntary hospitalization and treatment due to homicidal and psychotic thinking. This father needed intensive mental health treatment and was not an appropriate candidate for F4C. The clinician was able to advocate for the appropriate level of care that likely saved this mother's life.

JOSEPH

Joseph was a 38-year-old, White, father of three biological children and one stepson. He was referred following an incident of IPV at his home, in which he was reportedly drinking and yelling at his wife and stepson. He pushed his wife, 44-year-old Julia, and she fell to the ground. His stepson called the police. When police arrived, there was broken furniture, and the house was in disarray. Joseph had a residential stay-away order in place but could see his biological children for supervised visits. During the F4C assessment, Joseph railed about "the system" and how it was "a woman's state." He was able to admit to the argument and yelling but felt the legal intervention was unnecessary. Joseph denied problems with anger or drinking and reported that he did drink recreationally on weekends to relax, but said he didn't have time for much of it because he worked an average of 80 hours per week. He reported psychological and physical abuse by his biological father and being abandoned by his mother, who had an addiction. He lived with his grandparents for most of his childhood. He had his General Educational Development (GED) degree and was proud of his work ethic; he owned his own business. He reported significant symptoms of anxiety and depression. He denied difficulties managing his emotions but reported that he often did not understand his feelings in the moment and felt the feelings he had were wrong. He had an avoidant attachment style and was very uncomfortable with closeness.

Julia had a significant history of trauma. She was from Guatemala and had been in the United States for 15 years. She felt that her husband mistreated her first son and did not parent him the way he parented their biological children. She reported that Joseph worked many hours and was hardly ever home. When he came home, he was often stressed and yelled at her and the children because the house was a mess or the kids were too loud. Julia said the kids did miss him and wanted him to come home; she was unsure whether she wanted to reconcile or file for divorce. She reported a score of 3 on the DAS (increasing violence, having a child that was not his, Joseph controlling most of her daily activities). She reported symptoms of anxiety and PTSD and was seeing an individual therapist (for information on coordination with other providers, see Chapter 10). Julia also reported that she and Joseph did not coparent well; she felt he was too strict, and she was more relaxed about rules at home. Joseph also acknowledged this difficulty.

Given that Joseph's visits with the children had to be supervised, his F4C play assessment was arranged through CPS. The clinician contacted the CPS social worker for the family after getting a signed release of information from the father. The CPS worker felt the assessment was appropriate and facilitated contact with the father's sister, who was providing supervision for his weekly visits. She brought the children for the assessment appointment. His wife did not attend. Joseph was happy to see the children, and he interacted in a warm way with them, but there was some discomfort. He seemed more comfortable with his youngest daughter (age 4) than with his two sons (ages 7 and 9). It was clear that they did not play together frequently. He asked lots of questions about what they had been doing since he saw them last and had trouble settling in to play a game with them.

This assessment reveals that Joseph is not taking responsibility for his behaviors, but his distrust of "the system" and concerns about legal repercussion for his business make this unsurprising. He is avoidant of feelings and ambivalent about change; however, he is very committed to fatherhood and admits that the dynamics at home are unhealthy. He would like to work things out with his wife for his children's sake. He reports that he would find individual therapy preferable to group therapy, and his history of trauma, avoidance, and distrust, make this program a better fit. F4C was recommended in this case.

Therapist and family match can also be an important consideration at the conclusion of assessment. Female therapists can and do successfully conduct F4C; however, there are times when assignment of a male therapist may be needed due to fathers' views about women and the likely impact it may have on the therapeutic relationship. There may also be times when modification of the one-therapist approach of F4C is needed to meet the needs of the family. See Chapter 10 for several examples of cases that might require assignment of two therapists (one male and one female). It is important to know that even if you agree to start a case with a father, you do *not* have to continue in the model past the individual focused sessions. Inclusion of coparents and children can be determined as you proceed, develop rapport, and determine whether a father is using the treatment to make changes for himself and his family. The phased approach in F4C allows for flexibility as clinicians attempt to make connections with fathers and gain their trust. How to proceed with the motivational aspect of this first phase of F4C is discussed in Chapter 6.

CHAPTER 6

Phase 1

Engagement and Motivational Enhancement

Now that you have determined that a father is eligible and have completed your comprehensive assessment, you both are ready to embark on the first phase of treatment. Engagement is a significant problem in programs for those who cause harm. This has led to research and strategies to try to better engage this population. As mentioned in Chapter 4, use of fatherhood as a motivational strategy is key to F4C. The motivational engagement phase of F4C includes four topics: Introduction to F4C; Fathers' Roles and the Importance of Fathers to Child Development; Reflecting on Father–Child Interactions; and Reflecting on the Family of Origin. Before introducing these topics, let us first consider the clinician's stance and reasons for fathers' ambivalence regarding treatment.

CLINICIAN STANCE

In F4C, the client must be *active* in the reflective process to gain the most benefit from the intervention. This process requires that a feeling of safety, curiosity, and support be established with the client. Clinicians should not approach fathers as the "all knowing" expert who is going to teach them a set of information and skills. This is not a psychoeducational experience for him to get through; this is a therapeutic process. Clients must have the opportunity to reflect on their own experience and come to understand themselves better through the sessions. The therapist takes a nonconfrontational stance, especially at the outset, with a goal of understanding the father. F4C clinicians listen to fathers and reflect back what they hear, so that fathers feel heard and understood. Clinicians must continually evaluate their own biases and assumptions to ensure that they are approaching fathers with an open mind and a curiosity about them as individuals. (Refer to the training and reflective supervision needed to successfully do this work as outlined in Chapter 4.)

When working with the father throughout treatment, the clinician must continually think about the reflective abilities of the father and how to help move him toward better self-reflective, coparent-, and parent-reflective functioning. The clinician must notice the patterns of development a father may take through this intervention. Some fathers may do very well developing a self-focus, but others may struggle more with mentalizing. Some may be better at mentalizing with the partner or child but less able to attune to themselves. Clinicians must think about each father holistically and support his development through the intervention—and provide feedback to the dad accordingly that helps him locate his areas of strength and those in need of further development. This intervention cannot be administered in a rote manner, without developing a clinical formulation of the client and developing a trusting rapport.

Using motivational interviewing strategies (see details below) is key to engaging this population of fathers. As the treatment progresses the therapist may decide to challenge a father's thinking patterns or stance, but it must be in a reflective and wondering way. A curiosity about the father's feelings, thoughts, or ways of coming to conclusions about a situation will lead to better engagement of the client than taking a challenging, expert stance. This in no way means that we do not hold fathers accountable for their behaviors or set clear boundaries when needed, especially if the father presents with high levels of personality traits like narcissism. In taking a supportive and interested stance, clinicians must be mindful not to collude with blaming of coparents or children or allowing fathers to excuse their violence. The goal is to help him understand himself and how he can take control of his thinking, feeling, and behavior.

KEY POINTS FOR THE FIRST SESSION FOLLOWING ASSESSMENT

The first phase of the intervention following the assessment is focused on the father's individual motivation and background. It is not uncommon for fathers to enter the assessment and initial session of the intervention in a very defensive way. They want to convince the clinician that they do not need this program. They are "not like the other guys referred to this program." They report, "I'm a great dad. I'm not violent." This is not the time to be confrontational or pull out a police or CPS report and read the charges or allegations. It is the time to ask open-ended questions and wonder about how a program like this might help him in some way. Fathers who are referred by CPS or the courts can have many worries: (1) that they will lose their children; (2) that they will lose their family (partner and children); (3) that they are seen as a monster, criminal, or some other horrible person; (4) that if they admit to their behaviors, they will forever be labeled and seen as a perpetrator, batterer, or abuser; (5) that the clinician is judging them and will have influence over their children's placement or their criminal charges and the likelihood of going to jail; (6) that they will be discriminated against and misunderstood/judged for being a person of color, undocumented, or from another marginalized group. It is crucial that these concerns are addressed during the first session. Persons who do not feel safe cannot share information about themselves or be vulnerable. It is your job as the clinician to make the client feel listened to and safe, to develop a therapeutic relationship that will allow them to acknowledge their unhealthy behaviors, the ways they have caused harm, and be open to change. This can take more than one session and clinicians must be patient and willing to build this trust over time during this initial phase.

F4C has four phases following assessment: (1) Motivational Engagement, (2) Reflective Functioning and Skills Building, (3) Coparenting Communication, and (4) Restorative Parenting. Each phase includes key concepts, or "Topics," covered with clients. In this chapter we begin with Phase 1 (Motivational Engagement), which includes Topics 1 through 4:

1. Introduction to F4C
2. Fathers' Roles and the Importance of Fathers to Child Development
3. Reflecting on Father–Child Interactions
4. Reflecting on the Family of Origin

These topics usually take one session each, but sometimes a father needs more time to become comfortable and develop rapport or think about his family background before moving forward. Phase 2 includes Topics 5 through 8 (reviewed in Chapter 7); Phase 3 covers Topics 9 through 12 (reviewed in Chapter 8); and Phase 4 includes Topics 13 through 17 (reviewed in Chapter 9). Topic 18 is the end to treatment and final step in F4C (reviewed in Chapter 10).

TOPIC 1: INTRODUCTION TO F4C

The aims of the first topic are to review the information attained in the assessment, further develop rapport, discuss goals of the program, and gain some commitment to participation. This first session typically begins with an appreciation for the time the father spent completing the assessment and acknowledging the personal nature of the questions and process. Engage the father in conversation about the assessment process to see how he feels about coming in at this point. Does he feel burdened and annoyed? Were there things that surprised him about the assessment or things he learned about himself from the questions and discussions? Clinicians might ask questions such as the following:

- "How was the assessment process for you?"
- "Were there things that surprised you?"
- "Are there things you would recommend changing to make it easier?"

These questions allow the father to feel that his opinions about the process are heard and that the clinician is interested in his experience and feelings.

Next, broadly review the assessment results that he reported pertaining to substance/alcohol misuse, aggression, emotion regulation, and coparenting concerns that brought him to treatment and the nature of his referral to the program. Review of assessment does not need to include specific scores or numbers from assessment measures, but instead an overview of the kinds of difficulties or areas of concern the father reported. Many of the fathers who engage in F4C are sent by the court or CPS. It is important to acknowledge this mandated order openly and begin to see whether the father feels forced and is not interested in participating in the program. The primary goal of this session is to develop rapport and to begin to build the father's motivation to continue in the program.

Using Motivational Interviewing Techniques

Rapport can be built using motivational interviewing (MI) skills (Miller & Rollnick, 2023). Rolling with resistance (not arguing back or confronting the person) is a main approach in this first session. Many fathers have been marginalized, and they feel defensive when they come in; they need to feel heard and to have the clinician empathize with their experiences of the "system." We also use the core skills of MI, called "OARS": Open Questions, Affirmations, Reflections, and Summarizing.

Open questions are used to help the client share their experiences, but it is important to keep the discussion focused on the client. For example, if the client says, "My problem is my wife and her constant nagging," you could respond, "Tell me more about what happens for you," or "Tell me more about your role during these discussions." These types of responses keep the client focused on their own experience and steers them away from their partner.

Some open statements or questions that might start off the discussion include the following:

- "What is your understanding of why you are here?"
- "Tell me about your family [partner and children]."
- "Are there areas of your life you'd like to change?"
- "Are there areas of your relationship with your child or the child's mother that you'd like to change?"
- "What might you find useful in our meeting together?"

These kinds of questions act as invitations for exploration and provide the client with a level of agency that can strengthen rapport. If the father reports no areas that he'd like to change or ways intervention might be helpful, some additional MI techniques can be useful, such as the readiness scale. You might ask, "On a scale of 1 to 10, with 10 being the highest, how motivated are you to be in this program?" If he says he is a "1," ask, "Why aren't you a zero? You are here." Responses to this question can take the form of change talk (an important concept in MI) that indicates the client's desire to change regardless of how small—for example, "I'm here because I want to get child protective services off my back." The father is motivated to get systems out of his life, which is a place to begin.

You may also try other statements that could elicit change talk, like "Are there no areas of your relationship with your child or your child's mother that could be strengthened?"; "It sounds like from your perspective everything is going perfectly for you now." Alternatively, a clinician may ask the father to talk about what he thinks is going well in his family and with his child, with a question such as "What are the areas of your life that you feel are going well?" or "What brings you joy in your family life?"

Affirmations are an MI approach that can help build rapport by giving compliments or affirming a behavior of the client—for example, "I really appreciate your taking the time to come in and meet with me today and explain your views on whether you need a treatment program or not." Affirmations show the client that you appreciate their time and effort in showing up to meet and talk with you, even if they did not want to attend.

Using *reflections* is another key MI strategy that is used to validate the client's feelings. These are statements such as "You seem really upset right now," or "That sounds very overwhelming." Reflections validate clients' feelings and empathize with their frustrations. However, clinicians should *never* reflect blame toward the survivor of FV. Keep the conversation focused on the person sitting in front of you, and not on the survivor. If a client is reporting that his problems are entirely because of his coparent, the clinician might say something like "It sounds like you feel the problem is with your partner and you have no role in the difficulties?" If he agrees and continues to blame his coparent, the clinician could interject and ask, "I'm wondering if there is any way that you could have an impact on this dynamic? The only thing you can control is your own behavior. I'm wondering if there are any ways you might do things differently that could help?"

Summarizing is another MI approach that takes all the information you have heard and provides a summary to let the client know you have been listening and you understand what they've said. It is a special application of reflective listening—for example, "OK, let me see if I can summarize what you've told me so far. You feel that your wife should not have called the police on you, and that you could have handled the incident yourselves. You are angry that child protective services are now in your life and that you cannot live at home before completing a domestic violence program. Did I get that right? What did I miss?"

If a father is ambivalent or adamant that he has not used FV, this may be due to a lack of understanding about the range of behaviors that are considered abusive. It may be necessary to do some psychoeducation about what behaviors are considered intimate partner violence. Men sometimes focus on whether they "put their hands on her." There are many ways that words and actions outside of hitting can be abusive. Clinicians can use materials describing the types of abuse—for example, the Power and Control Wheel or Equality Wheel (*www.theduluthmodel.org/wp-content/uploads/2017/03/powerandcontrol.pdf; www.theduluthmodel.org/wp-content/uploads/2017/03/equality.pdf*)—if they feel the father needs this educational approach to develop a shared language or complete Worksheet 6.1. How Healthy Is My Relationship? Again, the stance is not confrontational but is meant to provide information for him to consider as you continue to work together and discuss his relationship. These materials are typically *not* used in a first session but are presented after a session or two of MI continues to result in no ability to set goals or no acknowledgment by the father that any of his behavior could be contributing to the difficulties in his family.

Clinicians may also return to queries from the assessment to help understand the dynamics in his relationship:

- "Tell me about what happens when you disagree with your partner/coparent."
- "How do arguments end? Who makes up with whom?"
- "How do you know an argument is over?"
- "Tell me about how decisions are made in your relationship."
- "Who makes decisions about money, use of the car, raising the children, and so forth?"

These probes help to provide a clear understanding of the dynamics in the relationship. The clinician can then begin psychoeducation about power and control, and what constitutes FV. As an introduction, the therapist might say something like the following:

> "I want to talk with you about how abusive and unhealthy relationship dynamics are defined compared to healthy relationships. Sometimes we get focused on physical acts like hitting and we forget that other actions and words can be considered forms of family violence."

This discussion is not meant to have the clinician convince the father that he is abusive. It is meant to provide him with information, so that he can better understand the ways his relationship has been unhealthy.

Recall that in this topic the clinician works to establish the father's commitment to treatment and development of some initial goals. Covering this introductory ground can take more than one session if the client is in a precontemplation stage of change and is ambivalent about participating in treatment. Listen for change talk during the session and work toward open-ended questions, affirming, reflecting, and summarizing the change the client talks about during the session. These MI strategies can be used to help the client commit to treatment goals (see the example of Darius below; OARS strategies are noted there). This topic typically ends with the father signing an Assessment and Treatment Agreement (Form 6.1 in Appendix A) at the end of Session 1 or Session 2, as shown in the case example that follows. Figure 6.1 is a sample treatment agreement that clinicians can use to guide this discussion.

OARS in Action

CASE EXAMPLE: DARIUS

Darius, a 35-year old African American, has initiated treatment in F4C because he was involved in a domestic dispute with his wife in front of his 1-year-old son. He was arrested and is very worried, because he is on probation and this arrest violates that probation. He has no prior police involvement for FV but has served jail time for other criminal convictions. He is hoping that engaging in F4C will help him when he appears in court. He completes the intake assessment and reports no physical violence. He does acknowledge some verbal violence and breaking items during the argument with his wife that resulted in his arrest. He indicated that his wife was angry because he didn't pick up their son from day care; he thought she was picking him up, and stated that a heated argument ensued, and his wife called the police. He indicated that it was a one-time thing and they normally get along very well. He is guarded in his responses and reports minimal information about his background.

During the first session of F4C, the clinician uses open-ended questions to understand why Darius is in the program and what he hopes to get from F4C.

CLINICIAN: Tell me about what brings you to F4C?

DARIUS: I didn't do anything wrong. And I don't plan on getting anything out of this program. All these programs are the same. They tell you to attend these programs, but they already have ideas about you and who you are.

CLINICIAN: What do you mean? What kind of ideas? [Open-ended questions]

DARIUS: I've gone to other programs, and they have all these topics to go over, but they aren't made individual or they don't seem to care about my situation.

CLINICIAN: I appreciate you coming in to meet with me even though you feel like it's a waste of your time. That took effort. [Affirmation]

DARIUS: Well, I feel like if I don't, it's just going to cause me problems.

CLINICIAN: I can understand that worry. It sounds like you've had some past experiences that you have not found helpful. [Reflecting] I do have questions to ask you today, but they are for me to hear from you about your individual experience. This is an individual program where we meet one on one, so we can apply all the information directly to your experiences. When you answer questions based on your experience, then I understand your situation and what might best help you. It allows me to provide you with a program that is a fit for you.

DARIUS: I suppose that makes sense.

CLINICIAN: There are certain topics that we will cover, but we will tailor them to your needs. It sounds like you may have experienced discrimination and racism from other programs or systems, and you feel that this could be the same. [Reflecting] I'd like us to be able to talk about that when it comes up. As a White woman, I have not experienced what you have as a Black man. If there are times you don't feel I understand, I'd like you to tell me. That way we can be sure I understand. I'm here to help you, not help the system. What do you think?

DARIUS: (*quiet for a minute*) OK, that sounds fair.

CLINICIAN: (*Returns to goal setting, using what she has heard so far in session.*) It sounds like there was miscommunication with your wife around picking up your son?

DARIUS: Yes, that's what happened, and all couples have that sometimes.

CLINICIAN: Yes, it is true that miscommunication is common in relationships, and I wonder if there might be ways to strengthen your relationship with your wife?

DARIUS: Yeah, I think improving communication might be a good goal and learning how to be a dad. [Change talk] I was locked up and I missed out on some early parenting. I don't know how to be a dad. [Change talk]

CLINICIAN: OK, so there are two really good areas to focus on. Improving healthy communication and developing new parenting skills. [Summarizing]

Please read the guidelines below carefully, list several goals you have for yourself, and sign the bottom of the form.

1. I understand that I will be asked to complete assessment tools and questionnaires.
2. I agree that I will be asked to submit to random urine and Breathalyzer screens during my assessment and treatment.
3. I understand that this treatment will be 4 to 6 months in duration, and I agree to participate for this length of time.
4. I agree to attend the sessions and to be ***prompt!***
5. I understand that this treatment is intended for people who want to remain abstinent from alcohol or drugs, to manage their anger, to be violence-free, and focus on their roles as parents and coparents.
6. I understand that I must participate and practice the exercises to be most effective.
7. I understand that I *may* be asked to attend sessions with my coparent and/or children as part of the treatment.
8. I understand that my coparent and/or child may participate in sessions where I am not present.
9. I agree to work on the following goals during the program:
   a. *Learn to manage my emotions better.*
   b. *Improve my communication with my coparent.*
   c. *Understand my son's experience and support him.*

Darius Jones	*Darius Jones*	*4/19/2023*
Client Name Printed	Client Signature	Date
Dr. Stover	*Dr. Stover*	4/19/2023
Clinician Name Printed	Clinician Signature	Date

FIGURE 6.1. Sample Assessment and Treatment Agreement.

In this example, the clinician was able to focus on what she was hearing from the client about fears of discrimination and racism, and how he could be treated in the program. He also was presenting as ambivalent about making any change, but by using MI, the clinician was able to elicit change talk to find two goals for the program and begin to build a positive rapport with him to begin working. Because of the clinician's reflecting and summarizing, the client felt heard.

Parallel Session with Coparent

Individual parallel sessions with coparents for Topic 1 should cover similar content. Review assessment findings and the reason for recommending F4C, as well as how each phase is intended to help the father and family.

Several key areas to cover with coparents include the following:

1. Review the importance of their involvement and how that will look. Can they participate weekly? This is ideal, but it is up to them. At this point, do they wish to work toward conjoint coparenting-focused sessions with the father? (This would take place in Phase 3.)

2. What are their wishes and ideas about what will happen in their relationship with the father? How do they envision coparenting? Do they have current safety concerns? If so, be sure to safety plan and address them immediately in session using suggestions outlined in Chapter 5, including use of the VIGOR (Hamby & Clark, 2012).

3. Review the open-ended relationship questions with her that were used in the assessment (see Chapter 5) to get an idea from her about the dynamics in the relationship—for example, "Tell me about what happens when you disagree with your partner/coparent"; "How do arguments end? Who makes up with whom?"; "How do you know an argument is over?"; "Tell me about how decisions are made in your relationship"; "Who makes decisions about money, use of the car, raising the children?" Worksheet 6.1. How Healthy Is My Relationship? can be used to discuss the dynamics in their relationship that may be unhealthy. This discussion is not meant for the clinician to convince the coparent they are in an abusive relationship, but instead to provide an opportunity to look at the balance between healthy and unhealthy characteristics and what they may be striving for in the future both from their partner and themselves. Are the totals greater in the healthy or unhealthy column? How does the coparent feel about their scores in each area? The goal is to have them reflect on the health of their relationship and consider what changes might be needed.

Note: If it is clear that both parents have used violence and this is truly a mutually violent couple, then it is important to engage the mother in parallel sessions weekly when possible, and to have her set treatment goals related to improving her emotion regulation, reducing her use of FV, and improving her communication skills using Form 6.1.

TOPIC 2: FATHERS' ROLES AND THE IMPORTANCE OF FATHERS TO CHILD DEVELOPMENT

This topic, usually covered in Session 2 of F4C, is broken into several parts. The first part is to get an idea of what the father thinks it means to be a father. The second part is to talk about the development of his children: to introduce the potential impact of FV and substance misuse on children and explore any concerns he has about his parenting or his children.

Fathers' Roles

Start this topic by asking questions such as "What does it mean to be a father?" and "What is a father supposed to do?" Write a list of the client's ideas about his role as a father in his child's life. *What does he think he should do for his child? What areas does he find the most challenging?* The goal is to understand from his own background and culture his beliefs about his role as a father. Another great question to further this conversation is "What would you like your children to say about you when they are grown?" Following the father's response to this question, the clinician can ask, "Do you feel you are on track for your children to say those things about you?" This follow-up question can stimulate change talk if fathers feel there is a gap based on their current circumstances.

Some men have difficulty with these questions, especially if they did not have a father in their lives when growing up. Feel free to prompt and guide the discussion related to the following topics:

1. Financial support—"What is your view on a father's responsibility to provide for his family?"
2. Education—"How do you feel about education and the education of your child(ren)?"
3. Discipline—"Do you discipline your child(ren)? If so, in what ways?"
4. Love—"How do you show your partner love? Your children? How do they show you love?"
5. Role modeling—"How do you think your child(ren) view you as

a role model? What are the things you try to role-model for your children?"

If a father is not engaged in this conversation and does not appear invested or is struggling to talk about the importance of fathers, the video documentary *Show Your Love* (*www.samkauffmann.com/ordering-show-your-love*) may be used to stimulate conversation. The video is just under 20 minutes and presents children from different backgrounds talking about what their relationships with their fathers have meant to them.

Parallel Session with Coparent

A parallel session with the coparent covers the same areas. *What do they think a father's role is? What are their wishes for the father's involvement with their children going forward? What were their own experiences of being fathered growing up? How would they like the experience to be the same or different for their children?* If a coparent feels a father is not important, the documentary video *Show Your Love* may be helpful to review and discuss as a way to illustrate how children experience both involvement and lack of involvement of their fathers. It is possible that a coparent who did not experience a father growing up may have a strong reaction to the idea of a father's importance to child development. Careful exploration of this topic and what it will mean for their children could really benefit the family going forward.

CASE EXAMPLE: JOANNA

Joanna was attending her second session of F4C with her clinician. During the session, the clinician was exploring the importance of fathers and how her children might be impacted by the current lack of contact with their father.

CLINICIAN: How has not seeing their dad in several months affected your children?

JOANNA: My kids are fine. I'm their mother *and* their father.

CLINICIAN: (*Begins to talk about ways fathers contribute to child development.*)

JOANNA: (*abruptly*) My kids don't need their father. I didn't have my father and I'm fine!

CLINICIAN: (*realizing she had touched on a painful topic for Joanna and that her approach was triggering*) You have done very well without your father, and it must have been painful that he was not available. If you could have had your wish as a child, what would you have wanted from your father?

JOANNA: I didn't need nothin' from him.

CLINICIAN: Maybe you didn't *need* anything, but what did you wish for or want from him? Think back.

JOANNA: I just wanted him to show up once in a while and want to be there.

CLINICIAN: You missed out on that father–daughter relationship. You are doing fine without it, you're right, and it also seems like it means something to you that he was not around.

JOANNA: Yes, I guess it does.

In this example, the clinician recognizes the mother's personal reaction to the loss of a father and first addresses her pain, so that she can be more open to her children's experiences and needs. This kind of conversation can open the door to exploration of how her children might have a different experience and her potential worries about it.

Normal Child Development and the Impact of FV

Now that the clinician has an understanding of how the father sees his role, it is time to introduce behaviors he might expect from his child(ren) given their ages. What is typical for the child's overall development at this stage? Use of normal child developmental handouts can be helpful to this discussion, such as those available from the Centers for Disease Control and Prevention (*www.cdc.gov/parents/infants/milestones.html*). The clinician can start by asking, "Tell me about what your children like to do. What are some of things they enjoy doing?" This allows for a discussion of their development and what is typical. As stated earlier, clinicians who are providing F4C need to have a strong knowledge of child development, including normal developmental stages and children's physical, emotional, and social development during infancy, toddlerhood, preschool, school age, and early and late adolescence. During this discussion, ask, "Is there anything you find challenging about parenting right now?" or "Do you have any concerns or worries about your children?"

These questions can lead to a conversation about the potential impact of FV and, if indicated, parental substance misuse on his children. Handout 6.1. Impact of Exposure to Parental Violence and Substance Misuse on Children, can be a means of discussing symptoms at different ages. Assist the father in identifying any symptoms or difficulties he has noticed in his children. Refer to assessment/intake information if needed.

Did he or his coparent identify symptoms or behaviors of concern that may be associated with FV or other family issues? Are there other developmental concerns? It is important not only to be assertive about the role of FV and its impact on his child(ren), but also to use person-centered therapy approaches. This father was a child who grew up in a family and learned how to be a partner and parent from his own family. During this discussion, help him reflect on the following: *What kind of modeling did he get from his parents? What kind of empathy did he receive in his own family? What were the expectations for closeness?* This reflection can help the father begin to think about areas where he lacked support or modeling in his own childhood and what he might gain from therapy to change in ways he wants to be different for his children.

Again, F4C is not intended to be confrontational, especially in the early stages of intervention. Continue to use MI skills during this session as needed to elicit change talk (for further reading and guidance in MI, see Miller & Rollnick, 2023; Hohman, 2021).

Fathers may have concerns about disclosing symptoms of their children, because they think it may result in a CPS response or that they admit to using FV. It can be helpful for a clinician to reiterate their role as distinct from CPS, the courts, and legal systems:

> "I believe you are important to your children, and my job is to help you be successful. If I understand how your children are doing, I can best help you in your relationship with them. Parenting is a very hard job, and we can all use support sometimes. My role is not to determine whether you are guilty of any crime, to comment on any legal action, or to give guidance about your CPS case. I am merely here to provide support and help you have the healthiest family possible. The more open we can be, the better I will be able to assist you in meeting your goals."

TOPIC 3: REFLECTING ON FATHER–CHILD INTERACTIONS

This topic continues the focus on the client's role as a father and his relationship with his children. It requires the most preparation out of all the topics in F4C. The clinician should review the video recording of the videotaped play assessment during the assessment process. Select segments of the video that you would like to watch with the father. These should be short segments of only a few minutes each. The primary focus of this exercise is to highlight successful moments of connection between the father and child, not to sit and watch the entire play assessment recording. Examples of good things to highlight include the following:

- Bids the child makes for the father's attention
- Successful exchanges that include affection, play, or cooperation
- Times when the child copies the father or is trying to please him
- Any caretaking behaviors the father performs

You can introduce this activity by saying something like "You may recall that during your assessment, you did a play session with your child(ren). Today we are going to return to that session. I have highlighted some moments I liked that I want to share with you and get your thoughts on them. Let me ask you first, what was it like for you to do the play assessment?"

To begin, allow the father to reflect on the experience. Many will say they were anxious or worried about what it was all about or what the clinician was looking for or wanted. Others might comment that it was strange. Acknowledge how strange it must have felt and that dads often feel anxious or strange playing during the assessment. Next, watch the first segment you selected and ask what he noticed. You might say something like "What did you notice about [child's name] and yourself?" Another option is to ask the father what he was feeling at the time and explore what he thought his child was feeling: "How do you think [child's name] felt while you were playing in this video? How do you know?" It is a good opportunity to assess the father's capacity for RF. What is he able to communicate about his own feelings and experiences? Can he differentiate his feelings from those of his child? How does he understand his child's feelings and experience? It is essential to help the father see moments when his child is well connected to him or is seeking closeness. You may have to point these out, as they may be subtle and may have gone unnoticed by the father. *The goal is for the father to leave the session feeling that he is important to his child, and that he has at least some beginning parenting skills.*

Clinicians can comment on any emotion they noticed, shared joy, or distress not brought up by the father. It is key to let the father know you *see* the good he can bring to his child and that you are there to support him in his role as a father. It is imperative that the clinician not come across as an evaluator of the father's parenting or relationship. Instead, the father and clinician look together at the selected moments from the video, then reflect on what the parent is doing that makes this particular interaction go well. These moments are often times when the father has responded in an attuned way to the child's action or initiative using a combination of nonverbal and verbal responses. This is not intended solely as a time for clinicians to find "good" video clips, then praise the parents. Therapist "praise" confirms to the father that the therapist is an evaluator of his parenting; this is not the intention. The goal is to involve the parent as a collaborator in reflecting together on the segments shown. Less use of praise and more focus on the naming of what is in the clips and the effects of what is named, enables a cumulative collaboration between the therapist and parent. Parents are not being taught how they should interact with their children, but they are learning how they can actively develop a joyful relationship. This approach is similar to those used in video interaction guidance (Kennedy, Landor, & Todd, 2011).

If there are striking areas of disconnect or difficulty, these can be reviewed after first examining moments of connection to begin planning ways you can assist the father in gaining further mastery of parenting skills. The following example details this kind of discussion.

CASE EXAMPLE: TYREK

Tyrek, a 30-year-old African American, is the father of 18-month-old Kareem and stepfather to 6-year-old Tanasia. During the play assessment, Tanasia continually attempted to engage Tyrek in play. She watched him carefully and tried to involve him in several activities. He criticized her play choices several times (kitchen and doll play) and encouraged her to play on her own while he sat next to her and watched. He then used several long, thin blocks to make drumming noises on a plastic bin. Initially Kareem was interested in this activity and tried to copy his father. Soon he lost interest and became overstimulated by the constant noise. Tyrek appeared not to notice and continued to drum and attempted to get his son to participate. The clinician watched several sections of the video with Tyrek.

CLINICIAN: What did you notice watching that clip?

TYREK: They didn't have appropriate toys for my son. These aren't the kind of toys we have at home.

CLINICIAN: You felt that the toy selection was not what you would want to play with your children. I can see how that would make it harder. [Reflection] What kind of toys do you play at home with the kids? [Open question]

TYREK: I enjoy building with large Lego blocks with Kareem when we have time. I'm unsure how to play with Tanasia and feel she should play with her mother.

CLINICIAN: Tyrek, do you notice the ways Tanasia tried to play with you and how interested she seemed in doing so?

TYREK: I hadn't at the time but watching it now, I see how much she wanted to play with me. It feels good. I've often felt that Tanasia did not really like or respect me as a father figure.

CLINICIAN: Let's come up with some things you would feel comfortable playing with Tanasia that you might try. It looks like she would really enjoy that and you would like it, too. What did you notice about the drumming?

TYREK: (*shrugging shoulders*) I thought Kareem liked it.

CLINICIAN: Kareem was interested in the drumming initially and it was a fun idea. Can you think about how the drumming and noise might have been for Kareem?

TYREK: It did get loud and he looks like he wanted me to stop. I guess I didn't notice at the time, but I was irritated watching it just now.

CLINICIAN: You can see what Kareem's experience is when watching the video. It's common for us as parents to miss the subtle cues our children send us sometimes.

This video viewing allowed for a discussion of cues to look for, and the clinician encouraged Tyrek to play with his children and be an observer of their clues. The clinician is a curious observer with Tyrek. She highlights connection (ways the daughter is trying to play with and be connected with him), and she encourages Tyrek to reflect on what he sees and assesses his ability to reflect on the experiences of his son. Tyrek felt seen by the clinician as valuable and encouraged with some new ideas to try to strengthen his relationship with his stepdaughter in particular.

This topic concludes with discussion of Handout 6.2. Good Role-Modeling Tips for Dads. The clinician should review this handout with the father and ask him if there are areas he thinks he'd like to focus on in particular.

TOPIC 4: REFLECTING ON THE FAMILY OF ORIGIN

This topic is focused on the development of a genogram to aid in discussion of the father's own family of origin and multigenerational patterns of trauma, FV, substance misuse, negative/conflicted relationships, CPS involvement, and so forth. A genogram is also known as a schematic or family diagram; it is a pictorial display of family relationships and patterns of behavior. Sometimes, there are patterns that are passed down generation to generation. There are standard symbols and guides for creating genograms, as they have been a standard practice for family therapists since they were introduced by Murray Bowen and popularized by Randy Gerson and Monica McGoldrick (1985). Using these standard symbols is not essential, but it is important for the clinician to be comfortable creating a genogram in front of the client. Drawing it in session in collaboration with the client is the most effective way to do the work.

There are computer programs available to assist in generating the genogram too (e.g., *www.genopro.com, www.edrawmax.com/genogram/genogram-maker*), but creating a large picture on paper with markers and use of colors can create a shared activity that works very well.

Clinicians introduce the activity to the fathers as a way to think together about the kinds of fathering and relationship role models they have had in their lives. Clinicians might say something like the following:

> "We are all influenced by the people in our lives, especially our families. Today we are going to draw a family map together so that we can talk about who is in your extended family and what everyone's relationships are like. We talked a little bit in our previous sessions about your parents and the kind of parent you would like to be; we are going to talk more about that today. I'm also interested in learning more about who provides you with support and the culture within your family."

The clinician should then create a genogram in collaboration with the father. Sometimes using large paper on a table is helpful or putting the paper up on the wall to create a visual focus for the discussion. It is important that the father can see what the clinician is drawing, and that they feel like it is a shared activity. The clinician should position themselves in an open posture to communicate collaboration. The genogram should include a minimum of four generations (the father's children and partners, his parents, the father and his siblings, and his grandparents). When creating the genogram, elicit information about relationships (i.e., who was close or distant), substance misuse, IPV, child maltreatment, significant traumas (including racial trauma), and use of corporal punishment. It is vital to take note of the nature of relationships in his family of origin. Were his parents married? Did he have a significant father figure in his life, either biological or step? Who did he live with growing up? With whom did he spend the most time? What were the cultural traditions in his family? How has his family been impacted by trauma, discrimination, racism, poverty or other factors? Fill in as much information as he knows about his child's mother's family as well. After the genogram is created, allow the father to look it over and ask, "Are there any patterns you notice in your family map?" or "What stands out to you when you look at it?" Be sure to point out and discuss the following:

- Patterns of IPV, substance/alcohol use, child maltreatment, homelessness, lack of marriage or father roles, and so forth.
- Ask with whom he spent the most time and what those relationships were like for him.

- Ask how this family history or environment impacted him as a child. Try to inquire about feelings (fear, worry, sadness), as well as outcomes (divorce), behaviors (adultery), and so forth.
- What is one thing he has noticed that he learned from his own family growing up that he has brought into his current family that he is worried or unhappy about?
- What traditions or aspects of his family culture does he want to bring forward?
- Who were his supports? From whom did he draw strength?

This exercise is an opportunity to explore further his relationship with his own father and how he would like to be the same or different from him or other father figures in his life. This can lead to a discussion about how his own behavior now (specifically, substance misuse, aggression, and negative coparenting) is impacting his child(ren) and how the work you will do together over the coming weeks can help him make the changes he would like in his family and prevent the same patterns for his own children. The genogram session is usually empowering for fathers and helps them recognize the opportunity they have to stop intergenerational FV and the significance of that opportunity. Fathers are often very responsive to this activity. Even those that have had very difficult family histories engage well in the genogram exercise and respond to the challenge of knowing they change the trajectory of their children's lives through their own actions.

CASE EXAMPLE: JAVIER

In discussion with his therapist, Javier shares the genogram pictured in Figure 6.2. He shares that he did not really know his father or the paternal side of his family because they lived in Puerto Rico.

CLINICIAN: What do you know about your mother and stepfather's relationship?

JAVIER: They fought a lot.

CLINICIAN: What was that like for you as a child?

JAVIER: I was always worried about what was gonna happen. I would ask, "Are we gonna leave now? Are we gonna be homeless again?" I don't want that for my son. That messes a kid up.

CLINICIAN: It sounds like the fighting and worries were very stressful for you. You said you want it to be different for your son. How do you think you can make it different? What can you do to be sure G doesn't see you and Amber arguing and things getting violent?

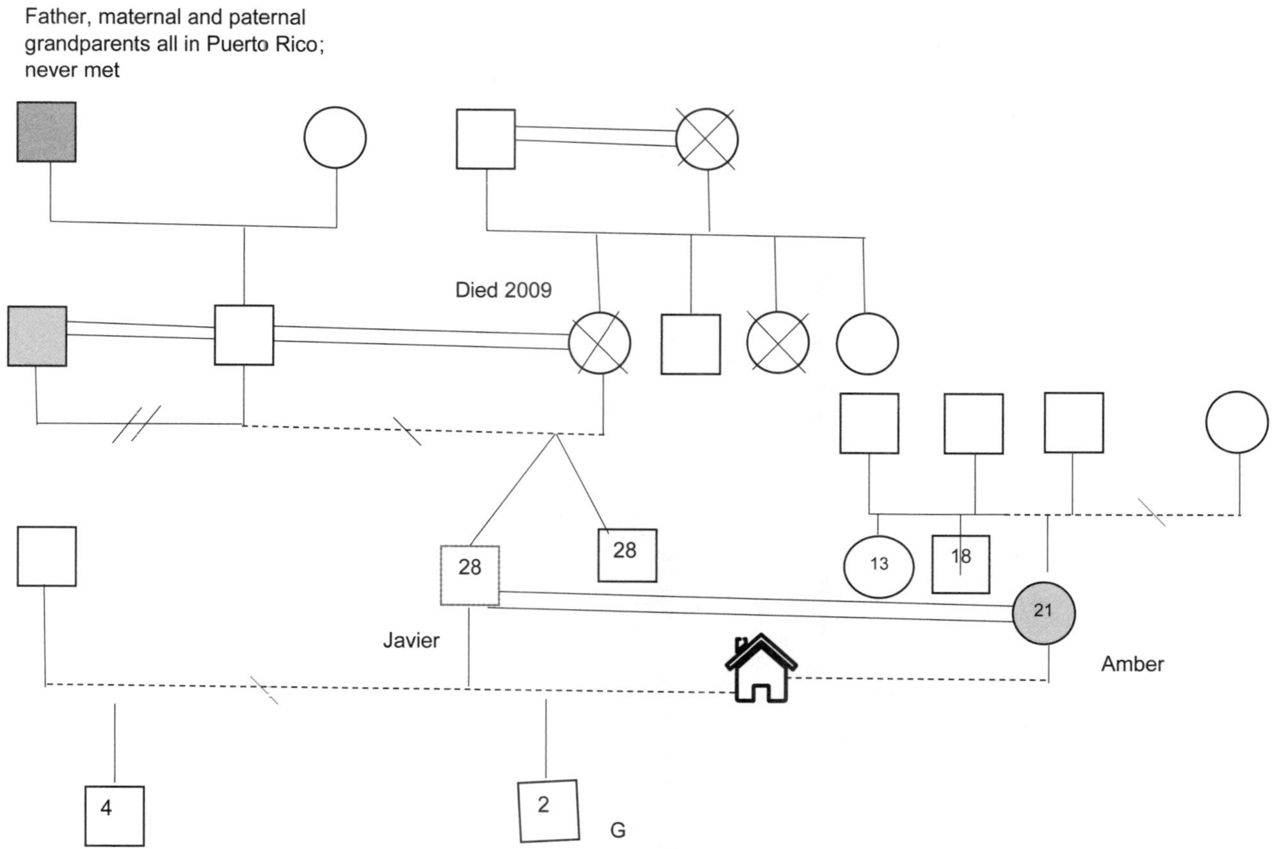

FIGURE 6.2. Sample genogram for Javier. Numbers inside shapes are ages. An X through the shape indicates the person is deceased. Double lines indicate domestic violence. Gray shading within a shape indicates a substance use problem.

JAVIER: We have to talk to each other like adults. We can't be yelling and hitting. If we can't figure out how to do that, then I think I need to leave so that it's better for G.

CLINICIAN: It sounds like you want to learn new ways of communicating with each other and to manage your emotions when you are in discussions.

JAVIER: Yeah, yeah, I do. Amber has to learn, too.

CLINICIAN: You can only control your own behavior. I can meet with Amber, too, so she knows the same skills you are learning, but it's important for you to know that often when one person in a relationship changes the way they talk to and treat their partner, the other person responds differently, too. Let's look at the change plan and write down some of these things we've just discussed.

The last part of this topic is to complete the Form 6.2. Change Plan, which reviews reasons for making a change and ways the father can make such a change. This is an opportunity for the father to reflect on the motivational work you have done so far and refine the goals he has for participation in F4C. This is also an opportunity to do safety planning with the father for high-risk situations, so that he is participating in safety planning, showing his own responsibility to keep the family safe from FV. This is highlighted on Form 6.2 in the final question: What specific strategies can he use now to prevent violence from happening (e.g., take space when he feels overwhelmed, talk to a trusted friend when he feels upset)? Write these down together. You will add to this list as he continues to learn skills through F4C sessions (see Figure 6.3).

Parallel Session with Coparent

Like the other topics in this phase, meeting with mothers for a parallel genogram session can be very helpful for multiple reasons. The clinician gains a better understanding of the coparent's experiences and her family patterns. Understanding their background and experiences with men in their family, where they draw support, and cultural norms and expectations around family roles and traditions can be helpful in understanding how they view relationships, coparenting, and parenting. As with the father, the clinician can use the genogram to have a discussion with the coparent about what they would like to see change in their current relationship with their coparent or dynamics with their coparent and children. If they are still in a relationship with the father or plan to resume the relationship, what could they see differently to show that they are making changes? What patterns or behaviors does he need to change? Are there important things that they are bringing from their own family

I understand that verbal and physical aggression, yelling, screaming, and controlling behaviors are unhealthy for my family.

Why is it important to make changes now?

I don't want G to grow up like I did. I do not want to mess him up like I was messed up watching my parents fight all the time.

What will successful change look like?

Amber and I will be able to talk to each other calmly without yelling or hitting. We will not fight in front of G. I'll do what's best for my son even when I'm angry.

What resources and strengths do I have that can help me reach these goals?

I am a good father. I took good care of G when his mother was using.

What barriers stand in my way?

I have trouble controlling my anger sometimes. I get so angry at her because she left us to use drugs.

What are specific ways I can ensure there is no physical aggression, yelling, screaming, and controlling behaviors in my family? How can I plan for high-risk situations?

I can leave the house if I am agitated before a fight starts. I can separate myself from Amber until things calm down.

I can control my own behavior even when I cannot control hers.

Javier — Client Signature

11/10/2020 — Date

FIGURE 6.3. Sample Change Plan for Javier.

of origin that are unhealthy or that impact the current family dynamics to consider in working with the father?

CASE EXAMPLE: BECKY

Becky and her F4C therapist are discussing her genogram. Through creation of the family map, Becky shares that her father was addicted to drugs and he had sexually abused her while he was high. She said, "I'm over it. I forgave him." It is clear from the genogram that Becky had no models for healthy relationships in her family. Addiction and abuse were common throughout the family. She felt a strong need to always protect her children. It was hard for her to be separated from them and she worried about them while they were at school/day care, and even leaving them with her mother for the therapy appointment was causing her distress. She admitted that she never left the children alone with her husband.

> BECKY: I can't trust no one. I don't want no one to hurt them. My husband drinks. What if he sexually abuses the kids?
>
> CLINICIAN (*gently*): That must be exhausting, worrying about your children all the time.
>
> BECKY (*crying*): I'm so tired.
>
> [*The therapist was then able to talk more with Becky about her worry, whether she had ever talked to a therapist about her anxiety about her children's safety, or her past sexual abuse. She had not.*]
>
> CLINICIAN: How do you think your children understand your worry about them being without you?
>
> BECKY: I don't know. I guess maybe it makes them think everyone is dangerous and scary.
>
> CLINICIAN: Right. You are teaching them that the world is unsafe, and no one can be trusted not to hurt them, including their teachers, family members, or their father. Tell me more about your worries about Tom being with the children alone.

This discussion helped clarify for the clinician real worries (e.g., Tom's drinking and the IPV that had occurred when he was drunk) and worries that were coming from Becky's sexual trauma (e.g., worry that Tom would sexually abuse the children). Becky didn't really think he would sexually abuse them, but she felt she couldn't risk it. When asked what she would need to see from Tom to trust that he could be alone with the children even for a short time, she said he would need to show her he was not drinking. She felt maybe with support she could allow him to be with the kids for short periods when she knew he didn't have time to get drunk.

In this example, the clinician learns important information about Becky's family history and her trauma. Tom's drinking is a trigger for her because of her father's behavior when he was using substances, and Tom has also shown that when he drinks, he can cause her harm. It is understandable that she would fear for her children's safety given her own experiences. At the same time, this hypervigilance about her children's safety is exhausting for her and is teaching her children to live in fear of everyone and that the world is unsafe. Becky feels heard and supported in this discussion, because the therapist validates her exhaustion and perpetual stress responses that result from her traumatic experiences. The therapist can continue to talk with Becky about these issues in parallel sessions and also suggest that treatment for PTSD could be very helpful for her and connect her with an individual therapist or agency that can offer her such treatment. Clinicians doing F4C should be educated about resources in their area for other forms of therapy or treatment so they can assist coparents in attaining needed services during or at the conclusion of F4C.

The goal of this phase is to work through the father's ambivalence and set clear goals for change to benefit his family, without allowing feelings of guilt or shame to prevent him from engaging in the therapeutic work ahead. In Chapter 7, Phase 2 of the program is presented—Reflective Functioning and Skills Building—which covers Topics 5–8.

CHAPTER 7

Phase 2

Reflective Functioning and Skills Building

Having worked on topics related to individual motivation and family of origin in Chapter 6, we now begin Phase 2. The individual reflective functioning and skills building components of this phase start with examining triggers for strong emotions and identifying the range of emotions fathers may experience. Clinicians help fathers begin to reflect on their emotional lives and what emotions trigger conflict and FV. These may include shame, guilt, anxiety, or fear, in addition to anger or frustration. In this phase of treatment, we provide clinical strategies to help fathers (1) identify emotions, (2) describe what emotions feel like physiologically, and (3) implement both physiological and cognitive coping strategies. The topics in this phase include Exploring Triggers for FV, Need for Control, and Use of Substances; Understanding Emotional Arousal and the Body's Stress Response; Physiological Reactivity and Management Skills; and How Thinking Impacts Behavior.

TOPIC 5: EXPLORING TRIGGERS FOR FV, NEED FOR CONTROL, AND USE OF SUBSTANCES

This topic is intended to help the father focus more specifically on his behaviors that have caused harm, including physical, psychological, and verbal aggression and misuse of substances. This topic can begin with a discussion of situations that have resulted in incidents of FV in the past (verbal, psychological, and physical) or have triggered his misuse of substances. The clinician can ask the father to describe the last time he and his coparent had a disagreement that escalated to verbal or physical aggression. This event could be the incident that prompted the referral to F4C, his most recent arrest, CPS involvement, or other recent incidents of high conflict. The occurrence should be focused on his aggression toward his coparent/partner or children when possible and not general aggression toward others. Ask him to tell you about the incident in detail, describing what led up to it, and what he was feeling and thinking at the time. Use of functional analysis can be very helpful during this session. Functional analysis assists in understanding a specific target behavior (e.g., FV) and identifying the triggers and reinforcers that cause and maintain the behavior (Iwata, Dorsey, Slifer, Bauman, & Richman, 1994; Yoman, 2008). It is a key aspect of cognitive-behavioral therapy and there are many published resources available. Worksheet 7.1. Functional Analysis of Behaviors is one tool that could be used to facilitate this work.

Functional analysis can be done by first exploring what, when, who, and where an incident happened and breaking down thoughts and emotions that accompanied the situation, then exploring the short and long-term consequences of the behavior. What reinforces the behavior? Are there also negative consequences? The clinician should try to elicit multiple examples of things that cause the father to be reactive or to withdraw. The goal is to identify underlying themes (consistent triggers or emotional states) that result in FV or use of substances to cope. The clinician may have ideas about trigger themes based on information from the genogram developed during the last topic. Common themes leading to FV are feelings of disrespect, guilt, shame, or abandonment. See Figure 7.1 for an example of functional analysis.

Emotions

CASE EXAMPLE: JORGE

Jorge is the 35-year-old Hispanic father of 5-year-old Carlos and 2-year-old Gabriella. Jorge gets into frequent verbal arguments that quickly escalate to violence both at home and in the community. In session, he describes an incident in which his partner is in the kitchen. He has just returned home from work and is sitting in the living room watching a sports channel. His children are in the living room making lots of noise while they play. Jorge calls to his partner, Ashley. She does not respond. Jorge yells louder to her and she still does not answer. He gets up from the couch and goes to the kitchen. He yells and swears at her that he is calling to her to deal with the kids because he needs some peace and quiet. He says she needs to take the kids out of the living room. Ashley gets angry and yells back that she has

Fill in the boxes below to examine what led up to behaviors you'd like to change (e.g., yelling, lashing out, aggression).

What and Where	• Where was I? • What was happening? • Who was with me?	*In the living room after work* *The kids were playing loudly and my partner was in the kitchen.*
Thoughts	• What was I thinking?	*I just need some time to unwind.* *Why are these kids being so loud!* *Why doesn't my wife know that she needs to give me some quiet space when I've had a long day at work?*
Feelings Sensations	• What were my feelings? • What sensations did I have in my body?	*Agitated and stressed* *Fidgety like I need to get away*
Behaviors	• What did I do?	*I yelled at the kids to go play somewhere else and then at my wife for not giving me some peace and quiet when I get home.*
Consequences	• What happened right after? • How did other people react? • How did I feel? • Any other consequences?	*The kids started crying and my wife got upset, but then everyone left me alone.* *I felt angry but was glad to have everyone leave me alone.*

FIGURE 7.1. Sample Functional Analysis of Behaviors for Jorge.

been with the children all day and it wouldn't kill him to play with them for a few minutes while she prepares dinner. The yelling escalates for several minutes until Jorge storms out of the house. The clinician breaks down the argument and asks Jorge what he was thinking and feeling when he called to Ashley.

> JORGE: I was feeling annoyed and thinking, "She knows I just got home, doesn't she know I need some time to myself?" When she didn't answer my calls, I was thinking she was ignoring me.
>
> CLINICIAN: What else were you feeling or thinking?
>
> JORGE: I was feeling stress from my workday and needed some time to relax, and I felt like my needs were not being met. I was thinking my wife didn't care about me, and she was purposely trying to get me upset.
>
> CLINICIAN: Were there other times in your life you remember feeling that your needs were ignored?
>
> JORGE: I often felt ignored in my home growing up. My parents were frequently unavailable or unresponsive to me because of their drug use.
>
> CLINICIAN: Might there be other explanations for why your wife did not answer you in that moment?
>
> JORGE: She said was in the middle of cooking dinner and doing some dishes in the kitchen. She may not have heard me over the noise in the kitchen combined with the TV and the kids. She may have been trying to finish what she was doing before she answered.
>
> CLINICIAN: It sounds as if you've thought about this situation again and changed your thoughts about your wife's intentions.
>
> JORGE: I am feeling much calmer and understand why she did not answer.

This example details how the clinician could use functional analysis of the scenario and elicit thoughts and feelings in the given situation while also helping the client understand why that issue may be particularly sensitive for him. Jorge frequently felt uncared for and ignored as a child, so when he perceived his wife to be ignoring his needs, he was reactive and hostile. Helping him begin to understand those underlying feelings will allow for generation of coping skills for how he can get his needs met differently in the future. The clinician could talk with Jorge about how he might take time to de-stress before coming into the house by using some relaxation or grounding techniques in the car before entering the house or revising his thinking about how he might enjoy play with his children to relax and reset. This topic sets the stage for that work.

Triggers

CASE EXAMPLE: KEITH

Keith is a 29-year-old White male and the father of two boys, 4-year-old Keith Jr., and 1-year-old Conner. Keith is in treatment due to substance misuse and FV. The mother of Keith's children, and previous partner, struggles with addiction and has not had extended contact with their children in months because of her recent relapse. Both of Keith's children are in the care of his father's long-time partner, Tammy, because of both parents' substance misuse and IPV. She brings the children to visit Keith for his supervised visits on the weekends for a few hours at a time. In session with his therapist, Keith recounts an incident when Tammy calls the night before to explain that she cannot bring the kids to see him on Saturday because Conner is sick. Keith is upset and argues with Tammy over the phone, stating that it is the second weekend in a row that she has been unable to bring the kids. Keith tells Tammy that she is making excuses about why she cannot bring them to see him. Tammy denies this and explains that she didn't think it would be a good idea to bring a sick toddler over to his friend's home where he is staying. Tammy says that she will bring them next week, when Conner is feeling better. Keith then yells at her and accuses her of purposely avoiding him because she thinks she is a better and more experienced parent than he is and doesn't trust him with his own children. Tammy responds that she is too old for this and has no reason to make up excuses. Keith then ends the conversation abruptly by hanging up the phone. The clinician breaks down that conversation.

CLINICIAN: What was going through your mind when you were speaking with Tammy?

KEITH: I was thinking that she doesn't like me because of my history of drug use and thinks I'm a bad influence on my own children.

CLINICIAN: What other sorts of thoughts did you have during the call?

KEITH: I'll admit I think my kids feel more comfortable with Tammy and may not want to come and see me. It makes me feel guilty and ashamed about not providing a stable environment for them because of my addiction and fights with their mother. My own father was not around much, and I'm resentful of that and wouldn't be surprised if my kids became resentful of me for the same reason.

CLINICIAN: Are there other, alternative reasons or ways you can view the situation?

KEITH: I think since I feel ashamed of my own problems, that makes me feel like a bad parent. I know Tammy is older and does not want to raise kids again; she's not trying to take my kids away from me permanently.

CLINICIAN: Let's reevaluate the conversation with Tammy. When she told you she could not bring the kids, that was a trigger for feelings of shame. I'm wondering what feeling started that though?

KEITH: I felt disappointed and sad. I've missed out on so much with them that I do not want to miss any more time. I feel so ashamed that I can only have a few hours a week supervised with them because of everything I've done.

CLINICIAN: So those first feelings of disappointment and sadness lead to feelings of shame about yourself as a parent, which led you to think that Tammy was trying to keep your children from you [meaning she must think you're a bad parent, too], when really it sounds like she was trying to care for them since Connor was sick?

KEITH: Right. When I think about how great Tammy has been and all she's doing for my kids and I know she does not really want to take them from me, I feel less angry and stressed about the situation. When I think about how Tammy must feel, and talking about it now, I know that she is not trying to keep the kids from me. She wants me to get better so I can parent them full time. She's not the one that thinks I'm a bad parent. In that moment I felt ashamed of myself and I felt I was a bad parent.

Through these conversations, the clinician goals are to develop a list of "hot button" issues or underlying feelings for the father, such as feeling unvalued, disrespected, abandoned, shamed, or ignored, and produce a list of topics and underlying feelings that accompany them. In this example, Keith was feeling shame for the time he had missed out on with his children. Shame typically leads to negative feelings about the self instead of a focus on actions. He felt shame and therefore assumed Tammy did not value him as a father, and underneath his shame, he felt he was a bad parent. Once a clinician uncovers shame responses in a father and talks about them in session, they can continually look for this pattern and encourage the father to reflect on when it is happening during interactions and how it shapes his behavior.

It is important for the clinician to explore feelings the father has other than anger and talk about the ways that anger can be the "tip of the iceberg," and that other feelings are often underneath the surface. Explore these underlying feelings that accompany anger; use these discussions to look for consistencies. Can the father make connections between his current "hot button" topics and his past experiences in his family-of-origin, childhood or teen experiences, or previous romantic relationships? Are there traumas from his past that are resulting in triggers within his current life? The overall goal is to help the father better understand his emotional experiences related to FV and misuse of substances, and to begin to understand the feelings that underlie his strong reactions and develop empathy and compassion for himself.

Uncovering Shame

As with the earlier case of Keith, shame is a frequent trigger for aggressive responding in fathers who have caused harm. When individuals feel shame, there are two very common responses: withdrawal/avoidance or reactive/defensiveness. Shame shuts down a person's ability to reflect on their behavior and take responsibility to make amends. Helping clients distinguish between feelings of guilt and shame can be very important during Topic 5. Handout 7.1. Shame versus Guilt can be used to help fathers think about how shame feels different from guilt and how shifting away from shame and into guilt allows one to take accountability, make amends, and work toward changed behavior.

If we return to the example of Julio from Chapter 2, we can see how his shame prevented him from engaging in therapy to reunify with his daughter despite his longing to see her and be an active parent. If Julio had not responded to the clinician eliciting his feelings to help him move forward, as in the example from Chapter 2, they might have decided to do some psychoeducation about shame and guilt with him in the moment using Handout 7.1 to assist him in thinking about how shame was impacting his decision making. For example:

JULIO: I'm going to get a lawyer and go to court to fight this. I don't need anyone to help me reconnect with my daughter. I'm a good father!

THERAPIST: How does it make you feel when you think about having someone supervise your visits with your daughter?

JULIO: I feel bad. I don't know, I just don't think I need it.

THERAPIST: You feel bad. I'm wondering if that bad feeling is shame?

JULIO: I'm not ashamed. I'm a good father!

THERAPIST: You feel like no one can see that. I see how much you miss your daughter and want to see her. Sometimes when we feel shame, it makes it hard for us to take any responsibility or action. Let me show you the difference between two feelings: shame and guilt. (*Reviews Handout 7.1.*) When we feel shame, we feel that we are bad. We think, "I'm a bad person. I'm a bad father. I'm a monster." That causes us to be defensive or to withdraw because it feels so terrible. But when we can shift to feeling guilt for our actions and think, "I did something wrong. My actions were hurtful," then we can acknowledge them and make amends. People can make mistakes, and those are wrong, but that does not make them bad. I hope that shame is not preventing you from doing what the court is asking so that you can see your daughter as quickly as possible.

Homework Practice

Ask the father to keep a list during the upcoming week of times he notices himself having unhelpful thoughts (especially shame thoughts) or strong emotions such as anger/hostility toward others or feelings of anxiety. Ask him to write down the situations and his thoughts about them using Worksheet 7.2. Emotion Triggers. It is helpful to work through an example in session so that the client has a guide on the worksheet to help him do this at home. (The worksheet includes an example.)

TOPIC 6: UNDERSTANDING EMOTIONAL AROUSAL AND THE BODY'S STRESS RESPONSE

Once the father and the clinician have started to examine triggers with Topic 5, it is important to check in about how the week has gone at the start of each subsequent individual focused session to assess for triggers. Worksheet 7.2. Emotion Triggers is used the first time you do this and can be reassigned for fathers to track emotional triggers week to week, or clinicians can choose to be more informal at the start of the session, asking the father to reflect back on his week and any times he was triggered, even if the worksheet was not assigned that week.

Start by assessing whether there were any high-risk situations, conflicts with partner or children, or use of substances/aggression during the past week? *Aggression* here is broadly defined to include any yelling, swearing, manipulation, controlling tactics, or physical violence. This opening discussion can lead directly into review of his homework using Worksheet 7.2. Emotional Triggers. Clinicians can expect that fathers may not do the homework, or they may have filled it out just before the session. Either way, the homework can be done in session if needed, with the therapist helping the father fill out Worksheet 7.2 with any incidents of emotional arousal and follow with functional analysis, as outlined in Worksheet 7.1. Functional Analysis of Behaviors.

The goal is to explore emotional triggers, especially within the coparenting and parenting areas. Continue to make connections between these situations and a father's underlying thoughts/beliefs/feelings (guilt, shame, fear of abandonment, feelings of disrespect, feeling overwhelmed, anxiety, etc.). The key is to focus on RF skills. How did he *feel*? Help the father reflect on the situations and what was going on for him in those moments. The more he can be in touch with his own experiences in these moments, the better he will be able to consider the feelings and thoughts of others. Focusing only on anger will not allow the father to fully understand himself and sets up the idea that anger is a "bad" emotion.

Occasionally, fathers report that they do not get angry or have strong emotions. In this instance, the therapist can ask the father to explain more about this view and how he contains his emotions. Some fathers do not have explosive responses, but instead withdraw or work to overly control situations and responses. The withdrawal can be equally as damaging to their relationships as physical or verbal aggression. Taking space to calm down and be able to have healthy communication about an issue is important, but many fathers state that they "just leave." They withdraw from the conflict and do not return to discuss the issue later. They pretend that nothing happened. When asked how they behave when they return, they state, "I just act normal, like nothing happened." This behavior can lead to bottling up of emotions and a greater likelihood of an explosive outburst down the road or, alternatively, disconnection in relationships and lack of closeness.

Emotional Thermometer Activity

In this activity, the therapist helps the father understand levels of emotion and how they feel physically in his body. You can use the analogy of a thermometer: Does he feel his temperature rise or lower with different emotions? For other fathers, it may be more helpful to focus on feelings of anxiety, because anxious worry is driving their FV. This is often the case for fathers who use a lot of controlling tactics. Their control is not driven by anger, but instead, for example, by worry that they will lose their partner. In this activity, Worksheet 7.3. Emotion or Substance Misuse Thermometer is a helpful tool. The clinician can introduce the activity by saying something like the following:

> "We all have a range of emotions. Innate emotions like joy, anger, fear, sadness, and disgust are universal. Everyone has them, and we can experience different levels of these core feelings. We can feel a little bit angry or very angry or rageful. In this activity, we are going to think about your levels of anger and how you feel them in your body. This is a thermometer. Just like temperature, our emotions can be cool or hot, high or low. Let's focus on the emotion of anger. What is a word to describe a 1 level of anger?"

The therapist explores the early physiological indicators of emotion words such as *frustration* or *annoyance*. How does he know he is frustrated? What are the physical sensations in his body? Try to let the father answer first, but if he does not, you can ask probing questions such as "Do you feel anything in your hands? How about your face? What are your heart rate and temperature like?" Create the hierarchy of physiological/physical indicators that go up the thermometer for different levels of anger from frustration through rage (see Figure 7.2 for an

List types of anger or other emotion (e.g., anxiety) next to levels from 1 to 10 (with 10 being the highest level) on one side of the thermometer, along with substance use craving levels from 1 to 10 (with 10 being the highest level). Include physiological body sensations at each level on the thermometer.

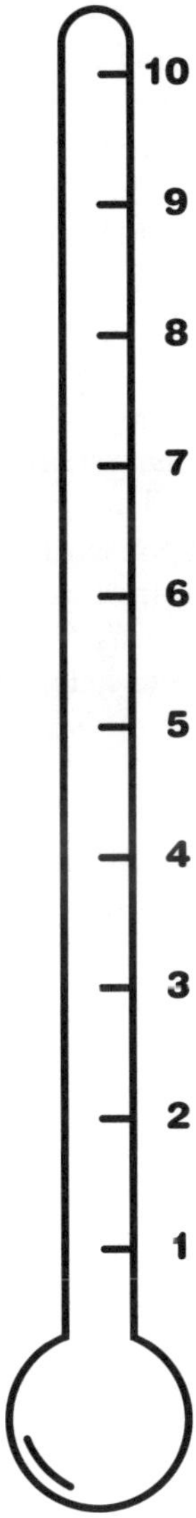

Physiological Sensations	Level	Descriptive Word	Craving Thoughts?
I just "white" out. I'm not thinking and I get physical	10	*Rage*	
	9		
	8		
	7		
I start breathing quicker and pacing, my hands are sweaty	6	*Angry*	*I need a drink*
	5		
My heart rate picks up and I start to feel hot	4	*Irritated*	*I really wish I had a drink now*
	3		
I start to feel tension in my muscles, especially my face, I bounce my leg up and down	2	*Frustrated*	*I could use a drink to calm my nerves*
	1		

FIGURE 7.2. Sample Emotion or Substance Misuse Thermometer for Keith.

example). The goal is to help the father identify early that he is becoming angry and interrupt the progression. Some fathers may have a very quick trigger to rage. Others may have more of a slow progression. It is important that the father describes physical sensations associated with these emotions. How does he know he's feeling them? It is also helpful to tie in other emotions that may be underlying anger. Does anger feel different than shame or guilt? How does it feel different? If the father also has a problem with using substances or alcohol, it is helpful to ask him about substance craving thoughts he has when his emotional thermometer rises, because these often happen simultaneously.

Following the Emotion Thermometer activity, the clinician should introduce the fight-or-flight response and diaphragmatic breathing, saying something like the following:

> "We all have two parts to our nervous system: the sympathetic and the parasympathetic nervous system. The sympathetic side controls what we call our fight-or-flight response. This is the part of our nervous system that reacts when we are faced with something that triggers strong, intense emotions such as fear or anger. The parasympathetic side relaxes your body and helps you remain calm and think clearly.
>
> "I'm going to tell you how this triggering works so that you can learn to be in control of these parts of your nervous system. Now that we have identified some of your early physiological signals, we need to talk about what to do to stop them from rising up your thermometer to risky levels."

The clinician should describe what happens when the fight-or-flight system is engaged, using Handout 7.2. Impact of High Emotion/Stress on Brain Functioning.

Here is a way to explain the response:

> "We have three parts to our brain. The lowest part of our brain is our animal brain, or survival brain. This is the part that keeps our organs functioning and works to keep us alive. The middle part of our brain is our emotional brain, where we process emotions, and the highest part of our brain, is our thinking brain. That's where our cerebral cortex is located, and it helps us think and solve problems. It is the part that makes us human. When our fight-or-flight response kicks on, the top two parts of our brain turn off and we are functioning only with our survival brain. We aren't thinking clearly, processing information, or understanding emotions or reactions of

others. We are only reacting to what we perceive as a threat and not thinking things through. This is not a good place to be unless we are in danger of being hurt or killed. Can you think of a time you might have been in your survival brain?"

Take some time to allow the client to react to this information and possibly think of examples. Some men describe getting so angry that they "blank out" or "everything goes white, and I just act." These are extreme examples of responding from the survival brain. These can be great examples when discussing how the father can be in better control. The next step is to introduce breathing skills to help him get control of his nervous system. You might say something like the following:

"There are ways for you to be in charge of your stress response system and get your thinking brain back in charge by doing a very simple breathing technique. We are going to try it right now. Have you ever been on a sports team or worked with a coach or seen how professional athletes take deep breaths before an important shot in basketball? They are using breathing skills to control their stress response. Let's try it."

Controlled Breathing Exercise

"Make yourself comfortable in your chair. Place one hand on your stomach and the other on your chest. [Demonstrate.] When we breathe in, the hand on our stomach should move up, and when we breathe out, it should move down. The hand on our chest should stay still and not move the whole time. This means we are breathing correctly. If you take shallow breaths into your chest, you are not getting the air into your diaphragm and oxygen to your body. What happens when you take shallow breaths rapidly into your chest when you are anxious? Try it now. What does that feel like? [Demonstrate and have the client take several shallow chest breaths.] You can hyperventilate, right? You feel very tense. That is what happens when our stress response system is activated. You don't get oxygen to your brain, and you can't think clearly. So, let's try taking a nice deep breath in through our nose, and let it out slowly through our mouth. [Give the client a chance to take a few breaths and check to see that they are bringing the air into their abdomen and not shallow breathing just into their chest. Provide guidance as needed.] OK, now that you're getting the hang of it, let's try to breathe more slowly when we breathe out than when we breathe in. I'll count the first time for practice, and let's see if I can count higher when we're breathing out than when we're breathing in. Breathe in 1-2-3-4, hold 2-3-4, breathe out 2-3-4-5-6. [Repeat this at least five times.]"

After this exercise ask the client how they feel. Do they notice a difference in their body after doing the breathing? Some highly traumatized fathers or coparents may struggle with controlled breathing. Focusing on their breath is challenging and triggering for them. In this instance, it may be necessary to spend more time on grounding techniques with the father. These are described below in the discussion on mindfulness.

Homework Practice

Ask the father to practice the breathing exercise once a day. Bedtime is a helpful time to do this, because it is usually a nonstressful time, and it can help with settling in for sleep. It is very hard for clients to implement this strategy when they are emotionally aroused without prior practice. Controlled breathing is a new skill that the father will need to practice to be good at it. They can try using it at times of stress, but it's important to also practice at other times to gain mastery.

Fathers Who Are Emotionally Detached

Some fathers who are referred to F4C report that they don't get angry or have strong emotions. There is a subset of fathers who are very disconnected from their emotions. They do not feel that exploring their emotions has value. They may have learned a long time ago that men should not have strong emotions, and that they are stronger if they keep their emotions under wraps. It is important in these cases to try to explore both the benefits and the costs of such emotional control. The clinician may need to explore whether the father is bottling his feelings and whether this behavior may lead to an explosion eventually, or whether the father is showing symptoms of depression and alexithymia or dissociation. *Dissociation* is a disconnection within a person's sensory experience, thoughts, or sense of self. Dissociation can range from a father feeling a mild sense of detachment (similar to daydreaming) to more severe disconnection from reality (feeling like his life or the world is not real). Fathers who have had significant trauma may be having subtle dissociation that they do not even recognize. They may feel detached from their experiences, feel numb to their emotions, or "blank out" for brief periods they cannot explain. They may report that they "feel nothing," which indeed can be their experience of what is happening. Clinicians may interpret fathers' reports of detachment from their feelings as resistance to treatment, when, in fact, it may be their genuine experience and a coping strategy they developed to manage trauma in their early life. This issue of types of emotional repression and expression is further explored in Topic 7.

TOPIC 7: PHYSIOLOGICAL REACTIVITY AND MANAGEMENT SKILLS

This topic is intended to further enhance the father's understanding of how his nervous system works and physiological indicators of arousal. Before beginning this topic, the clinician can check in regarding the diaphragmatic breathing homework assigned the previous session. Did the father practice breathing at bedtime as suggested? Did he have any incidents in which he got upset, angry, or anxious, or started to get upset, angry, or anxious? Did he use the diaphragmatic breathing at that time? Why or why not? How did it work for him if he tried it? Use this check in as an opportunity to problem-solve reasons why he may not be open to trying the breathing or what is getting in the way. Encourage him to practice the breathing daily at times when he is not angry or upset. This will get him into the practice of doing it and make it easier to implement at times when he is emotionally aroused. Before you move into the activity of this topic, practice the breathing exercise from the previous session for at least five breath cycles with the father to help him get into a relaxed state, ready for the session. This can become a weekly practice to start sessions going forward, to encourage focus on the session, and to further teach its benefits.

Use of an emWave2 or Heart Rate Monitor

This activity is designed to help the father better understand physiological arousal and how subtle it can be in the body. It's particularly helpful for those fathers who indicate they do not feel emotions or are very out of touch with their feelings. Use of an emWave2 developed by HeartMath (*https://store.heartmath.com/emwave2*) is very helpful. If it's not available, another heart rate monitor with good responsivity can be an alternative option. Let the father know that for this activity, the device will help signal changes in his heart rate and synchrony, so that he can see for himself how it works. Ask him to put on the device and explain how it works:

> "This device measures heart rate and physiological synchrony. It is sensitive to changes in how in sync your body systems are and can show us small changes in physiological response to situations. During our activity today, we are going to notice what the device is showing us about changes in your physiological responses."

Depending on what device is used, additional explanation about whether it beeps or has lights that change colors when there are physiology changes can be explained to the father.

Steps to Re-Create a High-Arousal Scenario

1. Ask the father whether new situations this week resulted in high levels of emotional arousal such as anger or anxiety. If they did, use that situation, since it is most recent. If not, you can use an older scenario that was particularly upsetting to him. On a scale of 1 to 10 (with 10 being highest level of emotion), his scenario should be at least a 5 or higher to be effective.

2. Ask him to put himself back in the situation and try to visualize it as if the situation is happening now. As he visualizes, ask him to tell you about the situation in detail (as if recounting a scene in a movie) and you write it down. Be sure to ask what happened (who said what, etc.), and about his physiological sensations, feelings, and thoughts as he details the situation ("What were you thinking then? What were you feeling in your body? What feelings were you having?").

3. Assess whether his heart rate or physiological arousal increases as he visualizes and describes the scenario (be sure he is choosing an incident that was very emotionally provoking to him). Ask him to describe how he feels now. What physiological arousal signals can he detect? Has the emWave2 changed from green to blue or red? Did his heart rate increase? The clinician can jot down changes in the emWave2 colors or heart rate changes if using a heart rate monitor alongside the description of the scenario (then review these changes with the father after Step 4).

4. Ask the father to lower or close his eyes and *imagine he is back in the situation when the event was happening*. Use the script you developed while he was telling you what happened to detail the event to him out loud while he visualizes it. Ask him to begin diaphragmatic breathing as you lead him through a guided imagery exposure to the stressful incident that you're reading to him. Use this opportunity to ensure that he is doing the breathing properly. His heart rate/arousal should decrease and be indicated on the monitoring device you are using.

5. Ask him how he feels after doing the controlled breathing while he listened to you read the scenario. Discuss the changes he felt and how he can take control of his anger or other strong emotions physiologically. You might say:

> "Controlled breathing relaxes our bodies. It keeps us from being tense and acting quickly by slowing us down. How did you feel and what was your heart rate like while you were focusing on your stressful situation? How do you feel now, and what is your heart rate like now? This kind of controlled breathing puts you back in control of your thinking and behaviors, and doesn't let your emotions take over. The situation did not change, but your body's reaction to it did. When you first told me the story, your heart rate was elevated and the emWave2 was blue and red. This time, while using the breathing, it was mostly green."

Note: For those fathers who report that they do not get to a level of 5 or above on the thermometer, you may have to choose a lower-level situation to try. It is likely they are having physiological reactivity of some kind without awareness because they are cut off from their emotional experiences. In this instance, have them think of a situation that got them to the highest number possible. As mentioned earlier, there is also the potential that some fathers may really struggle with the controlled breathing. If the father struggled last week and continues to have difficulty connecting with his breath, the clinician can switch to a grounding technique instead (see the discussion of mindfulness below).

Teaching and Practicing Additional Coping Skills

The remainder of this session can be used to introduce and review additional coping skills the father can use when he is feeling, tense, anxious, agitated, stressed, and angry, or when he withdraws or dissociates. Any coping skills that you use in your practice to help with emotional arousal or trauma triggers can be very helpful to fathers. These strategies can help him better cope with his emotions. Examples of activities include the following (see the resource list in Appendix B):

- Positive or guided imagery
- Urge surfing
- Taking space (see Handout 7.3)
- Mindfulness/grounding techniques
- Techniques to stimulate the vagus nerve
- Exercise/physical activity

It is important that clinicians help fathers develop a toolbox of strategies. Start each session going forward with diaphragmatic breathing for a couple of minutes and/or introduce additional relaxation or mindfulness/grounding techniques. Repetition of the breathing and grounding skills in session reinforces them and helps the father begin to see their utility. Many of the fathers seen in F4C have significant trauma histories that require a trauma-informed approach to introducing relaxation and grounding skills. Fathers may be dissociating during interactions and need help with grounding skills to be in the moment rather than responding from a place of past trauma. Being *trauma-informed* means understanding how trauma can impact responses to relaxation and mindfulness. Those who have experienced substantial trauma may have difficulty with mindfulness or mindfulness mediation. The focus inward can lead to traumatic reminders, reexperiencing, and reactivity (Treleaven, 2018). Clinicians must be thoughtful about the kind of mindfulness they introduce. For clients (both mothers and fathers) who are highly traumatized, with an overly active nervous system, a focus on activities to quickly help them calm their nervous system is needed before they can use the cognitive strategies introduced in Topic 8.

Grounding techniques help clients become more focused on their surroundings and bring them into the present and help them feel safe. A very simple technique is to slowly look around the room, turning one's head from one side to the other, then looking behind and noticing what is in the room. This can be an especially important technique to teach parents who often argue and become explosive in front of their children. Noticing that their child is playing nearby could be a signal that they are in a safe environment and do not need to act hostilely or aggressively in that moment. Grounding can be accomplished by using the five senses. Sight is often the easiest, but having a client focus on their environment and what they can see, hear, smell, touch/feel, and taste can be very helpful in accomplishing a present focus. This technique will be unique to each client. If clients report that breath work is not working for them, focus on helping them identify one of their senses on which they *can* focus. For example, they may be able to focus more easily on touch (e.g., "What does your butt feel like in the chair? Focus on how it feels on the chair"). Many clients find comfort in tactile objects that are soft or rough, and they can focus on how the object feels ("What does the sea shell feel like on your fingers?").

Clients who have experienced long-standing, repeated trauma, often called *complex trauma,* and have not healed can have a perpetually activated stress response. They need continued practice and exploration of how to turn the volume down on their overactive threat response. Helping them reflect and identify when this is happening and how to regulate are necessary before they can move ahead effectively in the therapy. These clients may benefit significantly from incorporating activities that stimulate their vagus nerve, which is a key part of the parasympathetic nervous system. Diaphragmatic breathing is one way to simulate it, but there are other ways to stimulate and strengthen this nerve, including humming or singing, gargling, cold stimulation (chewing ice, splashing cold water on the face, turning the water to cold for the last minute of a shower), yoga, prayer, meditation, or massage. Some resources related to polyvagal theory and activities for clients are provided in Appendix B.

Urge surfing is a technique that is often introduced in substance misuse treatment. It is a mindful approach to distress tolerance. It is used to manage one's own unwanted behaviors. Instead of giving in to an urge to use a substance or to become aggressive, the client "rides the wave" of the urge. Urges or cravings are usually very strong at the outset, but like a crashing wave, they peak and dissipate. The client is instructed to acknowledge the urge or craving, then implement some form of coping (imagining they are riding the wave through guided imagery, distracting themselves with some other activity they enjoy, etc.). A list of resources and references to an array of grounding and mindfulness techniques can be found in Appendix B.

Exercise or physical activity is a very effective regulating strategy. Clinicians can explore with their clients the kinds of exercise or physical activity they enjoy now or have enjoyed in the past. Do they have a place within their home, neighborhood, or community where they can exercise? When they feel dysregulated or emotionally escalated, are there some quick exercises they can do within their home (push-ups, sit-ups, etc.), or go out for a brisk walk or run in the neighborhood or community? Do they have a gym membership? Can they regularly schedule exercise into their day? Regular exercise reduces anxiety, depression, and stress, and improves mood, which may help reduce aggression, irritability, and violence.

Taking Space

Sometimes it is very difficult for fathers and their coparents to use their coping strategies while in each other's presence. They are too activated and triggered by their coparent to use the strategies they are learning. Teaching both fathers and their coparents how to appropriately take space apart from each other gives them a tool that can increase the chances that they will remain nonviolent. Handout 7.3. Steps to Taking Space should be reviewed with both parents individually, and parents should be encouraged to discuss this strategy and make a plan to implement it together at a time when they are both calm and can discuss how it can work best for them.

Although the directions may seem straightforward, coparents may struggle. Help them in session to think through possible pitfalls and reactions to this strategy.

CASE EXAMPLE: DAMION

Damion and his clinician were reviewing Handout 7.3. Steps to Taking Space.

DAMION: I don't think Melanie is going to go for this.

CLINICIAN: Can you say more about why you think that?

DAMION: Well, back when I was using, I would try to get in an argument with her so I could leave and go use. I would start a fight and then say I needed a break and leave.

CLINICIAN: So in the past you have used taking a break from an argument as a way to go out and use drugs.

DAMION: Yeah, I would go out with my friends and use, and not come home until the next day.

CLINICIAN: I can see how it would be hard for Melanie to trust that you are using the time to calm down if this is what happened in the past. I wonder if we can come up with a strategy that would be acceptable to her? We can try to think of a proposal together and you can talk with her about what would feel comfortable to her. A way to give you some time to calm down and return to the conversation without her worrying that you are using again.

DAMION: I don't know. Maybe.

CLINICIAN: Is there somewhere in your house that you could take space apart from Melanie? Do you need to physically leave your house? Is there a backyard or porch you could sit on?

DAMION: Yeah, we have a back porch.

CLINICIAN: OK, so could you say to Melanie, "I need to take some space to calm down. I'm going to go sit on the porch for a little while. I will come back in 30 minutes and we can try to talk about this again." What do you think? If you are on the porch, she can look out and see you and know you have not left, but it also gives you the physical space you would need to try the mindfulness and breathing we've been practicing.

DAMION: Yeah, that could work.

In this example, prior experience with the father's behavior may have impeded his coparent's ability to accept it as a strategy, so the clinician helped him to problem-solve. In an individual meeting with the coparent, the clinician in this case could have a similar discussion and help the mother think of ways she could accept the temporary physical separation to prevent FV.

Homework Practice

Select a strategy that you taught during the session and assign it as homework practice. Depending on what stress response reduction strategy you and the father identified, ask the father to practice it once per day and check in about how it went in the following session.

TOPIC 8: HOW THINKING IMPACTS BEHAVIOR

This topic focuses further on standard CBT skills by teaching cognitive processing. The goal is to assist the father (and coparent, if they come in for an individual session of their own) how thoughts, feelings, and behaviors are linked. It is important to use examples of thoughts and feelings leading to FV, aggressive or hostile responding, anxiety, or problematic parenting behaviors. First introduce an example of how the cognitive triangle works by providing the father with an example. You could say something like "Let's say you walk into the breakroom at work and there is a group of guys laughing. You think to yourself, 'they are laughing at me.' That makes you feel angry and then you ask them in a harsh tone, 'What's so funny?' Now let's say instead of thinking 'They are laughing at me' you think 'Someone told a funny joke.' How does that make you feel and act? You can see from this example how a person's thought about a situation can impact how they feel and then their behaviors. Now let's think of a situation from your own life and see if we can apply this."

Using Worksheet 7.4. Cognitive Triangle Exercise (see Figure 7.3), practice going around the triangle several times with the father: "What is your first thought? What is your first feeling? What is your first action?" Then try changing his thought to something more helpful, to illustrate how changing his thoughts can lead to different feelings and actions. It is important to relate this session's topic back to the emotion thermometer exercise and how positive self-talk (using positive interpretations and language to describe oneself) and relaxation skills as coping strategies can interrupt FV. Positive self-talk or changing one's thoughts about a situation can help calm the parent's elevated emotions. Positive self-talk can assist the parent in gaining positive control of their anger, hostility, or other overwhelming emotions before intervening with their child or discussing a hot topic with their partner or coparent. Importantly, though, this technique is usually helpful only at the lower levels of the emotion scale, before feelings reach high levels and clear linear thinking skills are lost.

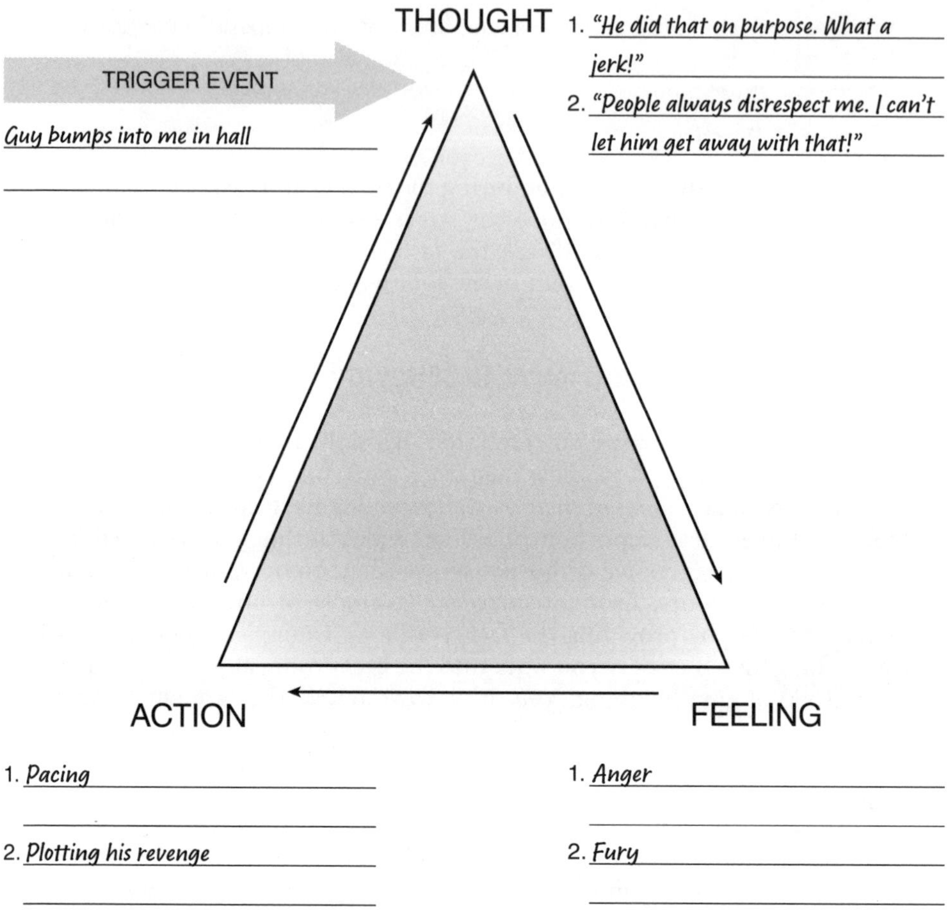

FIGURE 7.3. Sample Cognitive Triangle Exercise for Jim: Unhelpful thoughts.

CASE EXAMPLE: JIM

Jim describes an incident in which another client in a substance use program bumped into him in the hallway. When Jim tells him, "Watch where you're going," the guy glares at him and says, "F*** off!" Jim is thinking the guy is a jerk, and he is furious. This is a situation in which the incident would cause most people to become angry. The therapist asked Jim to continue walking around the triangle. His first thought was "The guy is a jerk." His first feeling was anger, and his first action was to begin pacing. His next (second) thought was "People always disrespect me. I can't let him get away with that." His anger escalated (second feeling), and he was planning to try to get back at the guy (third behavior). The clinician learned through continuing to understand Jim's thought process going around the triangle a second time that his thinking was escalating. This scenario would easily make anyone angry, but Jim's thoughts were not helpful and spiraled into a maladaptive core belief he has about himself: "No one respects me." These kinds of thoughts are usually associated with clients' beliefs about themselves. Deep down, Jim may feel he does not deserve respect.

The therapist was then able to ask Jim what some alternative thoughts might be for the situation. Jim realized that if he thought, "The guy is acting like a jerk. Maybe he's having a bad day," he would feel less angry. Instead of internalizing the situation and making his thoughts self-centered, he turned them outward and made them about the other person. He found that this made him less angry and volatile, as shown in Figure 7.4.

It is best to try to elicit situations in which the client has thinking that is distorted or unhelpful. The best kinds of situations involve unhelpful thinking about others that can be altered to ensure the client understands the concept of how his thoughts are connected to his feelings and emotions, and what strategies he can use to adjust his thinking.

CASE EXAMPLE: MALIK

Malik described an incident on the city bus going to work. He observed a man making sexual advances on a teenage girl. He was making sexualized comments and eventually leaned over and kissed her on the ear. Malik described yelling at the man to back off. He said he was thinking about how the girl reminded him of his sister and how he wanted to protect her.

This example is not the kind of situation that is helpful for this exercise. It is a situation that would make most people upset, angry, or compelled to act. Malik's thinking was not distorted or inappropriate. Empathize with his reaction and try to help him locate another example or continue to have him go around the triangle. Does his thinking become global with something like "All girls are unsafe and most men are sexual deviants." If it does, then the clinician can help him to stay focused on the man on the bus and respond thoughtfully ("He may be a perv, but most men aren't") rather than based on escalated views of most men in the world, for example.

Neither of these examples involves the coparent or children of the clients. When possible, using examples related to coparents or children is best, but sometimes clients have had an incident within the previous week that involves others, and using a very recent event can be helpful to illustrate how to use the skills.

Homework Practice

Worksheet 7.5. Changing Your Unhelpful Thoughts is given as a homework assignment after teaching the cognitive triangle in session. It is important to fill in an example with the father before he leaves the

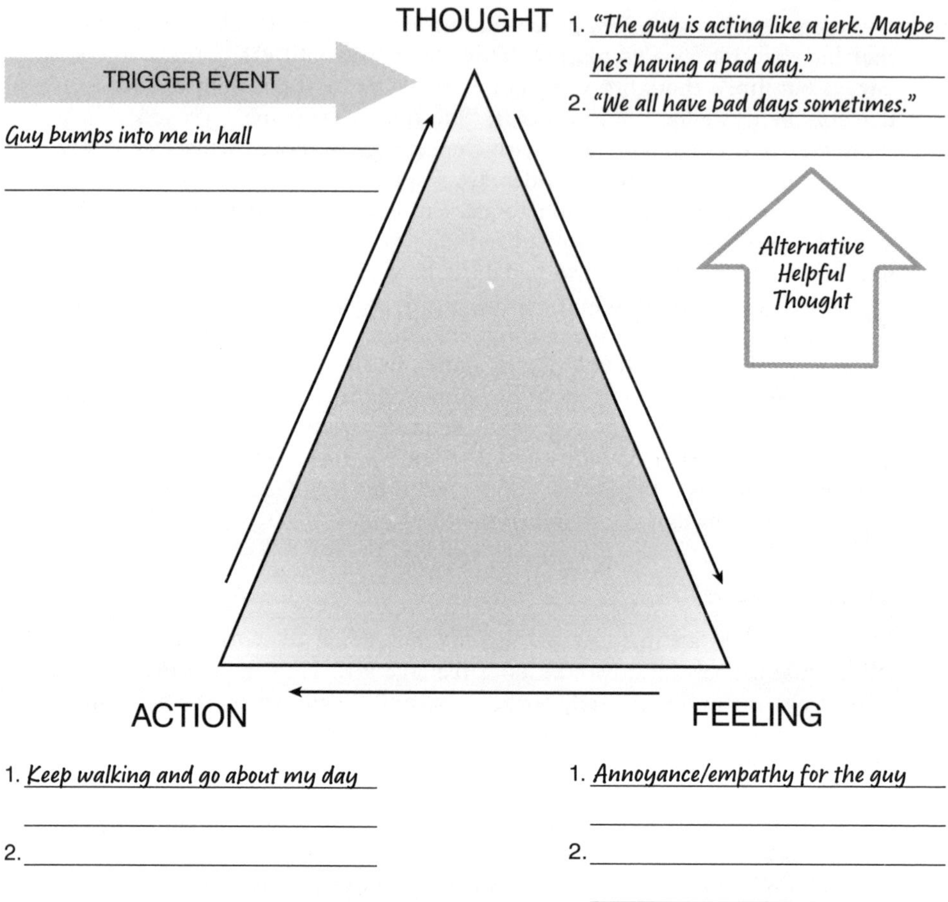

FIGURE 7.4. Sample Cognitive Triangle Exercise for Jim: Alternative helpful thoughts.

session to be sure he understandings how to change his thoughts. Otherwise, he will struggle to fill this worksheet out on his own. An example is provided on Worksheet 7.5 to get you started.

RF and Skills Building with Coparents

If coparents are also using FV, then the topics can be implemented in parallel, in the same way they are done with fathers. Helping coparents understand their triggers for aggression or substance use using functional analysis, understanding their stress response system and coping strategies, are all helpful for changing their behaviors. If coparents are survivors of the FV and are not using violence themselves, they can still benefit from meeting with the clinician in parallel to review these topics, but with a different emphasis. The clinician can focus the sessions on coparents' symptoms of PTSD, depression, or anxiety related to the FV and other traumas they may have experienced. Topics 5, 6, and 7 can all be implemented with a focus on triggers for symptoms of their trauma or anxiety and coping strategies to manage those symptoms. Helping coparents manage trauma triggers and reduce their symptoms will have significant benefit for them and their children. Furthermore, their knowledge of the same coping skills will allow them to know what the father is learning for skills and be able to assess whether he is making any changes. They can notice whether the father has been using breathing strategies, grounding techniques, or is taking space appropriately. Their understanding of taking space is often key to its success. If coparents do not support the fathers' use of taking space, then it is unlikely to be a successful approach.

Importantly, parallel sessions with coparents can also be used to understand survivor coparents' sense of self. This can be important to helping them reflect on why they might remain in a relationship that is unhealthy and harmful. Coparents may say they want to remain separate from the father who caused harm; they want to discontinue the relationship, but they worry they will return to the father. Help them understand the feelings they have about their relationship ending by using questions such as "What does it mean to you that your relationship is ending? What feelings does that bring up? What do you think it says about you that you are getting divorced?" Understanding the way coparents view the separation in relation to their sense of self can help them process the feelings of grief over loss of their wish for an intact family or feelings of shame about being unable to make their relationship work. These underlying emotions can contribute to both parents' continuing to return to a relationship they know is unhealthy.

CASE EXAMPLE: JANEL

JANEL: I really do not want to go back to Peter. I feel better about myself when we are separated and there is much less stress, but I'm worried I'll take him back. He started calling me and is being really nice and saying all the right things about how we can be together again as a family, but I know it's better for me if we aren't together.

THERAPIST: When you think about your marriage ending. What feelings come up?

JANEL: I feel relieved.

THERAPIST: Relieved, OK. What else?

JANEL: I feel bad for my kids. I got to grow up with both my parents, and I want my kids to be able to have an intact family.

THERAPIST: When you think about your boys living with divorced parents, what feelings come up?

JANEL: I feel bad that I cannot make it work. Like I should try harder. I feel like a failure.

THERAPIST: So getting divorced makes you feel like a failure.

JANEL (*crying*): Yes.

THERAPIST: I can understand those feelings, and you may also be feeling like others will judge you, and maybe even people in your own family?

JANEL (*continuing to cry*): Yes, they think, "There's that single mother who couldn't make her marriage work."

THERAPIST: We do get a lot of messages that children need and do best with both parents together, but it is also true that it is damaging for children to live with parents who are together when they are exposed to lots of tension, conflict, and violence.

JANEL: I know. I know it's been awful for them to see their dad and I fight. I know deep down it's better for them if we separate, but I just keep thinking maybe this time it will be different. We can do better.

THERAPIST: OK, I can understand those feelings. You really wish it could be different this time around. Have you seen any changed behavior from Peter since you both started this program?

JANEL: I mean, a little, but when we separate, he often acts nicer until he moves back in. Then after only a few days, he goes back to his usual ways.

THERAPIST: All right, so it sounds like you cannot trust his behaviors, and this is a usual pattern. Let's continue to talk about what you notice about his behaviors, and if you feel a pull to have him move back in, let's talk it through in our next session. That way we can see if it is these feelings of being a failure that are pushing you to allow him back home, even though you feel it is still unhealthy for you and the kids. Can we do that?

JANEL: Yes, that would be helpful. I just get so sad, and then I want to try again, even though I know it is going to probably be the same.

THERAPIST: Our sessions will allow us to evaluate whether Peter is doing anything differently and changing his behaviors or repeating the same patterns again.

In this example, Janel's underlying feelings about herself as a failure (which is shame responding) are pushing her continually to take her husband back, a pattern that has happened many times in the past. The therapist in this example highlights that pattern and the feelings Janel has that are causing her to continue the pattern, so they can keep processing each and assessing whether Peter is making any changes. Working with both parents in F4C allows the clinician to see what is happening from both coparents' perspectives. Although, the therapist may feel that the father is working hard in F4C sessions, it still may be that the dynamics in a relationship are unhealthy for the family, and separating safely is a good outcome of the F4C work. Considering the needs of both parents as individuals and the safety of everyone in the family is one of the most challenging parts of this work and why reflective supervision is necessary.

Both parents can benefit from the topics in this phase of F4C so that they understand their triggers and emotional responses, allowing them to react differently in the future. The third phase of treatment, Coparenting Communication, is covered next in Chapter 8.

CHAPTER 8

Phase 3

Coparenting Communication

Phase 3 of F4C focuses on coparenting communication. The techniques and skills covered in this phase are not unique to F4C. Many of them are used in other couple therapies such as behavioral couple therapy (O'Farrell & Fals-Stewart, 2000) or the Gottman method (Gottman & DeClaire, 2001). The skills presented here are put together in a structure that can be useful for coparenting, but they are *not* for rebuilding the couple's intimate relationship. These sessions also do not have to be with biological coparents. It is possible that the coparent for a child is the father's own mother, who has been caring for his child and is the legal guardian. It is appropriate to consider including others who are serving a significant coparenting role if improving communication is a needed and helpful goal of F4C.

The four topics in this phase include Increasing Coparent Positive Interactions; Positive Communication Skills; Coparent Problem Solving Part I; and Coparent Problem Solving Part II.

PREPARING FOR CONJOINT SESSIONS

Coparent communication sessions can be delivered with the father individually or in conjoint sessions with the coparent. Fathers who are going to meet with a coparent require preparation for those sessions. The clinician must discuss participation of the coparent in subsequent sessions if it is unclear whether the father wants that, or the clinician is unsure that the father will be able to have productive sessions with the coparent.

These discussions can happen during the assessment and during Topic 1 of F4C, as well as prior to initiating the coparenting communication phase. Ask a simple question such as "In F4C we can have some coparenting sessions together. How would you feel about including your coparent in some of our sessions?" A similar conversation can happen with the coparent to assess their interest in having joint sessions, giving the clinician an idea early in treatment about how each parent feels about meeting together.

As the clinician is finishing up Topic 8, if there was indication early in F4C that the father wanted to participate together with the coparent *and* the coparent has been participating in at least some parallel sessions, then it is important to revisit their joint sessions and discuss how each feels about it now that you are reaching that phase of the treatment. The clinician does not want to repeat the coparents' hostile, negative, or unhealthy interactions outside therapy in session, so they must feel that coparents can have some positive interactions with their guidance. A clinician might start this conversation with a father by saying, "How do you feel sessions with your coparent to improve communication would go?" or "Tell me some things that you appreciate about your coparent or things you appreciate they do for your children." If a father or coparent is unable to say anything positive about their coparent to you, they will be unable to say anything positive to each other in session together. In this instance, conjoint sessions should not be scheduled. Coparent topics should be done individually.

To proceed with conjoint sessions, the clinician *must* have had ongoing contact with the coparent through weekly parallel sessions or have met with her a minimum of three times in individual parallel sessions to get to know her and prepare for coparent sessions (as stated earlier, it is recommended that coparents be seen in parallel sessions throughout F4C, especially if the coparent has also used violence, but if they are willing, they can participate whether they used violence or not). This therapeutic contact with coparents will allow you to assess their level of comfort about participating in coparent sessions with the father and understand underlying issues and concerns they may bring to the coparent sessions. If they indicate they are fearful or report coercive controlling behaviors or increased agitation of the father after his individual F4C sessions, use your clinical judgment to determine if bringing up coparent sessions is appropriate. Safety of coparents and all members of the family is crucial. It is also important that the clinician have a solid clinical understanding of the coparents' symptoms and functioning before holding conjoint sessions. Fathers may be ready for conjoint sessions, but coparents may have not yet met the individual goals needed to prepare them for the conjoint work. They may need more time in individual sessions due to their own

FV use or their symptoms associated with experiences of trauma either at the hands of their coparent or others in their life. This may be in parallel individual session with you as their clinician or it may be beyond what F4C can offer. If a coparent has mental health symptoms that need further focused therapy, like an evidence-based PTSD treatment, then referral to that treatment would take precedence over continuing in F4C. Clinicians should use their judgment about the readiness of both parents to participate in productive conjoint coparenting sessions.

If the clinician feels it will be clinically appropriate and both parents are in agreement to have coparent sessions, ask the father's permission to call the coparent while you are in your final meeting before coparent sessions will begin, to schedule a time that is mutually agreeable. If he agrees, make the call and allow the father to hear your invitation. You might say something like "Hello, Ms. Smith. This is Dr. Stover from the Fathers for Change Program. I'm with John now, and we would like to plan for our first coparent session together. We are starting the part of the program that will work on coparenting communication. Would you be able to come in next week?" Given the therapist's prior contact with the coparent, they should be anticipating your call and have already indicated interest in participating in these sessions. *If they do not want to participate, or it is not appropriate based on your clinical judgment for them to meet together, you can proceed with the coparenting topics with the father individually.*

Prior to the first conjoint coparent session, discuss with each parent any information they have revealed to the clinician that they want to keep confidential during coparent sessions (e.g., what do their coparents know about their family history?). The clinician should use a session to prepare each parent for what is planned for the conjoint coparenting sessions. This discussion should include the topics and skills that will be covered in Phase 3 and those that will be off limits. Both parents must be appropriately prepared for the conjoint sessions. Many coparents have been anticipating these sessions and hope to use them to address intimate couple-related issues. These sessions *are not couple therapy*; they are not intended to address intimate relationship issues about sex or infidelity. If parents are able to have successful coparenting communication sessions about their children's needs, this indicates they may be ready for couple therapy and could be referred for such intervention as F4C treatment is ending. It is imperative that clinicians delivering coparenting sessions of F4C are managing sessions well. These sessions are not intended to be used to discuss whatever the parents want; they are focused, with specific topics and skills to be learned. If coparents are unable to stay on topic and continually become emotionally dysregulated, hostile, or inappropriate, then sessions should be discontinued. Coparents who insist on bringing up couple-related issues, or who continually verbally attack their partner and are unable to be redirected, cannot continue in coparenting sessions.

Be sure to have a plan for how you will handle potential escalation by each parent during coparent sessions. Ensure that you have a strategy to assist a coparent to leave the building safely, if needed. This likelihood is small, since you have been working with these parents and know them well at this point in the therapy, but it is better to be overprepared than to have an incident arise that you are unsure how to safely manage. Ensure that another colleague or the reception staff in your office is aware that you are holding conjoint sessions, and be sure someone else can be available if you need assistance in calling Uber or a taxi to assist another parent in leaving the session safely, or even to sit with a coparent if the emotions of both are too escalated to allow them to sit alone.

CASE EXAMPLE: JORDAN AND MOHAMMAD

CLINICIAN: Our session will focus on coparent communication related to your children.

JORDAN: I really wanted to talk about text messages I saw on his phone from someone named Maria.

CLINICIAN: It sounds like that is an important topic for discussion, but it is not what we will focus on today. As I mentioned when we met in our individual session last week, we are going to work on some specific coparenting skills. I know these may be things you want to discuss and work through, and when we finish our coparent sessions together, we can talk about whether seeing a couple therapist is the next step for you. The communication skills we are going to work on together can be used for you to talk about some of these other issues, too, but we will not be discussing them here.

JORDAN: Yeah, but isn't his cheating on me important to our coparenting?!

CLINICIAN: Your intimate relationship is separate from your coparent relationship. No matter what happens in your intimate relationship, you will still need to figure out how to parent your children, whether together in a relationship or separately.

MOHAMMAD: See, this is what I always have to deal with. She's accusing me of cheating and I don't even know who Maria is! This is why we are always fighting!

CLINICIAN: I can see this is a sensitive issue for both of you. Let's try doing some of our breathing exercises that I did with both of you separately to calm things down a little bit. Can we do that?

JORDAN: I don't even want to talk to him right now. He's denying those texts.

CLINICIAN: Jordan, can you press your feet into the floor and hold the bottom of the chair with your hands and press them into the seat of the chair like we've practiced in our sessions together? Let's try to begin some controlled breathing, too.

JORDAN: I can't.

MOHAMMAD: See, she's impossible!

CLINICIAN: OK, it seems like we are not going to be able to focus on the topic I had planned for today, and we are getting agitated, so I think we should take some space. I'm going to ask you, Mohammad, to go in the waiting room. I'm going to talk with Jordan for a few minutes and then I will come and talk with you. Mohammad, if you can practice your controlled breathing while you wait, that would be terrific.

MOHAMMAD: Yeah, sure, I think we need some space. (*Exits to the waiting room. He is calm so the clinician feels OK allowing him to go to the waiting room on his own.*)

CLINICIAN: Jordan, I can see that you are really upset. It's important when you feel like this to use the skills we've been practicing. We are here to try to use them to be able to communicate better.

JORDAN: I just want to talk about those texts!

CLINICIAN: I know that feels very important to you right now, but that is not why we are here. We are here to work on communication related to your children. So let's use our grounding skills. Press your feet into the floor and grab your chair and press into it. I'm going to start counting for our controlled breathing.

JORDAN: (*Follows the clinician's prompts.*)

In this example, the clinician was not able to get the coparents to focus on the planned topic, and they were not able to engage in coping skills together. Therefore, it was important to separate the parents so the temperature in the session would not escalate further (modeling effective taking space). The clinician did some processing and coping practice with Jordan while instructing Mohammad to take space and use his controlled breathing. After Jordan is calm, the clinician can talk with Mohammad to do the same processing and ensure that he is deescalated so that they can leave the session calmly. If it seems unsafe to have the parents leave together, the clinician should problem-solve with the coparent or father about getting an alternative ride home if they drove to the appointment together. The clinician could say to Mohammad, "I'm going to spend a bit more time with Jordan. Why don't you head home. She said her sister can come pick her up to take her home later." This way, both have more time and space to calm down, and if there are ongoing safety concerns, the clinician can help the coparent determine whether they should stay somewhere else for the night or if domestic violence emergency services should be contacted. There was no indication of that need from the vignette presented; however, further assessment may reveal more issues than those presented in the conjoint part of the session.

In this example, the mother needed the clinician's attention first because she was more escalated and unresponsive than the father. If the father is becoming hostile, raising his voice, or not responding to clinician prompts in session, then the clinician would choose to ask the mother to step into the waiting room to take space and practice some coping skills while the clinician works with the father to utilize coping skills (grounding, breathing, or other strategies) they worked on during Phase 2 of F4C.

The clinician could opt to retry a conjoint session with this coparenting pair again with continued clear boundaries, but if they are unable to follow the clinician's prompts again, then the clinician should revert to individual parallel sessions in lieu of conjoint sessions going forward. The clinician would still go over the topics in this phase but deliver them individually and practice them using role plays.

SELECTING COPARENTING TOPICS

The coparenting topics are in an order that has made sense in clinical practice with families seen through F4C; however, the exact order of these sessions is not prescribed. Therapists can use their judgment about which topics are appropriate for each family and when. If partners have been actively participating in parallel sessions and are living together, they may be ready to discuss areas they want to work on as coparents and examine their genograms together. Other coparents may be divorced or newly separated, and their ability to talk about problem areas is lacking, leading to concern that the sessions will deteriorate into arguments. The goal is to ensure that coparents have a different experience in session than they do normally. This means they can talk and be heard. For some coparents, it is necessary to teach the communication skills in Topics 10 and 11 individually to help parents learn how to give compliments, use "I statements," and actively listen prior to bringing them together to try these skills. Other couples do well learning these skills together. Clinicians should use their judgment about the order of the sessions and whether to cover the topics only individually in parallel, individually first and transitioning to conjoint, or conjoint only.

CONJOINT SESSION RULES

As mentioned earlier, it is important to meet individually with each parent to outline the goals of the coparenting sessions (to increase positive interactions, improve coparenting communication, and strengthen problem solving) and the topics to be covered outlined in F4C, and to review the following coparenting session rules (see also Handout 8.1. Coparenting Session Rules):

1. One person talks at a time.
2. When it is not your turn to talk, listen to understand what the other person is saying.
3. Stay on session topic.
4. The clinician will interrupt to help provide feedback, correct, teach a skill, or redirect a conversation as needed.
5. Yelling, interrupting, or demeaning your coparent or the clinician is not allowed.
6. Topics for discussion are focused on coparenting and raising your children together and not on your intimate relationship or past wrongs done by the other person.
7. Stick to the goals of the coparenting sessions:
   a. Decrease conflict/aggression/violence in relationship
   b. Improve communication related to coparenting
8. If needed, the session will be stopped and the clinician will meet with each partner separately.
9. Phones should be silenced and put away.

You will also review the rules at the start of each coparenting session to ensure that everyone is on the same page. Clinicians need to be prepared to interrupt clients and refocus them, if needed, to ensure the sessions do not turn volatile or move into topics that are not appropriate for these sessions (e.g., intimacy issues).

Each parent can add any rules they think are needed, and both sign the handout showing commitment to following them during sessions.

TOPIC 9: INCREASING COPARENT POSITIVE INTERACTIONS

After reviewing the rules for the conjoint sessions (if meeting conjointly), review the overarching goals for coparenting sessions that are designed to (1) decrease conflict/aggression/violence in the relationship by increasing positive interactions, and (2) improve communication and problem solving related to coparenting.

Clinicians must be sure the parents understand what is meant by coparenting relationships and how they differ from intimate relationships. Furthermore, provide psychoeducation about why coparenting is so important. You might say something like the following:

> "Our focus in these sessions is on your coparenting relationship. Coparenting refers to the ways that parents relate to each other in the role of parent. Coparenting happens when two people have shared responsibility for a child. It consists of the support and coordination that parents display during childrearing. It *does not* include romantic, sexual, emotional, financial, and legal aspects of adult relationships that do not relate to raising your child. So even though your romantic relationship can change, you will always be coparents to your children. All coparents have disagreements or areas in which they may not see eye to eye; however, using aggressive or controlling behaviors is no way to resolve them. In these sessions we focus on improving your coparenting relationship and communication."

The reason to focus on coparenting is that even in families with high couple conflict and hostility related to their intimate relationship, good coparenting, which is protective and leads to better child adjustment, is possible. Once it is clear that both parents understand the domains involved in coparenting, the clinician can introduce how to give compliments. The goal for this activity is to increase positive interactions between coparents that can improve their feelings about the coparenting relationship.

Giving Compliments Activity

This activity should only be initiated if the clinician is sure that each parent will be able to name something positive they appreciate about the other person's parenting or coparenting behaviors. In the individual sessions prior to beginning the conjoint sessions, the therapist should assess what the other parent appreciates or likes about the way their coparent interacts or behaves relative to parenting. Having this information provides an indication that the person will be able to name something when you meet jointly. If the parent is unable to name anything they appreciate or like about their coparent during individual sessions, this activity should not be done jointly.

In session, ask each parent to name something they think the other parent does well as a parent or with their child. After each parent has had a chance to respond, ask, "Did you know what they would say?" Explore whether they typically give each other compliments related to parenting. The therapist might ask, "Do you tell your partner the things you appreciate that they do?" Ask for examples of how they give compliments.

Review in session the difference between a simple compliment and a compliment with criticism—for example: "I liked the way you helped Johnny get ready for bed" (compliment). Why can't you do that all the time?" (criticism). When you give a compliment with a criticism, the person does not hear the compliment; they only hear the criticism. Discuss with the parents how to give compliments: words and body language matter.

Once compliments have been clearly defined, with examples from the clinician of both the correct way and incorrect way to deliver them, have each parent practice giving the other a compliment: "Han, I'd like you to turn to Janina and give her a compliment about her parenting, and Janina, I'd like you to accept the compliment." Review how to receive a compliment, because many parents are uncomfortable hearing positive feedback or are unsure how to accept it. They may reject the compliment out of discomfort, which spoils the moment and makes the parent who gave the compliment feel silly, hurt, rejected, or angry. So the therapist should facilitate giving *and* receiving compliments in healthy ways.

Positive Interactions

CASE HEAD: JANINA AND HAN

Janina and Han were uncomfortable in the conjoint sessions. They sat at opposite ends of a couch, and she hugged a couch pillow. Both talked directly to the therapist and they made little eye contact.

CLINICIAN: Have either of you ever told each other things you like about the other's parenting?

JANINA: No.

HAN: No. I do appreciate that Janina makes dinner much of the time, packs the children healthy lunches, and plays with them a lot.

JANINA: You've never told me that.

CLINICIAN: Han, turn to Janina and give her a compliment about her parenting using some of the things you just shared.

HAN (*turning to Janina*): I like the way you take good care of the kids while I'm at work.

JANINA (*giggling*): That sounded silly.

HAN: (*Appears embarrassed and looks down at the floor.*)

CLINICIAN (*turning toward Janina*): Does hearing the compliment make you uncomfortable?

JANINA: I don't really know how to act when people say nice things to me.

CLINICIAN (*addressing both Han and Janina*): It was hard for you. Han, to give the compliment and it was also hard for you, Janina, to know how to receive it. Janina, would you like for Han to tell you when he appreciates what you do?

JANINA: Yes, I would like that.

CLINICIAN: Han, how did you feel when Janina reacted the way she did to your compliment?

HAN: I felt stupid. It already felt weird and then she said that, and I felt even worse.

CLINICIAN: When coparents are not used to giving and receiving compliments in their relationships, it can be hard at first. Han, I'd like you to try giving the compliment again, and this time, Janina, I'd like you to simply say, "Thank you." Then you can try giving Han a compliment and he will receive it.

Homework Practice

This homework assignment can be given over several weeks. The first time it is assigned, provide Worksheet 8.1. Catch Your Coparent Doing Something You Appreciate to each coparent and ask them to notice the ways they are a good parent to their child and write them down for the next session. They do not need to share the compliments with each other at home this first time but will do it in session with therapist support, especially if they have really struggled to give compliments during the current session. The goal with this homework is to increase each parent's ability to notice the things their coparent is doing that they appreciate or that is good for their children's well-being.

When the parents return the following week, begin the session by reviewing the homework assignment to write down things they noticed about their coparent. What did they notice about the other parent? Did they offer any compliments? The therapist can use the things each parent wrote down to facilitate practice of giving and receiving compliments in session. If a parent did not do the homework, ask them to think of something they like that the other parent did during the previous week and have them tell the other person. Facilitate good compliment giving by modeling and coaching how to give pure and specific compliments without criticism—for example: "I love the way you pack lunches for the kids and me each morning. I especially like when you put a note in telling us to have a good day." After each parent has given the other at least one good, specific compliment, encourage them to continue focusing on the positive things they notice about each other and their children in the upcoming week and to give these compliments to the coparent during the week as homework. Close out this activity by asking each coparent to respond to the following question: "How do you think your coparenting relationship might be different as a result of these compliments?"

TOPIC 10: POSITIVE COMMUNICATION SKILLS

The goals of this topic are to (1) facilitate active listening skills, and (2) teach and practice use of "I" statements to express emotions and needs. This topic can take from one to three sessions with coparents depending on their skills and abilities, and how quickly they are able to understand and begin using the skills taught. This may also be a topic that must be taught individually first in parallel sessions, bringing the parents together after they have some mastery of the skill. The clinician can judge this need based on their experience with each of the parents in parallel sessions during the individual phase and how the parents did together around giving compliments. If they were able to learn to give compliments and worked well together in session, learning this topic's skills together in a conjoint session is usually possible.

Teaching Active Listening Skills and Using "I" Statements

This topic is meant to convey the importance of positive, healthy communication and parent roles in teaching this to their children. This is a good time to return to how parental conflict and aggression may impact their children. Give to each parent to take home Handout 6.1. Impact of Exposure to Parental Violence and Substance Misuse on Children, which lists signs and symptoms commonly seen in children living in high-conflict homes. You might say something like the following:

> "We have talked together about how high conflict and violence, both verbal and physical, can impact children. It not only causes symptoms and difficulties that are concerning, but it also teaches children that using aggression and violence is appropriate and an OK way to handle difficult feelings they have. As parents, you can help them learn other ways to express their feelings to you, other adults, and friends. You have shared that you did not learn positive ways of

coping with and expressing your difficult feelings such as disappointment, sadness, and anger. We are going to practice some ways of communicating that will help not only the two of you but also your children. Once you learn them and start to use them at home to communicate, your children will learn them too."

Active Listening

Below is a suggested progression of how to teach active listening to parents during a conjoint session.

1. Use Handout 8.2. Steps to Active Listening to review with parents what active listening is and how to do it. If they are able, have parents take turns reading aloud sections of the worksheet. This will allow for active engagement in the didactic part of the session. Next, the clinician should model with one of the parents what active listening looks like. Ask one of the parents to tell you what they had for breakfast. Model active listening so the parents can *see* what it looks like.

2. Have each parent practice active listening with their coparent. Have one parent, say the dad, pick a neutral topic such as describing his favorite TV show or a recent sports game he watched while the mom actively listens. The clinician must pay careful attention to the listener's body language and coach them as needed on what they are nonverbally communicating to the other person. Follow these steps:

- **a.** Speaker talks about their favorite TV show.
- **b.** Clinician asks listener to repeat back what they heard.
- **c.** Clinician asks speaker whether the listener accurately heard what was said. If the answer is "no," the speaker should repeat what was said again. This may also be a time when the clinician gives feedback on any nonverbal communication (e.g., lack of eye contact) that may be hindering the speaker from feeling heard.
- **d.** Clinician asks listener to repeat what they heard.
- **e.** Parents repeat these steps with clinician coaching until the speaker feels that the listener heard and understood what they said.
- **f.** Switch roles so that each parent has a chance to be the speaker and the listener.

Note: The clinician is very active during this activity. It is not helpful to let "bad" listening behaviors continue. Stop the activity and make adjustments/corrections if needed. This active corrective approach is needed for all communication skills training sessions.

Making "I" Statements

After practicing active listing with neutral topics, it is important to teach the use of "I" statements before going on to practice listening with more challenging topics. Using Handout 8.3. How to Make an "I" Statement, the clinician first reviews the steps of making an "I" statement. It can be helpful to say something without an "I" statement, then deliver it with an "I" statement and ask the parents to reflect on how they experienced each statement. For example, the clinician could ask the parents, "If I say, 'You are always late to pick up the baby,' how does that make you feel?" The idea is that this kind of statement makes people defensive and less likely to listen or want to change their behavior, and it is very likely to lead to an argument. The clinician could then say, "Instead, if I say, 'I feel anxious that I'll be late for work and get fired when you don't get home as planned. I'd like it if you could send me a text when you are running late so I know if I need to call out of work or find someone to watch the baby,' how does that make you feel?" The clinician can explore the ways both words and body language and tone of voice can lead to different responses. The second approach is more likely to lead to a discussion, because the other person hears the impact or feeling their behavior evoked and what would help the coparent feel less worried.

It is also helpful to ask parents how they explain discipline or limits to their child. Do they use "I" statements with their children (e.g., "No, you can't play near the street. It is dangerous and I'm worried you might get hurt"; "I don't like it when you throw your food on the floor. That makes Daddy angry. Food is for eating. I want you to help me clean it up"). This allows for a discussion about the importance of expressing the worry and concern behind an action or limit and not just the anger or annoyance. It feels different to a child (and coparent) when they feel the discipline or comment comes from a feeling of concern or love rather than anger alone or just a need to control them.

It is key to have each coparent practice making "I" statements in session while the other coparent uses active listening skills to respond. Have each parent choose an area of coparenting they would like to discuss from Handout 8.4. Areas of Coparenting. Have them form their "I" statements to communicate their concerns. Instruct each parent to use an "I" statement to communicate. The other parent should use active listening skills to respond to their coparent and be sure they understand the message being relayed. The clinician can facilitate conversation toward problem solving. The clinician must correct poorly formed "I" statements and poor active listening during this exercise.

Positive Communication

CASE EXAMPLE: JOE AND GLORIA

JOE (*turning to Gloria*): I feel you coddle the children too much, and I want you to be more firm with them.

[*Gloria looks tense and folds her arms across her chest as she prepares to respond.*]

CLINICIAN: That was not an "I" statement. You used the word "I" to start it, but then you immediately criticized Gloria. You just added "I feel" to the beginning of the criticism. The second part where you requested what you wanted instead was good, but the first part wasn't quite right. Can you identify what is missing from your "I" statement? [Joe looks confused and unsure.] What do you feel when Gloria coddles the children?

JOE: I'm worried they will misbehave and not listen to adults.

CLINICIAN: So, it worries you. The feeling you have is worry. So, you would start your statement with "I feel worried" or "I worry . . ." What do you mean by "coddle"? What does that look like?

JOE: When she sets a limit with them or gives a consequence but does not follow through. Like, if she said, "Jimmy, you can't watch TV because you misbehaved," but then she lets him.

CLINICIAN: OK, so how could you make an "I" statement that starts with your feeling, is very specific to what causes the feeling—Gloria might not know what you mean by "coddling"—and then says what you would like to have happen?

[*Joe thinks for a minute and starts to form the sentence with some support from the clinician.*]

JOE: I worry when you set a limit with Jimmy and then do not follow through. I would like it if you could be more consistent with your consequences, so he learns from them.

CLINICIAN: Gloria, what did you hear Joe say?

GLORIA: He thinks I'm too soft and not strict enough.

CLINICIAN: Joe, is that what you said? Did Gloria get it right?

JOE: She's defensive, and she didn't hear my worry or what I would like. She made it general.

CLINICIAN: Yes. Joe, can you try again? And Gloria, this time I'd like you to try to summarize what Joe said to show you understand him.

JOE (*repeating his "I" statement*): I worry when you set a limit with Jimmy and then do not follow through. I would like it if you could be more consistent with your consequences, so he learns from them.

CLINICIAN: Gloria, what did you hear Joe say?

GLORIA: He feels worried about Jimmy and what he is learning when I give a consequence and don't follow through with it. He wants me to follow through on what I say. I get it, but sometimes it's so hard. I get tired and sometimes I let him watch TV even when I said he couldn't, because I need a break.

CLINICIAN: Joe, did Gloria hear you this time?

JOE: Yes, she did, and I know it's hard and sometimes she is tired.

CLINICIAN: Gloria, is there anything you'd like to ask Joe about this topic to help clarify or further the discussion?

GLORIA: Yeah, does he have any ideas of consequences that might be easier to implement? Or can he help me with the consequences sometimes?

This case example illustrates how the clinician had to intervene to ensure that the parent was using "I" statements correctly and to assist the parents in moving the discussion along in a healthy way to try to solve a coparenting issue.

Examples of Incorrect and Correct "I" Statements

Often parents make "I" statements incorrectly. Here are some common mistakes parents make in forming "I" statements and their corrected versions.

1. *Incorrect "I" statement:* "You stay late at work sometimes without texting me when you will be home and it's annoying. I think that from now on, you shouldn't do that, because you wouldn't want me doing that to you. If you cared more about my feelings, we wouldn't be in this situation."

Corrected "I" statement: "I get frustrated when you do not text me when you'll be late getting home. I'd appreciate it if you can send me a text when you'll be late and what time to expect you."

2. *Incorrect "I" statement:* "I feel you annoy me on purpose when I am trying to get the kids ready for school because you're probably worried I might forget something. I would appreciate it if you trusted me more and let me take care of the morning routine."

Corrected "I" statement: "I feel annoyed when you ask me lots of questions while I'm getting the kids ready for school because I feel you don't trust I can do it. I'd appreciate it if you could trust that I can take care of the morning routine."

3. *Incorrect "I" statement:* "I feel irritated when you don't tell me when you're picking up the kids at school, because we've talked about this before. I would appreciate it if you remembered the conversations we have had in the past about these issues."

Corrected "I" statement: "I feel irritated when you don't tell me you are picking the kids up at school, because then I show up also. I would appreciate it if you let me know in advance if you can get them."

4. *Incorrect "I" statement:* "I feel disrespected when you leave things around the house and expect me to do all the dirty work, because you're a grown adult who can put things where they belong. I would appreciate it if you could please be mindful of where you're leaving things and try harder to put things where they belong."

Corrected "I" statement: "I feel disrespected when you leave your things around the house (like your dirty laundry on the floor) because it makes me feel like you do not want to help keep our home clean. I would appreciate it if you could put your things away when you are finished with them."

5. *Incorrect "I" statement:* "I feel used when you say you can't help out with buying the school uniforms but spend a lot on cigarettes, when you know your mother had lung issues, among other things, because it puts pressure on me to buy food, gas, and pay bills, not to mention I'll have to take care of them once the cigarettes take over your health. I would appreciate it if you woke up to this dream you're living in and lend a hand."

Corrected "I" statement: "I feel used when you say you can't help buy school uniforms, because it feels like you are not putting the kids' needs first. I would like to talk about how you can lend a hand with expenses."

Homework Practice

If the parents have been able to construct "I" statements in session and/or effectively use active listening, they should be encouraged to try making at least one "I" statement to communicate something during the week and to use their active listening skills each day.

TOPIC 11: COPARENT PROBLEM SOLVING PART I

This topic focuses on setting rules for healthy relationships and further practicing problem solving with more complicated or higher-conflict topics. Clinicians should present this topic if they feel it is safe for both members of the couple and neither of them has used extensive coercive control to dominate the other parent. If the initial coparent sessions have proceeded well, without high conflict, use of coercive control or indications that either parent feels unsafe, then there would be significant benefit to covering this topic with the coparents. This topic can be reviewed with parents individually if coparent sessions are not safe or possible.

The clinician should first review the rules for healthy relationships with the parents using Handout 8.5. Ground Rules for Healthy Problem-Solving Discussions. After each rule is explained, parents individually complete and then discuss together in session Worksheet 8.2. Rules for Healthy Problem Solving. This is an opportunity for them to individually acknowledge the areas they need to improve. There may also be opportunities in the discussion for parents to give each other compliments on the rules they have followed well. After a review of these rules, parents can work together to complete the Worksheet 8.3. Planning for Disagreements and Form 8.1. Healthy Problem-Solving Contract. This gives parents an opportunity to commit to the rules they have discussed and bring a contract home with them to remind them of these important rules, even if they live separately.

Following review and discussion of these rules and commitment to follow them, the clinician can ask the coparents to bring up a subject from the previous week or recent past that has caused conflict. Ask them to discuss the issue using "I" statements, active listening, and the rules for healthy problem solving. The clinician can provide guidance to parents in using active listening, "I" statements, and positive nonverbal communication during these discussions. As in prior coparenting topics, the clinician must remain active and vigilant about correcting parents when they break any of the rules for problem solving, misuse "I" statements, or are not using active listening. Allowing them to continue to use poor skills is not helpful.

Homework Practice

For coparents who are living together, or who work to do joint activities with their children if they are not living together, help them choose one activity to do together as a family for homework. It's not acceptable that the coparents say they will think of these activities later. Help them identify a shared activity that is realistic and not costly, and nail down a day they plan to do it. This level of specificity will increase the likelihood that they can carry out the activity. (If coparents are not living together or each coparent is participating in the sessions alone, focus on activities they enjoy with their child and develop a plan for a new activity they can try in the coming week.) The activity could be playing a new game together, trying a new playground, going out for ice cream, and so forth.

TOPIC 12: COPARENT PROBLEM SOLVING PART II

Begin the topic by reviewing previous skills, homework, and how the week went in trying to use new communication skills. Did they engage in their family activity? If they did not, problem-solve what is getting in the way of spending positive time (work schedules, chores, etc.). Can they set aside just 30 minutes to 1 hour during the week to do something enjoyable as a family, such as play a game together, take a walk, eat a special meal together, and so forth?

Next, ask the parents to "take a look at Handout 8.4. Areas of Coparenting and think about areas that might be most helpful for us to focus on today." Give this handout to the father and his coparent, if they are present. Ask each parent to tell you which of the coparenting concerns they would like to address:

1. Differences in opinions on childrearing (e.g., moral values, discipline, behavioral expectations, emotional needs, educational standards, safety, and peer relationships).
2. Division of labor related to childrearing.
3. Supportiveness (how supportive is each parent of the other's parenting skills and relationships with their children?).
4. Family management.

After reviewing these areas, clinicians could reference the genograms that were conducted separately with each parent during Phase 1 and ask them to talk about what they learned from their families of origin or their own experiences of being parented, and how these might be influencing their parenting practices. The goal is to tie this discussion in with the areas of disagreement or difficulty in coparenting they identified. You might say something like the following:

> "When we met several weeks ago one on one, we made a map of your families and talked a bit about where you come from. We talked about how you were raised and what you learned about relationships

and parenting from your own upbringing. I'd like you each to say a little bit about your background and how you think it is impacting you as a coparent, and how it might be related to the differences in the way you parent or coparent?"

Some additional questions clinicians might ask parents during this discussion follow:

- "What are your main worries for your child(ren)?"
- "Are there differences in the way you were parented that led you to think about things differently?"
- "What dreams do you have for your children? How will you, as parents, help those dreams become reality? What are the roadblocks?"
- "What are the differences between the roles of fathers and mothers? What are your parenting expectations of what is your responsibility, and what is the responsibility of your coparent? Are your responsibilities different? Have you ever discussed these together?"

Your goal as the therapist is to find common ground on which the parents can agree and work toward the positive future they imagine for their child(ren), and how they might work together to achieve those goals. Be sure to reinforce use of active listening and use of "I" statements during this session.

Daily Routines and Rituals Activity

Discuss daily routines in the home (bedtime, waking, a typical day and what pitfalls come up). Using Worksheet 8.4. Daily Routines, review the structure of the day and who does what related to parenting of the children. Where are the areas of conflict? How can routines be increased? Start when the family wakes up in the morning. Who wakes up first? What is the routine? Write down the activities and who does what throughout the day. What are each parent's expectations of the other? Are there areas that could be altered to make the day run more smoothly? Are there routines that could be put in place to ease transitions? Help the parents develop plans to make changes to their routine as appropriate. What increased positive role could the father play (e.g., reading a book at bedtime, helping with bath)? Be mindful of cultural norms in families around male and female roles as you have this discussion, while looking for ways the father may have more positive time with his child and support his coparent.

CASE EXAMPLE: JOHN AND KAREN

The therapist has reviewed Worksheet 8.4. Daily Routines with clients John and Karen, who are parents to three children, ages 8, 4, and 13 months. Karen is now a stay-at-home mom after being laid off from work, while John works full time at a grocery store. The family was referred after an IPV incident that occurred when John was drunk. Karen and John are both Puerto Rican and they recently bought their first home, which is a point of pride for them. Karen was laid off just before the IPV incident, and the family was under considerable financial stress and worry about paying their mortgage without her income. The children saw their father arrested, handcuffed, and taken away in a police car. The family members were living together during treatment, and both parents were participating in F4C, working hard in the coparenting sessions together. Through completing Worksheet 8.4. Daily Routines, the therapist learned the following:

- Karen was largely responsible for the care of the children and their routine. She got the older children ready for school each day, while John went to work.
- Karen prepared dinner and helped with homework. When John returned from work, he often had a beer or two and watched television.
- Bedtime was difficult in the house. The two older boys watched TV in their room until they fell asleep (which was often close to 11:00 P.M.). There was no routine in place, except parents yelling for the children to get into pajamas and brush their teeth.
- The 13-month-old daughter slept in her parents' bedroom in a crib and was still waking up several times during the night to nurse. She also was staying awake until close to 11:00 P.M. (she typically napped while her mom made dinner from 4:00 to 6:00 P.M.).
- Both parents would watch TV separately in the evenings or hang out with the kids, or be frustrated that the kids were not yet asleep. They would go to bed exhausted and wake up to begin each day at 6:30 A.M.

In this case, there are many possible areas of the daily schedule and family life in which the clinician could intervene. The sleeping routines of the children are of concern. John reports being unhappy that the baby is still sleeping in their room and nursing during the night. He would like more time alone with his wife. These issues get into the areas of intimacy and the couple's relationship, but for these sessions, the clinician needs to stay focused on coparenting and the children. The clinician asks the parents what the hardest part of the day is for them. They report that the evening, from dinner through bedtime is the most challenging. This knowledge allows the clinician to attend to this part of the schedule and to focus first on the bedtime routine. The clinician helps the parents discuss and problem-solve how things flow in the house from dinner to bedtime, and how they might put more structure and routine into that time with both of them actively involved. The clinician writes down a schedule for the nighttime routine that the parents feel good about trying, and their assignment is to try the routine that evening.

Conducting Coparenting Communication Sessions Individually

Sometimes it is not possible to have conjoint coparenting sessions. This can be due to safety concerns, apprehension that the sessions will not be productive, or a lack of interest by either coparent in participating in these sessions together. If coparenting sessions cannot be held jointly, the topics should still be implemented individually so that fathers can learn the communication skills and healthy relationship rules presented. When presented individually, the clinician reviews the topic (e.g., active listening) and then role-plays situations with the father so that he can practice using his active listening and "I" statement skills. Without in-session practice, the father is very unlikely to learn to effectively use the skill, and even less likely to try using it outside of session. In role plays, the therapist can take on the role of the father's coparent or children. And, if meeting with the coparent in a parallel session, the therapist can play the role of the father or children. Practicing these skills with each parent individually will allow them to take these skills forward into other relationships in the future.

Chapter 9 covers Topics 13–17 in the last phase of treatment, Father–Child Restorative Parenting.

CHAPTER 9

Phase 4

Father–Child Restorative Parenting

Restorative parenting sessions should be designed to meet the needs of each family. If a father is unable to bring his child(ren) for sessions, the therapist can opt to focus solely on parenting skills or prepare the father to make amends with his children outside of session on his own. In this last phase of intervention (Topics 13–17), the number of sessions and the topics covered are based on the issues uncovered in the initial assessment, discussed in prior sessions with the father, and likely in coparent sessions with both parents. The topics in this phase are Parenting Skills; Preparing to Make Amends; Taking Responsibility: Conjoint Father–Child Session; Father–Child Play (optional); and Father–Child Feelings Identification and Expression (optional).

Note: Topics 16 and 17 are optional and their implementation should be based on clinical judgment. For example, some fathers need sessions focused on child-directed play and increased positive time with their children; other fathers already have nice play skills with their children and need more focus on how to intervene with their aggression or emotion regulation difficulties. For some families it may be determined that the sessions with father and child should focus on emotional coping skills, as this will benefit father and child most. The topics presented below are a guide. Clinicians can choose some or all of them based on family need and the father's capacity to successfully meet the needs of his children in sessions (this is discussed further under each topic below).

TOPIC 13: PARENTING SKILLS

This topic is intended to focus on emotional and behavioral concerns the father (and coparent) may have for the child. The clinician can begin with a return to discussing typical development based on the child's age. This may also be a time to revisit the impact of FV, parental substance misuse, and other chaotic home situations that may have an impact on young children. The clinician selects parenting skills that are most appropriate for a given family but should start with emotion coaching with the father. The parenting skills that can be covered are (1) emotion coaching, (2) praise, and (3) behavioral interventions such as time out and time in.

Emotion Coaching

Teaching fathers about emotion coaching is important and is a suggested topic for all fathers. They have been working on identifying, understanding, and managing their own emotions and now it is essential to focus explicitly on how to translate that into coaching the development of their children's emotional intelligence. John Gottman developed five steps to emotion coaching that are concrete and helpful for fathers to learn.[1] Emotion coaching is how parents coach their children to understand and manage their emotions. Even more than intelligence, research indicates that emotional awareness and ability to handle feelings has a significant impact on a person's well-being and success in life. This emotional intelligence is learned through interactions with others. Children learn directly from their parents how to understand and manage their emotions (through parents' modeling of these behaviors). Clinicians can introduce this idea to parents by referencing the reflective and coping work they have been doing themselves during F4C by saying something like the following:

> "Today we are going to discuss emotion coaching with your children. Emotion coaching is how you help your children identify, understand, and manage their feelings. It is important, because when children receive good emotion coaching, they learn how to manage their emotions in healthy ways. We've talked together about ways for you to identify, understand, and manage your own emotions. Today we are going to think together about how you coach your children in these same skills."

Gottman's five steps are as follows:

---

[1]Emotion coaching is a research-based tool that was developed by John Gottman (for further information and resources, see *https://emotioncoaching.gottman.com*).

1. Be aware of emotions.
2. Connect with your child.
3. Listen to your child.
4. Name emotions.
5. Find solutions.

Talk through each of these steps and ask the father to think of times he could have used these steps with his own children. What are times when his children have had big emotions and how did he help them manage them? What are ways the emotion coaching skills could be applied in those situations? How might he provide emotion coaching to a baby? What about a toddler? Preschooler? If the father has sons, what does he think about emotion coaching with a son versus that with a daughter? Does he think the response should be different? Why or why not? This is a good opportunity for fathers to reflect on the ways they were taught to manage their emotions (especially sadness or fear) and what the cost was to them for learning to suppress those emotions. There are some great TED talks by Tony Porter (n.d.) speaking about the "man box." These can be wonderful conversation pieces about the way we socialize boys compared to girls; these videos can be viewed together in session to promote conversation on these topics. Exploring a father's cultural experiences of the roles of men/fathers and emotions enables him to reflect on how they have helped or hindered him. What are the costs of learning to suppress emotions and fit into the "man box"?

Fathers have been working to label and understand their feelings during F4C sessions. The clinician can now encourage fathers to label their feelings in front of their children and explain emotions, and how to manage them to their children.

> "It is so helpful for parents to share all sorts of feelings with their children on a day-to-day basis, so that children begin to learn how to label their own feelings. If you are upset about something, it is OK to label that for your child: 'I am angry that you are not listening to me. I would appreciate it if you could get ready for bed like I asked' or 'I am upset because something went wrong at work today. I'm going to relax and watch my favorite show to calm down. I can play with you in a half an hour when I'm finished.' These kinds of examples help your children understand your emotions and teach them how to label their own feelings and share them with you."

Once the steps to emotion coaching have been discussed, along with their importance, the clinician should focus on practice in session by generating different scenarios and asking the father how he could use emotion coaching in those situations. It is best for the clinician to generate situations that are applicable to the father, so that the practice is immediately applicable to his own children. Some possible scenarios to get started are provided below.

Emotion Coaching Scenarios Practice

These situations could be used with the father to give examples of how to use emotion coaching skills like those outlined by Gottman. How can the father label emotions, provide support, and set limits as needed while encouraging emotional expression? When possible, make sure the examples you use are as closely related to situations with his own children. Examine closely the emotion coaching of sons and of daughters, and how the father may view each differently and why. Below are examples of emotion coaching scenarios a clinician could use:

1. Sasha is 2 years old and wants to be picked up. You are in the middle of fixing something. She starts demanding, "UP! UP! UP!"

• *Emotion coaching example:* "I see you want me to pick you up right now. How about if you hand me that tool over there? That would help me finish this project faster. Then I can pick you up [finding solutions]."

2. Ethan is 3 years old. His new baby sister has come home from the hospital. Many visitors are coming to greet her. When the family encourages Ethan to come over to see his new sister, he tries to bite her hand.

• *Emotion coaching example:* It is important for the parent to intervene immediately but gently. "No, Ethan, you cannot bite your sister. I know it is hard to share everyone's attention and you might feel jealous of your baby sister because you want me all to yourself [labeling feeling]. Why don't you tell your grandma and grandpa what you've been doing since we got home from the hospital with your sister [finding solutions/alternatives]?"

In this example, the family must intervene quickly, because the behavior of the child was aggressive. Talking with the father about how a quick intervention to stop dangerous behavior is appropriate, and is most effective if followed up with calm discussion of the feelings the child was having at the time and what alternatives they can choose instead to manage their feelings.

3. Ava is 6 years old. Her father comes home to find her sitting in the corner of her room on the floor with her head on her knees.

• *Emotion coaching example:* The father could go sit down on the floor next to Ava and ask, "You look like you might be upset. Would you like to talk about it [being aware of his daughter's emotions]?" If she does not answer or says no, he could respond, "It's OK. I'll just sit here with you quietly in case you change your mind. I know sometimes it's hard to talk about our feelings [providing support to his child]."

One mistake parents often make is to try and force their children to tell them what is bothering them. They badger the child and even get angry that the child is not telling them what is wrong. This sort of strategy only shuts children down further. Sometimes, all children need and want is someone to be with them when they feel sad or lonely, and if a parent sits quietly with their child in their emotions, the child will frequently start sharing what happened after sitting quietly for a while.

4. Four-year-old Carlo loves toy trucks. His dad brings him a new toy truck. He begins running around the room jumping up and down on the furniture and yelling, "Yay for my new truck!" He is so loud that he wakes his baby sister.

• *Emotion coaching example:* "Carlo, I know you are really excited about your new toy [labeling emotions]. But we need to use our inside voice, so we do not wake up your sister. You could get hurt by jumping on the furniture, so why don't we go play in your bedroom with the new truck [finding solutions/alternatives]?"

Sometimes happy or positive emotions can also lead to behaviors that are not acceptable. Parents need to coach children in understanding and managing all kinds of emotions, not just those that we label as "negative," such as sadness or anger. It is also important to help fathers understand that all emotions are normal and necessary. Sometimes we all feel sad, and allowing ourselves to feel sad can help us move through the sadness.

5. Antonio is 10 years old. He gets off the bus from school and enters the house. He throws down his backpack, ignores everyone who asks what's wrong, and storms into his room and slams the door.

• *Emotion coaching example:* His dad could approach Antonio's room and knock on the door and say, "Antonio, you seem very upset [being aware of emotions]. Can I come in so we can talk about it?" If Antonio says no, his dad could respond, "OK, I'm going to give you some space to calm down. I'll be downstairs if you need me [being available for support]. I'll come back and check on you in about 10 minutes to see if you are ready to talk then."

In this example the father is available for his son but recognizes that sometimes children need space to regain control of their emotions. The father acknowledges that he sees his son is upset and indicates that he is available and will check back; this lets the child know what to expect and to feel supported.

Praise

Just as attention was focused in the coparent sessions on showing appreciation and increasing positive interactions with coparents, it is essential to do the same with children. This skill encourages parents to focus on their child's efforts rather than outcomes to build self-confidence. Praising children helps them understand that the efforts they make are appreciated, not just their accomplishments. Children very much want to please their parents, so providing positive feedback about effort increases that behavior. It is very common for parents to focus only on what they consider negative behaviors or behaviors they want the child to stop doing. By focusing on negatives, parents miss all the times their children are behaving well and doing things that please them. To encourage effort, parents must tell their children specifically what they like that their children do. For example, say "Kelly, I love how you tried to put on your shoes. Good effort!" instead of "Good job!"

Praise is different at different developmental stages. Parents can praise infants through smiling, cuddling, hugging, and clapping. Toddlers need praise that includes words of encouragement, especially related to exploration. If a parent offers encouragement to their toddler to tackle challenges and try again, it will build the child's self-confidence and persistence. This encouragement should continue into the preschool years and beyond. Parents need to praise not only success but also efforts to do new things or to complete tasks. For example, "Nice work trying to zip your coat. Zippers can be hard" or "Good effort with your homework. I know some of those problems are challenging."

Clinicians should review steps to effective praise with parents in preparation for in-session role playing first with the clinician and potentially with the child during father–child sessions.

1. Praise effort and practice.
2. Give praise as soon as possible.
3. Be specific.
4. Be genuine.
5. Provide feedback about how your child's actions made you feel: "It makes me happy when you help clean up the toys in your room."
6. Have realistic expectations given your child's age.

It is imperative that the clinician practice with the father in session how he can praise his children. This can be done by having parents think of at least one thing they liked that their child did in the last few days, then role-play with the clinician the words they would say to praise their child about what they liked. If they have trouble thinking of something, ask them to think of a time their child was not misbehaving or was being quiet and describe it to you. Facilitate how the father might select something to praise and what words he could use. Encourage parents to watch for this behavior they would like to increase over the coming days and to praise the child when they see it.

Clinicians can introduce homework to continue this focus on child positive behavior and praise during the coming week. It's key to relate praising efforts back to the skills covered in previous sessions (catch your coparent doing something you appreciate) and how doing so will also make children feel noticed and loved for the good things they do.

Homework Practice

Assign Worksheet 9.1. Catch Your Child Doing Something You Appreciate. Instruct the father to focus on noticing the positive things his child does over the coming week. He should notice when the child listens, sits quietly, follows directions, or helps in small ways. The more the father encourages these things, the more the child will do them.

Behavioral Interventions Such as Time Out and Time In

Therapists should discuss with parents how they respond to their children's misbehavior. As discussed in earlier chapters of this book, there is significant overlap between use of IPV behavior and child maltreatment (physical and psychological abuse). Many fathers who have used IPV experienced maltreatment or the use of physical/corporal punishment themselves. They often describe them as whoopings, spankings, popping, and so forth. It is helpful to ask parents about their views on punishment, what kinds of strategies they have tried, and what has worked or not worked for them in the past. Some parents may report that they use "time out." If this is the case, ask them to describe how they use it. What behaviors do they use it to correct, and what steps do they follow to implement it? Parents often misuse time out; it is intended to be a strategy to curb serious behavioral problems by giving children a quiet space to calm down and regain control of themselves. When children have experienced FV, they often struggle with regulating their emotions, even more than is typical of children their age. Instead of time out, clinicians can suggest use of "time in" as a first line of intervention, as it is helpful in building connections between parent and child and providing space for good emotion coaching. Handouts on the implementation of time in and time out (Handout 9.1. What Is Time In? and Handout 9.2. What Is Time Out?) can be used to review the steps with parents, as well as Handout 9.3. Why Not Spanking? Other good parenting programs have developed and used these techniques with parents. Programs like Circle of Security (*www.circleofsecurityinternational.com/resources-for-parents*) have excellent resources on some of these topics for parents and were the basis of some of the guidelines provided in this book.

Sometimes parents believe that spanking is needed to teach children how to behave. Some parents feel that it worked on them; having this information opens the opportunity for an important discussion about *how* it worked. The F4C clinician's role is to wonder with the client about their views on various forms of punishment, including spanking. The clinician seeks to understand and provide information for the client to consider. The discussion below illustrates how a conversation of this sort could play out in session.

THERAPIST: Tell me about what kinds of discipline strategies you've used or that you think are best to use with kids.

DURELL: We use a lot of different things. Sometimes we take stuff away. We've tried time out, but that doesn't work. Sometimes you just have to pop a kid on the hand or butt.

[*Here the therapist has several possible choices to pursue. The dad indicated that time out does not work and that use of physical punishment is sometimes needed; both of these areas should be explored. Parents need to feel they have alternatives that work if they are going to change their use of physical punishment.*]

THERAPIST: Tell me more about how you've tried time out. What happened?

DURELL: Well, we used it a few times at the suggestion of Johnny's preschool teacher. He wouldn't stay in his room, or he would just play with his toys, and it didn't teach him anything.

THERAPIST: What kinds of misbehavior were you using it for, and how long did he have to stay in the time out? It sounds like you sent him to his room?

DURELL: Yes, he had to go to his room for an hour when he was not listening to me.

THERAPIST: I have some suggestions of things you might try that might make your use of time out more effective. When you send Johnny to his room, he has access to his toys and things he likes. This is not really the point of time out. Time out is meant to give children just a few minutes to calm down and regain control of themselves, so that you might then be able to talk calmly about their misbehavior. It can work best if you identify a time-out spot that does not have any distractions (toys, TV, etc.). For example, a chair in quiet corner of a room or the bottom step on the stairs. Johnny would then sit there for the same number of minutes as his age. Johnny is 4, so he would have to have a 4-minute time out. You could set a timer with an alarm so both of you know when his time is up. You can say something like, "I want you to sit in this chair for 4 minutes, until you hear the timer go off, and then we'll talk about what just happened together." That seems like a short amount of time to us, but to Johnny, 4 minutes will seem like a long time. What do you think? Is that something you'd like to try?

DURELL: Maybe. That seems like a pretty light punishment.

THERAPIST: I can understand that. You've told me about your experiences with punishment growing up. Let's talk more about how punishments worked for you. Tell me about how your mom's use of popping helped you behave better.

DURELL: Well, I learned what I was not supposed to do. I stopped doing stuff.

THERAPIST: OK, so you stopped doing the misbehaviors. I'm wondering how you felt about your mom when she popped you?

DURELL: Well, I would be mad at her. Sometimes I was scared. I would hide stuff from her.

THERAPIST: So, it caused you to keep stuff from your mom. Did you still do things she didn't want but you'd just hide it or lie to her?

DURELL: Yeah, I got sneaky with stuff.

THERAPIST: So, it sounds like the popping worked initially but then it made you feel like you had to hide things from your mom, and you got sneaky with doing things anyway.

DURELL: Yeah, I did. As I got older, I didn't care about the popping. I thought I'll just do what I want and if she catches me, I can handle the popping.

THERAPIST: So it sounds like the effects of it wore off, and it changed your relationship with your mom. If you were in trouble, would you have called your mom?

DURELL: No way! Anyone but her!

THERAPIST: So, I'm wondering how this experience fits in with how you want Johnny to feel about you.

In this example, the therapist not only provided corrections regarding use of time out but also used the father's own experiences to help him think through why the use of physical punishment may not be creating the kind of relationship he wants for himself and his son. Sometimes parents will present use of spanking or physical punishment as cultural. Clinicians can be open to hearing this perspective. Some black parents feel they must use physical punishment to ensure their children learn for their own safety. This dates back to slavery and is an important cultural context for clinicians to consider. For further readings on this important topic see Akbar (2017). This issue will be further discussed with an example later in this chapter.

TOPIC 14: PREPARING TO MAKE AMENDS

This topic is intended for all fathers. If a father has an infant (under age 2), then holding a conjoint Taking Responsibility session is not developmentally appropriate. However, it is still helpful to talk through with the father what he is accountable for and the ways his behaviors have impacted his baby (goals 1 and 2 below). For children over age 2, a conjoint session can be planned, as outlined below. As mentioned earlier, if a father is unable to meet together with his children in session, the issues discussed in this topic are still important and can be reviewed in the hope that he can discuss them with his children on his own in the future.

To have successful father–child sessions related to making amends, it is crucial for clinicians to prepare fathers thoroughly for these sessions. This means ensuring that fathers understand the importance of this upcoming session for their relationships with their children, and that there is a clear and concrete plan for what they will say and how the session will look. It is contraindicated for therapists hold these father–child sessions without individual preparation with the father first. In this work, you are holding the child's developmental and relational needs in mind and planning for relationship reconnection or the beginning of repair to harms caused by the father. The child's experience and needs have the highest priority.

The specific goals of this topic are listed below:

1. Review progress in treatment thus far and skills learned.

2. Review prior history of FV and plan with client how to talk with his child(ren) about past behaviors and changes he is making.

- **a.** What kinds of conflicts, aggression, substance misuse did his child witness or hear?

b. Review the reactions children can have even to minor disagreements and tensions between parents.
c. Reiterate the parents' roles to teach their children about how relationships work and how to be a partner and parent when they get older.
d. What do they think they have modeled for their children so far, and what do they want their children to learn from them about being a partner, coparent, and parent?
e. Practice reflective functioning by asking parents to describe how they think their child(ren) experienced their arguments or substance misuse.

3. Plan the goals of the initial father–child session and review these with the father to ensure that he is comfortable and agrees with the plan. This involves getting *very* specific about what he will say to his child(ren) about why he has been coming to treatment and why he is bringing them to meet his counselor/therapist. Discuss what the father hopes will happen in father–child sessions. Help him script what he can say, and *write it down* prior to bringing the children into session. You can assist him to develop age-appropriate language and practice *exactly* what he will say using Worksheet 9.2. Guidelines for Making Amends Session Letter; this can help guide the development of the script the father will use in session with this children. An example of a completed worksheet is shown in Figure 9.1. Some fathers will be able to fill this worksheet out in session. Others may want to think about it after your initial discussion and take it home as homework. Either way is acceptable. If fathers take it home for homework, clinicians can return to it the following week to continue preparation for the conjoint sessions with the children.

4. The final developed script is kept by the therapist when it is finished so that it is available when the father arrives next session with his children. The father may forget the letter at home and then not have it when he arrives, or he may decide to try to talk to his children on his own without therapist support. If a father has children of very different ages (e.g., a 3-year-old and an 11-year-old), it may be helpful and necessary to hold more than one father–child session. If children are close in age and development (e.g., a 4-year-old and a 6-year-old), then seeing them together will work well, but if children are in very different developmental stages, then offering separate sessions will allow the father to talk with each child at their developmental level. The questions and needs of an 11-year-old for explanations and discussion differ from what a 3- or 4-year-old can process. Think through with the father how to structure sessions if he has multiple children in different developmental stages.

1. What have your children experienced/witnessed that you need to acknowledge or for what behaviors do you need to take responsibility?

   They saw me breaking things and yelling at their mom. I was swearing and calling her names.

2. In what ways have these experiences or your behaviors impacted your children?

   I think they got scared when I raised my voice. They had some anxiety about being away from their mom to go to day care.

3. What are you trying to do differently now so your children do not have these experiences again? What skills have you learned or what behaviors are you changing?

   I'm trying to use the skills I learned here to communicate better with their mother so we can all get along.

4. Write a statement in developmentally appropriate language for your child/children that includes an acknowledgment of what they experienced, an apology for your behavior, and how you are trying to change:

   I know you saw me breaking things and yelling at your mom lots of times. I'm sorry that I did those things. It was not OK for me to act like that or to hurt your mom. I know you were scared. I've been learning some ways to manage my anger and to talk to your mom nicely. I'm working on it and will keep working on it so things will be better at home.

FIGURE 9.1. Example of Worksheet 9.2. Guidelines for Making Amends Session Letter.

Getting Ready to Restore and Rebuild

Research interviews reviewed in Chapter 3 with children exposed to IPV have revealed three things children want from their fathers after witnessing IPV: (1) acknowledgment that the violence happened, (2) an apology, and (3) a change in their father's behavior. There is no single way to talk to children about these issues. However, it is important to help the father be able to touch on the three areas of acknowledgment, apology, and change. Fathers should say something about why they are in treatment and why they are bringing the child to meet the counselor. Some examples of things fathers have been able to say to their children are as follows:

Father with Two Children, Ages 3 and 7

"I know you saw some scary fights between your mom and me. We were yelling and hurting each other. I should not have acted like that. Yelling mean things and hurting people is not OK, even when I'm angry. I'm sorry you saw and heard those things. I've been coming here to meet with Dr. Stover and she has helped me learn some new ways to handle my mad feelings. I have been working hard and I wanted you to come here with me so I could talk with you about what I did wrong and show you some things I have learned. Do you have questions for me about fights you've seen or the way I treated mom, or what I've learned with Dr. Stover?"

Father with His 5- and 8-Year-Old Children

"I know you remember when the police came and took Papi away that time when I was yelling and hurting mom after drinking lots of beer. That was wrong. I should not hurt mom, and you should not have to see dad act like that. Dad got in trouble with the police because what I did was against the law, and they said I had to come meet with Dr. Stover for help. She has been helping me learn new things that will help me when I get angry. I'd like to show you some of the things I've learned, but first is there anything you'd like to ask me about it?"

Father of a 4-Year-Old Son in a Family with Mutual Situational Couple Violence

"Your mommy and I used to get in really bad fights with yelling and hitting. That was wrong. People should not scream and hit each other, especially if they love each other. I'm sorry you had to see that. I have been coming to see Dr. Stover and mommy has, too. She is helping us learn new ways to talk to each other when we are mad or upset. We want to show you some of the things we have learned, because we know you get really mad sometimes, too, and it's hard for you not to hit people and scream. We do not want any more screaming, hitting, or hurting each other in our house. We are going to work together."

It is also important that fathers talk to their children (even very young children) about addiction, if that is part of the picture for the family. Handout 9.4. Talking with Your Kids About Addiction and Treatment can be a useful guide to discussion and help fathers think about what to say. Some sample language a father could use to describe his addiction to his young child is as follows:

> "I have a kind of sickness called addiction. It isn't a sickness you can catch. It means that I take drugs (or drink alcohol), and it is very hard for me to stop. I am getting help for my addiction. My counselor is helping me with my sickness, and I am getting better. My addiction sickness is not your fault. Nothing you did made me use drugs. There is nothing you can do to make me stop. I need to stop myself, and I am working very hard with the help of my counselor. I love you, and I'm sorry that I cannot be with you all the time, because I need to be in treatment for my sickness now. Do you have any questions?"

Practicing Amends in Session

It is important that fathers practice reading their statements relative to this topic and think about how their children may respond. The clinician will be serving a gatekeeping function during the father–child session to ensure that the messages the father is giving his children are both developmentally and clinically appropriate, and focused on restoration of their relationship. The clinician should have the father read the statement out loud and imagine that he is reading it to his children. Then ask him, "How do you think you'll feel when you read it to them? How do you think they will respond?" Fathers should *not* expect to be forgiven and not make promises that they will never use FV or use substances again. They can state that they will "work hard" or "try really hard," but stating FV will never happen again is a promise they may not be able to keep. Behavior change is hard, and making potentially false promises is not helpful to children. These sessions are for their children's benefit, not for the father to feel absolved of past wrongs. Clinicians must help fathers to anticipate how children may respond, state clearly that they are not to ask to be forgiven or to make promises they may not be able to keep. Some children will have many questions, while others will say nothing at all. Help prepare fathers for these possibilities and to accept that all responses from the child are OK. Also, select activities the father and children will do together after this discussion is finished. Teaching a child(ren) diaphragmatic breathing or some other coping strategy is suggested, as well as selecting toys or a game that the child(ren) would like to play with at the end of the session to increase their positive interactions and provide them with something fun to close the session.

If the father has more than one child, the clinician should consider the ages/developmental stages of the children. It is typically appropriate to meet with the father and children together. However, if a father has young children (ages 3–5) and also children who are older (11+), it may be better to plan two sessions to meet the needs of his children and allow for developmentally appropriate conversations with his very young children and then a more advanced discussion with his older children. The dynamics among his children may also play a role in how these sessions are structured. Let's examine a case situation and how a clinician might structure the father–child making amends sessions.

CASE EXAMPLE: HENRY

Henry is the father of a 12-year-old son in middle school (entering seventh grade) and his daughter has just turned 5 and will start kindergarten next month. The children witnessed a significant IPV incident in which the father was drunk, smashed up things in the house, and physically assaulted their mother in front of them. They saw him arrested by police, and he was unable to see them for several months due to a full no-contact protective order for the mother and children. The protective order has now been modified, and he is able to visit with them but still cannot live in the house due to a residential stay-away order from the court. The 5-year-old is highly anxious. She is very attached to her mother and prefers to be with her. She sleeps with her mom, and she avoids her brother. The 12-year-old son is angry and getting into trouble a lot at school. The father worries that his son is getting in with the wrong crowd and may be experimenting with marijuana and alcohol.

In this family, the son and daughter are in very different developmental stages and have different symptoms and difficulties following FV and the aftermath. In this case, it makes sense for the father to meet with his son and daughter individually to allow for conversations specific to each child. The father could still craft one making amends statement that he will say to both separately or he might add different information depending on his worries and what he wants them to know about his own treatment. The therapist can help him anticipate the questions, responses of each child (which may be quite different), and what discussion might be prioritized. For example, the discussion around his drinking and alcohol misuse may be more pointed and specific to spark discussion with his son about his possible substance experimentation. He might say something like the following:

> "The night I was arrested at the house for hitting your mother and smashing up everything, I was drunk, and my behavior was unacceptable. I have an alcohol problem and I'm getting help to stop drinking and learn to manage my stress and angry feelings better. I want us to be able to talk about alcohol and other drugs, because addiction runs in our family. Your grandfather also had an addiction to alcohol, just like I do. This means that you could also develop an addiction to alcohol or other drugs, and I do not want that to happen to you. Addiction is a sickness that means we cannot use alcohol and drugs because we are unable to stop, and after a while, all we care about is drinking. I am here to answer your questions, and I'm sorry that you had to see me hurt your mother and destroy our things. You deserve better. Do you have any questions about what I've said?"

The clinician can then help facilitate discussion between the father and son about addiction, the worries the father has for his son, and the treatment the father is getting both to manage his addiction and change his ways of coping with stress and emotions. With his 5-year-old daughter the father might slightly change his statement to something like the following:

> "The night the police came and took Daddy to jail for hitting Mommy and smashing up everything, I drank lots of an adult drink called alcohol and my behavior was wrong. I have an addiction to alcohol, and I'm getting help for it and learning to manage my stress and mad feelings better, so I don't hit your mom, yell, and break things. Addiction is a sickness that means I cannot use alcohol, because I am unable to stop. It is not a sickness you can catch. I am here to answer your questions, and I'm sorry that you had to see me hurt your mommy and break our things. I know you were scared, and I was wrong to do that. I will try very hard not to let that happen again. Do you have any questions about what I've said?"

Here the father gives generally the same message but focuses less on addiction running in families and more on what he did wrong and an explanation of what addiction means.

ASSESSING FATHER'S READINESS FOR CONJOINT FATHER–CHILD SESSIONS

Fathers are often uncomfortable with the making amends conjoint session goals. This is understandable. Fathers may be unsure what they should say to their children. They may feel self-conscious or indicate that their children do not need to talk about the past violence or substance misuse they have witnessed or experienced. A common response from fathers is "I don't think we need to talk about this. It happened a long time ago, and my kids never mention it. I think it's better if we just move on. I don't want to retraumatize them."

In this kind of instance, it is crucial that the clinician respond with reasons why doing this father–child session will help heal their family and their relationships with their children. The therapist can respond by saying the following:

> "I understand why you feel that way. This is a really hard thing to talk about. It is very common for kids *not* to talk about what they saw or bring it up. They may be scared to talk about it or think they are not supposed to bring it up. Since you haven't talked to them about it and probably no one has, they think it's not OK to speak about it. Without talking about it though, you have no idea what your kids are thinking and feeling about it. Kids often blame themselves for arguments and problems at home, even when it is not their fault. Without you telling them, your kids also do not know you realize what you did was wrong, and you are trying to change. They may be worrying that it will happen again."

From this explanation, the father and therapist can continue to talk about the father's worries about talking to his children in a session. The therapist can assure the father that they will be there to support him and his children during the session. Another approach is to ask the father to reflect on the absence of these conversations in his own childhood. The clinician could ask, "Did your parents ever talk to you about conflict, aggression, or substance use in your family? How did this affect you? How would you feel if your parent did talk to you about it back then?" Asking these questions can provide an opportunity for the clinician to state that the goal of the father's session with his child is to stop the patterns he himself experienced.

If a father is unable to write a making amends statement, continues to deny any impact on his children, or indicates that he will be inappropriate in a father–child session (e.g., blame the child's mother or talk about developmentally inappropriate aspects of the incident or aftermath), then attempting the making amends session together with his children is not appropriate. The goal of the session is to provide the father and his children with a beginning to repair their relationship and for the child to have a positive experience. If the clinician feels the father is unable to provide that for his children, then they should not proceed with this topic.

TOPIC 15: TAKING RESPONSIBILITY: CONJOINT FATHER–CHILD SESSION

The primary goals of this father–child topic are threefold:

1. For the father to talk with his child(ren) about his past behavior (acknowledge the FV and apologize)
2. To describe the work he's been doing in treatment and open the lines of communication with his child(ren)
3. To provide an opportunity for positive interactions between father and child(ren)

Note: As mentioned earlier, if fathers only have infants (under 2 years old) and no older children, they would not do this topic together with their child.

The session should begin with the therapist introducing themselves and immediately turning to the discussion the therapist planned with the father the previous week: "Hi, I'm Dr. Stover. I'm your dad's therapist. I've been working with him to learn new ways to manage his emotions and to get along better at home. Your dad has something he'd like to say to you to get us started." Spending time chatting about other things just prolongs everyone's anxiety about the point of the session; get right to it. You do not need to develop significant rapport with the children. They should be comfortable, but the focus is on the father–child relationship, not on the therapist–child rapport.

It is OK if the father reads the statement from notes, as some fathers are very anxious and reading makes it easier for them to stay on target with what was prepared. The conversation should include the father taking responsibility for his previous actions (aggression, substance use, or child maltreatment, as is appropriate for each individual father), a heartfelt apology, and some description of changes he is trying to make. After the father opens the discussion, the child should be given an opportunity to ask questions. The therapist should allow the father and child to talk together as much as possible, intervening only as needed to guide the father, assist him with answering questions, and provide encouragement ensuring that the interaction remains positive.

It is not uncommon for children to have no questions or response to the father's statement. This type of meeting is an unusual situation; it's not a topic they have discussed, and they are doing it with a new person in the room. It is appropriate for the therapist to ask a few questions as prompts or to summarize the reason for the visit to help guide. For example, Joe made his amends statement to his 11-year-old daughter. The statement included taking responsibility for not only his verbal abuse of her mother but also his harsh punishment and verbal abuse toward her. The father was genuine in his apology and in discussing things he was learning to do better in the future. His daughter sat silently under her sweatshirt hood and shook her head when the father asked if she had questions. Joe's therapist then interpreted the discomfort by saying, "It's understandable that you might not have questions now or that talking about your dad's behavior might feel strange, because you may not have done that before. I'm wondering what you thought about what your dad just said?"

If the child still shrugs or does not respond, the therapist could continue with the following:

> "It's OK not to have questions right now. The reason we met today was so that your dad could share some things with you, open the conversation about what has happened in your family, and to start to heal your relationship. Your dad understands that this will take time, but he wants you to know he takes responsibility for what happened and is open to talking about it with you when you feel ready."

It is also possible that the child will have questions that the father struggles to answer. These may be things like "How do I know you won't do this again?" or "What does it feel like to use drugs?" Fathers may be shocked by these questions and look pleadingly at the therapist for help. The therapist should be prepared to help the father respond to these questions. This may involve simple encouragement or outright interjection, if needed, to help the father respond in a developmentally and clinically appropriate way. Sometimes during these sessions, a father's shame will be triggered, and he will try to minimize his child's experience, as in the following example:

CASE EXAMPLE: SAM

During the making amends session, following his father's amends statement, 7-year-old Sam responded, saying there were some big fights and the walls were shaking. His father chuckled nervously and said, "I don't think it was that loud." The clinician interjected and said, "For Sam, the yelling was very loud, and it felt like the house was shaking. When you are 7, your parents' yelling can be very scary and feel very dangerous." Sam nodded. His father responded, "I'm sorry I scared you like that, Sam."

In this example, the therapist was able to gently shut down the father's minimization of the child's experience by interpreting it for the father, which allowed him to understand it from his son's experience and have more of an empathetic response.

After the discussion of the father's amends statement, he can share with his child some of the things he has been learning in treatment, such as coping skills he has learned. Again, the therapist will have planned this conversation with the father in advance and helped him to come up with ways of teaching the skills he's learned to his children. The father can teach his child how to do diaphragmatic breathing or progressive muscle relaxation, and they can practice together in session. It is helpful to end this session with a fun activity to increase positive interaction between father and child. This can be 10–15 minutes of free play or a game.

Homework Practice

At the end of the session, suggest that the father and child think of an activity or game they can play together over the upcoming week. Was there a game or play they enjoyed during session? Assign doing this activity once during the week at home.

TOPIC 16: FATHER–CHILD PLAY

This session is intended to provide unstructured, child-guided play time for the father and child. The clinician will provide direct modeling/coaching for the father in imaginative, nondirective play with his child. This session can be implemented with fathers who are struggling to have positive interactions with their children or who need more support in learning how to play with and spend time with their children. Some fathers have little experience playing. They may not have experienced adults playing with them as children or even remember how to pretend play. Supported sessions with a clinician can help them with ideas of developmentally appropriate play activities they can easily do at home. This topic is an opportunity to encourage father–child play and for the father to practice using praise directly with the child in session. The therapist should provide appropriate pretend-play toys or games depending on the child's age and direct the father to allow the child to be in charge of the play.

Note: Fathers who are observed to be very good at pretend or child-guided play during the play assessment at the outset of treatment may not need this topic. Clinicians can decide to skip this if it is not an area of need for the father.

Start this topic with a review of the goals of child-directed play, a concept described in detail by the developers of PCIT (*www.parentchildinteractiontherapy.com*):

1. Follow the child's lead.
2. Allow the child to control the content and pace of play.
3. The father should be attentive and responsive.
4. Encourage imagination.
5. Describe what the child is doing, but do not ask questions.
6. Encourage use of praise as you've discussed in prior sessions.

Role of the Clinician in These Sessions

It is essential that the clinician allow the father and child to play together. It is common for female therapists who have done a good amount of child therapy to feel the need to engage the child and build a rapport. The child should feel comfortable with the therapist in the room, but the therapist should not be overly involved or the primary focus of interactions. The following is an example of a therapist getting too involved in a father–child session:

CASE EXAMPLE: XAVIER

Xavier arrives to session with his 2-year-old son, Javier. The therapist, Julia, has set up age-appropriate toys for Xavier and Javier on the floor of the office. Julia welcomes them to the playroom, then sits down on the floor near the toys. Xavier sits on a couch. Julia begins talking to Javier about the toys and showing him the different choices. Xavier begins telling Julia about some interactions with the coparent over the week. Javier brings some toys over to Julia and hands them to her to begin to play, while Javier continues to talk from the couch.

This session is already set up for the child to think he will be interacting with the therapist, not the father. Julia incorrectly thought that if she modeled sitting on the floor with the toys for the father, he would automatically do that. Julia failed to explain to Xavier the expectations for the session and allowed him to begin talking to her about issues (as was typical when they met individually) rather than directing him to the focus of the current session. An appropriate way to set up this session would be as follows:

Xavier arrives for the session with his 2-year-old son, Javier. The therapist, Julia, has set up age-appropriate toys for Xavier and Javier on the floor of the office. Julia welcomes them to the playroom and sits on the couch. She motions for Xavier to sit on the floor near the toys and to explore them with Javier. She then tells Xavier the rules for the session today: "Today we are going to let Javier be in charge of the play. I'd like you to let him choose the toys and how you play with them. I'd like you to give him praise, like we've practiced, for the things you like that he's doing. Try not to ask him questions but just play. Any questions?" It is OK for the therapist to give these instructions in front of the child, since a young child like Javier likely will not separate from his father.

Xavier begins telling Julia about some interactions with the coparent over the week. Julia responds, "Today let's focus on playing with Javier, since he's here with you and we can find another time to talk about that." Javier brings some toys over to Julia and hands them to her. "Javier, it looks like you've found something you'd like to play with first! I think your dad might like to see; can you show him?" Javier walks over to his father and Xavier responds, "What shall we play, Javier?"

This example has set up a much better situation for the father and child to interact and spend time playing together during the session. The therapist's goal in this session is to be as uninvolved as possible. Providing encouragement to the father and child or suggesting ways the father can provide praise, or gently correcting if he becomes intrusive or takes over the play. The therapist might say, "Remember, today, Javier is in charge of what you play," or "Let's let Javier choose today."

Homework Practice

At the end of the session, give the father Handout 9.5. Child-Directed Play Guidelines. Have him set up a time during the week to practice play at home with his child(ren) for 15 minutes using this guide.

TOPIC 17: FATHER–CHILD FEELINGS IDENTIFICATION AND EXPRESSION

Teaching feeling identification in a session with a father's children can be a nice way to solidify this skill for the father. You might start the session by reminding parents of all the feelings they have discussed in prior sessions and say something like "Today, we want to play some games with your children to teach them all the feeling words. Just like we practiced how to identify feelings and what to do, as parents we teach our kids to understand their feelings, too." Reading a children's book about feelings appropriate for young children may be a nice way to introduce this topic (a list of possible children's books can be found in the list of resources in Appendix B). The father can read the book to his child(ren), allowing for some close contact and affection between father and child. Often in families with high hostility, there is very little affectionate touch, and harsh words and limited positive physical contact are common. Encouraging fathers to use affectionate touch with their children can be a vital intervention during their joint sessions. Practicing use of hugs, sitting close together or on his lap, and cuddling or back rubbing, as appropriate, can increase feelings of closeness for the father and his child. Reading a book together naturally elicits close contact and an opportunity for this touching if the child is comfortable.

Feelings Identification and Regulation Activities

Practitioners can use a few different games to assist parents and children to interact around different feelings. When possible, parents should model feelings for children first. Start by generating a list of feelings with the father and write them down (at a minimum, happy, sad, scared, mad, surprised, and disgusted should be there, but it's good to have a long list). It is helpful to have a mirror in the room for very young children. When a feeling is named, the therapist can say, "Let's all make a happy face. Let's all make a mad face," and so on. The children can make their faces and view themselves in the mirror. They can mimic the faces their parents make for emotions that may be new to them. This is also an opportunity to talk about things that make people feel different emotions. Another game the father and child can play using the list of feelings is called feelings charades. Parents and children take turns acting out different feelings and trying to guess the feelings the other acts out. This is a fun way for kids to practice identifying feelings and for parents to show their new knowledge in a fun way to their children.

It is also necessary to talk together with the parents and their children about what happens when our bodies have big feelings. You might say something like the following:

> "Sometimes when something happens to make us mad, upset, or scared, we can feel all mixed up, like we don't know what to do. Our feelings are so big, we are out of control. When that happens, we might cry really loud, kick our feet, or hit people. Your dad has learned some ways to manage big feelings, and he is going to show you the new things he has learned to help calm down and relax our bodies when we have big feelings."

Ask the father to show his children some of the coping strategies he has learned. These might include diaphragmatic breathing (if not already done during the making amends session), grounding techniques, mindfulness or guided imagery (as described in Chapter 7). If the father is unsure, you can guide the whole family in an emotion regulation activity.

For learning diaphragmatic breathing, children might find it easier to lie on the floor and watch a stuffed animal or small toy rise up and down on their stomachs as they practice.

It may be difficult for very young children to get the hang of this breathing technique. Talk about breathing in through the nose like you do when you smell something. "Let's smell the flower! Breathing out is like slowly blowing out your birthday candles. Let's smell the flower. Now blow out the candles!" If the clinician is guiding the father and children, they might use the following way to introduce the breathing to the family:

> "We are going to learn some special breathing that will help relax your body when you have big feelings. [child's name], make yourself comfortable in the chair or on the floor. Place my friend, the dog [use a small stuffed dog or other stuffed animal], on your stomach and put your hand on your chest. Dad, you can place one hand on your chest and the other on your stomach. [Demonstrate.] When we breathe in, our friend should move up, and when we breathe out it should move down. The hand on our chest should stay still and not move the whole time. This means we are breathing correctly. . . . Let's try it. Take a big deep breath in through your nose like you are smelling a flower and let it out slowly through your mouth like you are blowing out birthday candles. [Give the participants a chance to take a few breaths and check to see that they are bringing the air into their abdomen and not shallow breathing just into their chest. Provide guidance as needed. You might say to the child, 'Look how you are making Mr. Cat go up and down with your belly.'] OK, now that you're getting the hang of it, let's try to breathe more slowly when we breathe out than when we breathe in. I'll count the first time for practice, and let's see if I can count higher when we're breathing out than when we're breathing in. Breathe in 1-2-3, hold it, breathe out 1-2-3-4-5. [Repeat three to five times.]"

Homework Practice

Depending on what activities were done in session, the therapist can assign homework practice. For example, if controlled breathing was introduced in session, then assign home practice of the breathing for the father and child at bedtime. If discussion of feelings and feelings identification games were practiced in session, then assign the father and child the task to practice labeling feelings at home. Fathers and children can label feelings of those around them during the week.

CULTURAL CONSIDERATIONS

Sometimes parents may respond skeptically to some of the parenting techniques and suggestions provided in this phase. The most common issue that arises is use of corporal/physical punishment or views about how fathers treat their coparents or children that are described as cultural. It is important to be thoughtful about discussions around the issue of cultural norms or beliefs. The goal is not to put your cultural values on a client, but to help them consider whether a behavior is really necessary to be part of their culture and why. How does a particular discipline strategy or belief align with their culture? How would using an alternative approach impact their cultural identification or feelings of belonging within their cultural group?

CASE EXAMPLE: DEVON

Devon, the 36-year-old Jamaican American father of 11-year-old Anaya, was referred to F4C by CPS after a report was made by Anaya's neighbor that he had beat her with the buckle side of a belt after she posted a photo on social media that he found inappropriate. During the investigation, it was uncovered that Devon was very controlling with regard to his wife's access to finances, transportation, and contact with friends. He frequently belittled her in front of their children and threatened her with physical violence. When meeting with Devon and discussing the incident of physical abuse with his daughter, Devon reported that in Jamaica, this practice was common and it was cultural. He felt justified in the punishment and felt that children in the United States had too much power.

DEVON: Anaya knew better than to put that photo on social media. She had to be punished. She will not do that again. My father used to beat me with a switch, and it kept me in line. I am thankful to him for that.

CLINICIAN: You feel that your father's beatings were helpful to you as a child?

DEVON: Yes, that's how children learn, and as a father, it is my responsibility to ensure she learns how to behave.

CLINICIAN: You mentioned it was cultural. Can you help me understand what about that practice is cultural to being Jamaican?

DEVON: It's how we believe children should be raised. Spare the rod, spoil the child.

CLINICIAN: I agree that different cultures can have different practices around how to parent and interact with children. I wonder if it's culture or simply a belief you have that you were taught by your parents? Do all Jamaican's use this form of discipline?

DEVON: I think most do.

CLINICIAN: Is there any reason this approach might not be helpful to children?

DEVON: Well, someone could take it too far and really hurt their kid.

CLINICIAN: How do you think Anaya views you as a father after this incident? How do you think she feels about you?

DEVON: I think she's angry at me 'cause she knows she was wrong. She thinks I don't understand her.

CLINICIAN: Can you think back to being a child and how you felt when you got a beating with a switch? You said as an adult you are thankful, but I'm wondering if you can share how you felt and thought about it when you were 10 or 11?

DEVON: I knew to stay in line 'cause I didn't want to get the switch. I sometimes avoided my father if I had done something I thought he'd whip me for.

CLINICIAN: Why was that?

DEVON: I guess I was scared of him.

CLINICIAN: As a child, did you feel beatings were part of being Jamaican?

DEVON: No, I guess not.

CLINICIAN: What did being Jamaican mean? What felt part of your culture?

DEVON: I mean, I guess the food we ate and some of the family stuff we did.

CLINICIAN: I'm wondering if the beating is not really part of being Jamaican, but is what you learned as a way to discipline from your parents and if there might be other ways that could work, too? Will you feel less Jamaican if you do not use this form of punishment?

DEVON: I mean, probably not.

In this example, Devon describes a behavior as *cultural* to defend against criticism, and the clinician probes gently to try to open up his thinking about whether that behavior is about his culture and what it means to be Jamaican. Helping parents explore how they feel a part of their culture or family is an important consideration to help shift thinking. Discussions about discipline can be challenging. Some Black parents report feeling they must be harsh with their children in order to teach them to behave, so that they will not get hurt or killed. There is a fear among Black parents that must be acknowledged. It is strongly recommended that clinicians practicing F4C with Black families read about intergenerational transmission of racial trauma and approach conversations about discipline with the goal of understanding rather than criticism and judgment. This recommendation does not mean clinicians should not clearly define for clients what behaviors are considered abusive and illegal in the United States or the country they are living in now, but understanding cultural differences and where these practices may have come from is important for maintaining rapport. Some suggested readings on this topic can be found in Appendix B. White clinicians should seek consultation from Black or other minority colleagues to ensure cultural sensitivity and humility when addressing abusive behaviors that are presented as cultural or are a result of intergenerational racial trauma and viewed as necessary by parents. If clients feel misunderstood or sense there is a racial or cultural divide with the therapist, this can impede the therapeutic process and will not yield change.

When done well and with preparation, restorative parenting sessions can be rewarding and beautiful for everyone involved. Fathers and their coparents can see changes in the relationships with their children and reductions in child symptoms. Therapists have the honor of facilitating and bearing witness to very difficult conversations that can promote healing. Chapter 10 presents details on ending the treatment and provides useful referral information for your clients.

CHAPTER 10

Ending Treatment and Other Considerations

Ending treatment with fathers is just as important as beginning it. Setting up realistic expectations and planning for high-risk situations (e.g., substance relapse) that are bound to arise in the future are crucial. When fathers and their families end F4C, sometimes additional treatment is needed. This chapter first provides an overview of how to end F4C treatment, including recommending other services and treatments from which families may benefit following F4C (e.g., child–parent psychotherapy [CPP], couple therapy, interpersonal therapy, relapse prevention, and family therapy). Next, F4C is not a match for every father or family. Possible alternative interventions available in the field and when these might be preferable are reviewed. Last, a discussion of issues that may arise for F4C providers and the need for fathers to return to F4C-informed therapy is addressed.

ENDING F4C

As indicated in earlier chapters, there is no set number of sessions for F4C; however, in some court-ordered or other service setting contexts, it may be necessary to deliver the treatment within a given number of sessions (e.g., a course of 18 sessions is considered complete for a court-ordered diversion). In this context, it can feel more difficult to end treatment, especially if you are concerned that treatment goals have not been met. Often clients who have not committed well to the goals of F4C but are attending due to external pressures from courts, defense attorneys, or CPS try to attend the program and gloss through the topics without taking accountability or engaging fully in the therapeutic work. It is recommended that these clients not advance through the treatment; therefore, they do not end up getting to the last sessions of F4C, and the clinician is faced with trying to explain why they have not successfully completed the program even though they attended all of the sessions.

CASE EXAMPLE OF UNSUCCESSFUL TREATMENT: JONAH

Jonah, a 35-year-old White father of two sons, was referred by his local CPS to complete F4C as part of his case plan following an incident of IPV that occurred in front of his children and resulted in the police being called by a neighbor and Jonah's arrest. Jonah was reluctant to participate from the beginning and did not acknowledge use of IPV. He indicated that it was all a misunderstanding that was blown out of proportion. At the outset of treatment, this response from him was not unexpected given that he was facing criminal charges and had hired a high-powered defense lawyer to defend him in his criminal case. He was recently divorced from his wife, who wanted no part of the F4C treatment. She did agree to have his children participate, as she hoped they could have a healthy relationship with their father. Jonah attended all scheduled sessions on time and participated in session content; however, his engagement was on a surface, psychoeducational level. He could talk about triggers and coping skills in abstraction but did not acknowledge any of his own difficulties. He did not complete homework assignments, stating things like "I didn't have anything come up to write down." He would listen to session topics and respond with things like "I can see how this would be helpful for people who have anger problems" or "That is a useful skill for some people." His therapist continued to meet with him individually and to deliver coparenting topics. During this phase, he engaged in role-play practice in session, showing his ability to do active listening and make "I" statements.

When it got to the father–child-focused sessions, Jonah was willing to have conjoint sessions with his two sons, ages 6 and 8. However, it was very difficult for him to acknowledge any wrongdoing or develop a making amends statement. He felt it best to "leave the past in the past." The clinician was not convinced the conjoint sessions would go well for the children or meet the goals of F4C. Therefore, she provided parenting skills with Jonah individually. She was then faced with ending treatment. She was unsatisfied with his engagement in the therapeutic work. He had not taken any active accountability, did not engage with the material between sessions by completing homework, and had not met with his sons for restorative parenting sessions, yet he was at the end of the planned F4C program, and she felt uncomfortable providing him with a letter stating he had completed F4C for the court. Luckily, she had been straightforward with Jonah throughout their work together, indicating that she did not feel he was fully participating or making any changes to his behaviors due to treatment. During their last session together, she was faced with a difficult conversation with him.

CLINICIAN: We have now done the topics of F4C that are possible for you. As we've discussed, we did not meet together with your sons, which is the last phase of F4C. I know you have stated that the incident with your ex-wife was a misunderstanding that was blown out of proportion. I'm not here to dispute that, but it has been very challenging for you to take any accountability for ways you might improve your relationships or ways you may have contributed to difficulties in your marriage to your coparent. Although you have attended all the required sessions of F4C, I do not feel you have met the treatment goals.

JONAH: What do you mean? You were the one who said we should not meet with my sons. I'll meet with them. What does it mean if I do not meet treatment goals?

CLINICIAN: I did not think it was appropriate to meet with your sons, because you did not feel comfortable doing a making amends statement with them. Remember we spent two sessions together talking about that and you did not feel it was necessary?

JONAH: No, I didn't. So, because I didn't do that, I failed the program?

CLINICIAN: No, it's not only that. Remember that this program was to address conflict, aggression, and IPV that happened in your family. One of the goals was to identify your triggers and develop coping skills. This was only partially achieved, because it was very difficult for you to acknowledge your emotions or think about how to apply skills we were practicing. My plan is to let your case worker know that you attended all required session appointments, but that there were some aspects of the program we did not do and I think you would benefit from some additional therapy to address relationship difficulties after the courts have ruled on your charges. I think it is difficult to reflect and think about ways you might do things differently when you are concerned about legal or criminal repercussions to taking any accountability. I can understand the bind you may be in.

JONAH: So, what will that do for my case?

CLINICIAN: I'm not sure exactly, but since you have attended all the required sessions, it should not impact your criminal case. Your attendance at a program for domestic violence likely will help you in court. I would just like you to reflect on ways you might do things differently in your relationships and how changes you can make will benefit your sons. I do not see this as a failure but a beginning. You can choose to continue or not.

JONAH: Well, my case worker probably will make that decision, not me.

CLINICIAN: That may be true, but you get to decide how much you invest in the sessions after your criminal case ends.

In this case, the clinician is indicating compliance but not success of the therapy. This clinician felt that continuing sessions of F4C now would not be productive because the father was not able to be authentic in the sessions. He did not trust what would happen with the information, so he did not participate fully. Although the conversation the clinician had with him at the end of treatment was difficult, it may allow him to consider how he might benefit later in future therapy.

POSTTREATMENT ASSESSMENTS

It is recommended that families participate in a posttreatment assessment prior to the last session (Topic 18) of F4C. This can serve to provide excellent feedback to families on their progress through the program and identify continued treatment needs. It can also provide outcome data on the program for agencies looking for grant support to provide the treatment. It is recommended the following areas be assessed posttreatment:

- FV/dangerousness since intervention began
- Substance use during treatment (data can be reviewed from weekly urinalysis screenings if they were implemented as discussed in Chapter 5)
- Reflective functioning (RF)/emotion regulation
- Coparenting (conflict and support)
- Parenting/father–child relationship

The same measures used at the start of treatment (see Chapter 5) can be implemented at treatment end, along with a final father–child or family play assessment to share progress the therapist has seen in family interactions. Both parents can participate in assessment, and then the clinician can discuss changes in scores from the start to the end of treatment in their final session. Parallel individual final sessions can be held with each parent to review progress in treatment and provide further referrals and recommendations and to discuss exit safety plans as needed. Typically, postassessments take one or two sessions and include feedback and discussion of progress. The goals of this final part of treatment are as follows:

1. Review treatment goals and progress.
2. Plan with client for high-risk situations that might lead to substance use or FV.

3. Review skills.
4. Provide referrals for additional treatment/services as needed.

CASE EXAMPLE OF SUCCESSFUL ENDING OF F4C: HENRY

If we recall the case of Henry from Chapter 9, he had finished two making amends sessions. One with his 12-year-old son and another with his 5-year-old daughter. He was in recovery for alcohol dependence and had been violent toward their mother in front of them. He had engaged very well in F4C and had significantly improved his RF and emotion regulation. Father–child sessions focused on accountability and beginning to rebuild trust and communication at each child's developmental level. Postassessments indicated that Henry was maintaining sobriety, and his relationships with his coparent and children were much improved. His daughter's anxiety had reduced significantly, and she was now able to sleep in her own bed. Henry and his coparent decided to seek individual therapy for their 12-year-old son given his anger problems and concerns that he was beginning to use substances. Henry was participating in parent guidance and family sessions as requested by his son's therapist. His son had been resistant to attending therapy previously, but when he learned his father was attending therapy and that addiction ran in his family, he was able to understand why learning to manage his angry feelings and process what he'd witnessed with his father would be helpful. Without restorative sessions with his father during F4C he may have been unwilling to engage in therapy in this way.

RECOMMENDED REFERRALS AND TREATMENTS THAT MAY FOLLOW F4C

Following F4C, some fathers may need additional services or referrals. During the course of the therapy, it may have become clear that the father would benefit from ongoing individual therapy or psychiatric care. Referrals to other treatment can happen at any time during F4C; however, this decision must be made carefully. How much treatment can a father engage in at one time, both psychologically and logistically? Certainly, if a need for psychiatric medication comes up, these kinds of referrals should not be delayed. Since F4C is an individual therapy, other individual-focused treatments could happen simultaneously but often should wait until F4C is concluding. If a client has significant depression, anxiety, or PTSD that needs more immediate treatment that cannot be managed within F4C, then referrals may be made sooner. These referrals would be made in collaboration with the father's wishes. Clinicians can ask fathers to sign a release so they can speak openly with the other agency, program, or therapist about the reasons for referral and to coordinate care.

Referrals made at the end of F4C can serve to continue to explore issues addressed in F4C, like ongoing mental health symptoms such as depression, PTSD, or anxiety, or for general supportive therapy. Group therapy may also be appropriate. Fathers may benefit from a psychotherapy or supportive group with other fathers that is focused on parenting or some other specific topic. Again, asking a father's permission to contact a program, sharing your suggestions for how the program may benefit them, and reviewing areas of continued growth based on your work with them could enhance this next phase of work.

In terms of father–child and couple or family therapy, it is typically best for these therapies to begin at the end of F4C. This will allow the father to work on his own triggers and difficulties and develop basic communication and relational skills to continue in these forms of therapy. For example, following the few sessions of father-child work that happen in the last phase of F4C, some clients may be well prepared to continue in a dyadic parenting intervention such as child–parent psychotherapy (CPP; Lieberman, Ippen, & Van Horn, 2015) or parent–child interaction therapy (PCIT; Zisser & Eyberg, 2010) if further work on the parent–child relationship or interactions is needed. CPP is a dyadic treatment for very young children from infancy through age 5. CPP was developed specifically for children who had witnessed IPV between their caregivers and has since been applied to other trauma exposure types. CPP is an attachment-focused intervention that examines how trauma and the caregivers' relational history affect the caregiver–child relationship and the child's developmental trajectory. A central goal is to support and strengthen the caregiver–child relationship as the means to help the child with emotional recovery. Targets of the intervention include caregivers' and children's maladaptive representations of themselves and each other, and interactions and behaviors that interfere with the child's mental health. Over the course of treatment, the clinician helps the caregiver and child to create a joint narrative about the traumatic experiences and identify and address traumatic triggers that generate dysregulated behaviors (e.g., aggression and tantrums) and emotions.

PCIT, an intervention developed to treat children between ages 2 and 7 with disruptive behavior problems (*www.pcit.org*), is an evidence-based treatment for young children that places emphasis on improving the quality of the parent–child relationship and changing parent–child interaction patterns through a focus on child-directed play and parent-directed interactions. This intervention is usually provided when children have significant behavioral problems such as aggression. The child-focused play strategies outlined in Phase 4 of F4C are a large focus of

PCIT. If a father–child dyad needs additional support in this area, PCIT is an appropriate referral.

Another intervention for parents who cause harm and their children is Alternatives for Families–Cognitive-Behavioral Therapy (AF-CBT; Kolko, 1996). The intervention is designed to reduce or prevent the impact of exposure to child or family anger, aggression, and/or child physical abuse. AF-CBT (originally named abuse-focused CBT) teaches parents and children (ages 5 to 17) intrapersonal and interpersonal skills to enhance self-control, promote positive family relations, and reduce violent behavior. These skills include anger and anxiety management, how to challenge misattributions to support flexible thinking, child social skills, effective and safe discipline strategies, and healthy family communication and problem-solving skills to help maintain a safe and secure home environment.

Couple therapy may be recommended if the parents are interested in continuing to work on their relationship and the coparenting sessions were safe and successful. This referral could come at the end of the coparenting phase if parents are eager for this kind of therapy or be provided as F4C is ending. It is essential that any recommendation and referral for couple therapy is made to a therapist with experience working with high-conflict couples and those who have experienced abuse within relationships. Therapists must research providers in their area to ensure they can provide the most fitting referrals. F4C therapists in practices offering couple therapy could decide to continue with the couple themselves given their experience and understanding of the couple dynamics; this can provide a nice continuity in some cases.

Relapse prevention is another important consideration upon discharge. Fathers who have been able to greatly reduce their use of substances or remain abstinent would benefit from either individual or group-based relapse prevention programs. These programs take a variety of forms but typically encourage self-care practices such as relaxation and mindfulness, and support through connections with others in recovery. Providing connections and ensuring engagement prior to the conclusion of F4C is an important part of discharge planning for those with significant substance misuse problems.

Aside from therapy services, helping fathers with stressors in their lives and connecting them with resources both during F4C and at discharge enhances the likelihood of successful outcomes. As mentioned in Chapter 5, fathers who are unemployed or underemployed, are financially strained, lack education or vocational skills, have legal issues, and so forth, will continue to experience stress that can contribute to substance misuse and FV. To what helpful resources can you connect the father? Are there educational or vocational services in your area?

Are there fatherhood resources such as fatherhood support groups or fatherhood-focused agencies? Legal aid or low-fee legal services? When fathers feel supported and are not seen as criminals, they are more likely to engage in services and help.

MODIFICATIONS AND ALTERNATIVES TO F4C

As discussed in Chapter 5, F4C may not be appropriate for all fathers who are referred and assessed for the program. It is important for clinicians to know what other services are available in their area for fathers with FV behaviors (see Chapter 1). Many communities have group batterer interventions such as the Duluth model or some other CBT-focused program. It is necessary to know whether these groups are accessible to the community or can only be accessed through the court system. Many court-mandated groups can only take referrals directly from the court. Others will take both court-mandated and voluntary participants. Providers who offer F4C can take referrals from any venue as long as their agency allows for non-court-ordered services.

Consider carefully if you are going to refer a client to a group program instead of F4C; what is the reason you are doing it? Why do you feel this group program will be better suited to the father's needs? It is often felt that fathers who are more narcissistic or antisocial should be referred to group programs with other men; this can be true but is not universal. The composition of the group is important in this instance. If the group is filled with several men with high levels of narcissism and antisocial personality traits, there can be a group contagion that makes it hard for facilitators to hold participants accountable for their use of violence. Participants may feed off each other's negativity and blaming of women, the state, and the system without any acknowledgment of the problems with their own actions.

That said, as stated in Chapter 5, there are also some men who do better working with other men encouraging them to be responsible for their own actions. If you are a female therapist doing F4C, there may be occasions when a male therapist who can provide F4C or a men's group is a better match for a particular client. This often happens when a father has very gendered views or exhibits sexism, and it is hard for him to engage in the therapeutic work examining his feelings and behaviors with a woman. A male therapist can be assigned in this instance. There are also ways of modifying F4C to use two therapists. Generally, it is better for one therapist to work with a family, because it allows them to have more information and to understand the experience of the children in the family, who may be caught between two parents who are not communicating well. Still, there are times when each parent would benefit from having their own therapist. In this instance, therapists must work collaboratively, and if joint coparenting sessions take place, both therapists need to be present in those sessions.

CASE EXAMPLE 1. NEEDING TWO THERAPISTS: KHALID AND AMNA

Khalid and Amna were referred to F4C after their 12-year-old daughter, Iman, reported to her teacher that her father had hit her repeatedly because he was upset about her use of social media. During the course of the CPS investigation, the younger two children in the family reported that their father sometimes yelled a lot and hit their mother. Both parents denied these reports. Khalid admitted to disciplining Iman but said it was not abuse, and that it was within his right as a father to ensure that his daughter followed his rules. Amna agreed that Khalid had only been disciplining Iman for not obeying his rules about social media. Khalid and Amna were active in their local mosque. They had been living in the United States for 13 years. They had immigrated from Pakistan just after their marriage and before the birth of Iman. During the assessment process with his female therapist, Khalid minimized any issues in the family, stating that the therapist and CPS social worker were getting too involved with his family and that he knew how to handle the situation. He said he would attend F4C to get CPS off his back but felt it was ridiculous. Amna reported that her husband was a good provider, and he took her wherever she needed to go. She said he was sometimes stressed out by trying to care for her and the children. Amna did not have a driver's license or any income of her own. She had no access to the family's bank account. When the parallel sessions of F4C were described, Amna indicated she would participate if Khalid wanted her to, but she thought he probably would not. Khalid confirmed that he did not think his wife needed to participate in sessions.

In this example, there are client considerations that are both cultural and psychological. Khalid has very gendered views of women and a lack of interest in the therapy that will make progress with a female therapist difficult. A male therapist could work with Khalid if it were determined that working with both parents puts the mother at risk for further violence. In that case, only one male therapist would be needed to work individually with Khalid. Given the Muslim faith of the family and Khalid's gendered views, a male therapist working individually with the mother would not be comfortable for the family and not an appropriate approach. However, the best solution here would be to have a male and female therapist share this case: the male therapist working with Khalid and the female therapist working with Amna. This would allow mother space to share in individual sessions and for safety planning to occur, if needed.

CASE EXAMPLE 2. NEEDING 2 THERAPISTS: JAMAL AND SERINA

Jamal and Serina are referred by CPS for F4C following a domestic dispute that involved both partners becoming aggressive during an argument about Jamal's cheating behaviors. Jamal denied cheating, but Serina felt she had evidence from his phone. The father met with the therapist, Josephine, to begin assessments and seemed appropriate for F4C. He minimized his own behavior and focused on Serina's jealousy, but this is not uncommon during initial assessments.

When Serina met the therapist for the first time, she sat down and said, "You already met with Jamal?"

THERAPIST: Yes, in this program we meet with both coparents, as I mentioned to you on the phone when we spoke about you coming in today.

SERINA: I am not comfortable with you meeting with Jamal. You are exactly his type, and he will not be able to have you as his therapist! What did he tell you? I'm sure he made me look bad to impress you! You are young, and you look a lot like his ex!

THERAPIST: I can see that my meeting with Jamal has made you uncomfortable. That was not my intention. My role is to work with each of you individually and, I hope, together later in the therapy. We focus on coparenting communication as part of this program.

SERINA: Yeah, that's not going to work. You are too pretty and just his type. I won't be able to trust that there is nothing going on with the two of you.

THERAPIST: I can assure you that I am a professional with a job to do. I only want to help your family. Do you have questions about the work we'd be doing that might help?

SERINA: I'm gonna text him now. I just know he's probably so happy to have you as our assigned therapist.

THERAPIST: Serina, do you think we can spend some time getting to know each other? That might make you more comfortable?

[*Serina is caught up in texting with Jamal.*]

SERINA: He's denying it, of course, but I know better. I can't trust you.

THERAPIST: OK, it seems like my working with Jamal is causing you some distress and I do not want that. What if you and I work together and we assign Jamal to work with my colleague Darren? That way you and Jamal each have your own therapist?

SERINA: That would make me feel better, but I'm still concerned about you having contact with Jamal.

THERAPIST: Let's see if we have a session together—you and I—and

> see how you feel. If, after we talk more, you think it just cannot work, then we can try to find another therapist to work with you and your family.

In this case, Serina is so concerned about Jamal's contact with the clinician, Josephine, it is likely to result in additional domestic disputes. This sort of situation is never helpful. Josephine suggests two therapists in this case to ensure that the mother is not jealous of the female therapist, which is a clear concern. Josephine hopes to build a trusting relationship with the mother, but if she cannot, she understands that a new therapist may be needed, as the mother seems triggered by the way Josephine looks. If assigning new therapists does not help, it may be that Serina is unable to participate in this type of therapy program with Jamal. It is likely that assigning Jamal to a male therapist to continue F4C without Serina could be a solution in this case.

IF VIOLENCE OCCURS DURING F4C

FV episodes can happen during the time F4C is provided to a family. In Chapter 8, an example of how to deescalate a session and ensure safety if violence occurs in session is discussed. This is a rare occurrence. What is more likely is for clinicians to learn about an FV incident that occurred between sessions. Sometimes, it is an incident that resulted in police involvement. In this case, law enforcement would be notified and contact with CPS would be based on police involvement, so clinicians would not need to make any formal reports. They would, however, need to determine whether there is a change in protective orders, assess the safety of all members of the family, and determine whether F4C can continue. Sometimes a father who has caused harm will be arrested and incarcerated during F4C. In this case, the clinician would need to learn about the likely length of the incarceration. Sometimes jail stays are very brief, while individuals make bond and they are then quickly back in the community or back home. If they are facing multiple felony charges that will keep them incarcerated for at least 2 months, or if the nature of the violence now meets F4C exclusion criteria (he threatened to kill his coparent with a weapon or caused her serious injury resulting in hospitalization), then he would need to be discontinued in the F4C program. Clinicians can continue to work with coparents to ensure that they and their children are connected with the right safety and therapeutic supports. If, however, it was a more minor incident of situational couple violence or does not meet criteria for withdrawal from the program, then continuing to work with the father, and if safe, his coparent is the right approach. Relapse to use of violence is not uncommon as people attempt to change their behaviors. Using functional analysis of the incident, examining triggers, and exploring what the father could have done differently to prevent the incident would be the first steps in an individual session with the father once an incident is disclosed during treatment (see Chapter 7).

If an FV incident is disclosed in session that was not reported to the police or CPS and children were present, then a report will need to be made to the appropriate CPS office. It is most helpful to do this in collaboration with the family to try to preserve the therapeutic relationship. Explaining why the report needs to be made and offering to include fathers or coparents in the call can be helpful to preserving the relationship: "As we discussed early in treatment, I am a mandated reporter. When I learn of an incident of FV with children in the home, I must report it to CPS. Would you like to report it together or to listen in to my call with them? I will be sure to let them know you are in an FV program and we are working together to develop a safety plan."

Collaboration with CPS following a report can be helpful. This can only happen if the father and/or coparent sign releases of information for you to speak with CPS after the report is made.

FATHERS NEEDING ADDICTION TREATMENT

Fathers with a substance dependence that require inpatient detox will need to complete detox before engaging in F4C. As noted earlier, F4C has been implemented in residential treatment settings and has been helpful to fathers who have completed an initial course of their residential substance use treatment (Stover et al., 2017; Stover, McMahon, et al., 2019; and as discussed in Chapter 3, this volume). Implementation of F4C within residential or outpatient substance use settings can be a terrific addition to existing services. Fathers are often eager to have an opportunity to focus on their roles as fathers and to think about their family dynamics as part of their substance use treatment. It is best if F4C is provided after fathers have detoxed from substances and engaged in the initial milieu and group therapy components of a residential treatment. Once fathers have settled into the community and committed to treatment goals, F4C can be offered. Delivery in a format of one to two sessions per week is ideal, but this could be increased if the residential stay is briefer. A format of 12 residential and four outpatient booster sessions has been shown to reduce relapse (Stover, McMahon, et al., 2019).

As mentioned in Chapter 5, fathers who have a primary mental health diagnosis that is untreated may be better served in another form of individual therapy. For example, if a father has PTSD and is ready to address his symptoms related to his traumas, then a referral for evidence-based PTSD treatment could have significant impact on his functioning and use of FV.

Making connections and a warm handoff to the new provider (introducing the family and ensuring they make their first appointment with the new provider) will increase the likelihood of engagement in the referred services.

OTHER SYSTEMS CHALLENGES

F4C is a different approach to working with individuals who have caused harm that may be misunderstood by the systems with which clients are interfacing (e.g., justice system, CPS). Some states mandate that individuals arrested for domestic violence participate in a Duluth model type of group domestic violence offender program. This may prevent clients from enrolling in F4C even if they would prefer it and benefit from it, because they are required to do another program to complete court-mandated requirements. Therapists who are early adopters of F4C in their geographic areas may need to provide information about the treatment approach and the evidence for decreased FV and improved outcomes to stakeholders in order to engage referral sources and systems that interact with the client population. A presentation on the therapy approach and its benefits for judges, court support services, and CPS agencies can provide an avenue for referrals and allow clients to receive this mode of intervention to satisfy court requirements. These systems are often concerned that F4C will not hold offenders accountable for their actions and therapists will be manipulated. Discussing the ways F4C encourages clients to take accountability for their actions and make change may be important to this discussion. Providers of F4C are often tasked with trying to change the way other agencies view those who have caused harm. Systems often approach these clients with the goal of punishment rather than recovery or rehabilitation.

CASE EXAMPLE: RAMON

Ramon was a 33-year-old Latino father of two children, ages 5 and 3. He had a history of IPV with his partner Mariella. He was incarcerated for IPV when his older son was an infant. When he was released, he completed F4C at the request of CPS. He engaged well in the therapy with Mariella and his sons. His therapist, Jim, was disappointed when he received a phone call from Ramon about a year after his completion of F4C. Ramon had been arrested for another IPV incident, but this time with a new girlfriend. Ramon and Mariella had decided to end their relationship a few months after F4C concluded, but he had continued to coparent his sons. Jim felt this was positive, as previously when Ramon and Mariella broke up, his parenting role would stop. Ramon had maintained his commitment to positive parenting.

Ramon's new partner, Arianna, had six children from another relationship. Ramon was not living with her but frequently stayed over. Ramon often provided money to help support Arianna and her children. Their argument ensued when he asked her to cook him some dinner after a long day at work and she refused. He was living with his cousin, sleeping on a mattress on the floor and paying his cousin rent. He felt he had no real place to be. He was working full time as an electrician. He was very proud of his work ethic. He worked lengthy hours because he felt that making money was the best thing he could contribute to his family. Ramon contacted Jim because he knew he needed to reengage in therapy after the new incident with his girlfriend. He had a long history of anxiety and knew he needed to be reassessed for psychiatric medication. Jim began meeting with Ramon for individual therapy and connected him with the agency psychiatrist. Simultaneously, Ramon enrolled in a 26-week DV offender group program at the suggestion of the family relations counselor at the courthouse.

When he finished the DV offender program, Ramon pled guilty to the domestic violence charge and was given probation. At this point, he had been back in an F4C-informed therapy for 3 months and had resumed psychiatric care for his anxiety. At his first meeting with his new probation officer (PO), Ramon was told that he would need to do an additional DV offender program that was 52 weeks in length. Ramon reported to the PO that he had a certificate from the program he had just completed, was engaged in individual therapy focused on IPV, and was being seen by a psychiatrist. The PO stated that Ramon would need to do this additional DV program regardless. Ramon became angry and began swearing at the PO and stated, "Go ahead and lock me up. I ain't doin' that program."

In session with Jim, Ramon detailed his meeting with the PO. He was highly agitated and dysregulated.

RAMON: He doesn't understand everything I have to do! I work 10- to 12-hour days to make money to support my kids, and my mom is sick. I already did 26 classes and now he's tellin' me I have to do 52? I do not need that. All them classes are the same! I've already done those type of programs twice! I have sessions with you and with my doctor for medicine! That's what I need. I'll go back to jail before I do that class!

JIM: I can understand why you are frustrated and I'm concerned that if you go to jail you will not be able to provide for your family either.

RAMON: Yes, but at least I won't be exhausted!

JIM (*gently*): Oh, I see. You're saying jail would feel like a break from everything?

RAMON: Yes, I'm just so stressed all the time. I'm worried I'm going to get rearrested all the time. I work so much to try to be a good provider. I did all these things to try to meet expectations by doing the other 26-week group and coming back to therapy with you. If no one cares, then I don't either. I'll go sit in jail. At least I get a bed and three meals a day.

JIM: You feel your efforts are not being seen or acknowledged. It sounds like you are constantly stressed about returning to jail, so you might as well give up?

RAMON: Yeah . . .

JIM: Would it help if I talked to your PO, explained the work we are doing, and see if I might help him understand that you are working very hard to change your behaviors related to IPV?

RAMON: I don't' know if he'll listen, but yeah, I'd really appreciate it if you talked to him. He just wasn't listening to me at all and I do not trust him.

In this case, Ramon felt misunderstood and thought the system was against him. He felt they wanted him in jail. He felt exhausted from the requirements being placed on him despite his work to engage in services he felt would help him change. In this case, the therapist needed to have contact with the PO to explain the work they were doing. The PO did not know what F4C was and, understandably, felt Ramon needed ongoing intervention for domestic violence. Unfortunately, the PO's approach to Ramon was counterproductive. The stress he was putting on Ramon was unhelpful and likely to lead Ramon to behave in ways that would result in his rearrest rather than support his continued recovery and growth.

This case also highlights another important consideration for therapists implementing F4C. Changing FV behaviors can take a long time. Clients may need to return to therapy for a booster after some time has passed. New experiences or stages of life bring new stressors that may result in the father slipping back into old patterns. Providing them with a good experience in therapy through F4C, where they feel understood and supported, allows them to return to the treatment again if they feel they are in need. It is not uncommon for fathers to call their F4C therapist months or years after discharge from the program to say they need further help; this is a success. Change takes time. Recovery from years of trauma and learning not to use violence to solve problems can be a slow process. FV behaviors are wrong, but it's the behavior that needs to change. The father is a person who needs help to make that change. Therapists using the techniques in this book to build relationships with fathers can help them make those changes.

Epilogue

Developing an F4C practice can be simultaneously challenging and rewarding. Clinicians may face a variety of obstacles that are unique to offering individual treatment services to fathers who have caused harm. The clients served by this program are complex and are often entangled in CPS and legal systems that may view them differently or feel they deserve to be treated in a way that is counter to our therapeutic endeavors. Clinicians taking on this work must be prepared for some to view their work as negative or even harmful. There may be people who will say you are putting survivors and their children at risk or colluding with the offender. It is possible that some fathers who have caused harm seek out your services only to "look good in court" or to "trick the system." This does not mean that no one should be able to access this kind of help. It is always possible for individuals to lie to their therapist. This is true in any treatment. In my career, I've had all manner of clients lie to me about things during sessions. My job as a therapist is to do the best assessment I can of what is happening and provide treatment that I think will help the individual change their behaviors and recover from using violence, while also doing everything I can to ensure the safety of coparents and children. This is why I feel that working collaboratively with all family members is important and helpful. Are there times when a particular father is not a good fit for this program? Of course. This is true for any treatment approach.

Because there can be biases from others about this type of work, developing a stream of referrals and refining your practice with the population can take time. Be patient. Find your allies in the community and seek reflective supervision/consultation. I can guarantee that there are like-minded thinkers out there who will be interested in a new way of working. Once your community comes to see the value of the treatment you provide, you will see a shift in how the treatment is viewed and how important you are in the community you serve. The person-centered approach and focus on helping one family at time in the way they need is an important avenue to ending violence in families. Punishment and shaming will not help fathers develop the skills they need to break the intergenerational patterns of violence. We must approach this problem with an eye toward recovery and giving individuals what they did not receive (someone to see them as the person and parent they can be and not judging them for their past mistakes). We can simultaneously hold someone accountable for their poor behaviors and support them to be better.

It has been asked, "Why was this program designed for fathers, and could it be provided to mothers as well?" We already have offered the program to many families with mutual or bidirectional violence, with mothers participating in parallel with fathers to stop their use of FV. We have also offered F4C with some modifications to mothers and to lesbian and gay male coparents who have used violence. The combined trauma and parenting focus seem effective regardless of gender. I started the development of this intervention with a focus on fathers because of the systemic approach to men who use family violence as criminals and "monsters." Given how fathers' importance is often minimized, especially if they have caused harm, I felt a strong need to put the word *fathers* in the title of the intervention and to keep that focus as I wrote this book. That said, many of the same principles can be used with mothers who are using violence, and I plan to continue to develop the work for them, too, assessing what modifications are needed and whether it is as effective with mothers as it has been with fathers through research.

I hope you have found valuable tools within this book to help you work in a new way with fathers who have caused harm. I hope we build a community of like-minded practitioners who will change the way we approach intervention for fathers who have caused harm. I believe past colleagues who supported a coordinated community response to domestic violence had the right idea. I think we just need to broaden what *community* means to include individualized intervention approaches for those who cause harm, in addition to the array of services available for those who have experienced violence, and systems that are in place to protect from future harm. We are all working toward the same goal: cessation of family violence. Listening to one another and collaborating is the best way forward.

APPENDIX A

F4C Forms, Worksheets, and Handouts

FORM 5.1 Incoming Referral Form

Office Phone Number: ______________________________ **Fax:** __________________

Referral Date: ____

<table>
<tr><th colspan="4">INFORMATION ON PARTICIPANT</th></tr>
<tr><td colspan="2">Father Name:</td><td colspan="2">Date of Birth:</td></tr>
<tr><td colspan="4">Current Address:</td></tr>
<tr><td colspan="2">City:</td><td>State:</td><td>ZIP code:</td></tr>
<tr><td>Home:</td><td>Mobile:</td><td colspan="2">Work:</td></tr>
<tr><td colspan="2">Email:</td><td colspan="2">Number of Children Under the Age of 12:</td></tr>
<tr><td colspan="2">Insurance Type:</td><td colspan="2">Insurance ID:</td></tr>
<tr><td colspan="2">Ethnicity:</td><td colspan="2">Primary Language:</td></tr>
<tr><th colspan="4">REFERRAL SOURCE INFORMATION</th></tr>
<tr><td colspan="2">Referring Office:</td><td colspan="2">Name:</td></tr>
<tr><td colspan="2">Number:</td><td colspan="2">Email:</td></tr>
<tr><td colspan="2">Current Criminal Charges:</td><td colspan="2">Current Orders of Protection and Type:</td></tr>
<tr><td colspan="4">Reason for the Referral:</td></tr>
<tr><th colspan="4">CHILDREN INFORMATION</th></tr>
<tr><td>Name:</td><td>Gender:</td><td>Date of Birth:</td><td>Child Living with Referred Parent?</td></tr>
<tr><td>1</td><td></td><td></td><td></td></tr>
<tr><td>2</td><td></td><td></td><td></td></tr>
<tr><td>3</td><td></td><td></td><td></td></tr>
<tr><td>4</td><td></td><td></td><td></td></tr>
<tr><td>5</td><td></td><td></td><td></td></tr>
<tr><td>6</td><td></td><td></td><td></td></tr>
<tr><td colspan="2">Coparent Name:</td><td colspan="2">Telephone:</td></tr>
<tr><td colspan="4">Is coparent interested in participating in treatment? ☐ Yes ☐ No ☐ Unsure</td></tr>
<tr><td colspan="4">Is father referred for or involved in other treatment? ☐ Yes ☐ No
If Yes, what for and where?</td></tr>
</table>

Please note: If referred by DCF/Courts, please include a copy of the Police/DCF report, if possible.

FORM 5.2 Request for Coparent Contact Form

The father listed below has initiated participation in Fathers for Change. We are interested in contacting his coparent to explain the program to them and invite them to participate if they have interest.

Father's Name: ______________________ **Date of Birth:** ______________

Fathers for Change Clinician: ______________________________

Clinician Phone Number: ______________________________

Clinician Email: ______________________________

Please contact the coparent to determine if they would like to have contact with our program and then complete the information below.

Victim's Advocate Name: ______________________________

Advocate Phone Number: ______________________________

Advocate Email: ______________________________

Contact with coparent was made to ask about contact? ☐ Yes ☐ No

Is coparent willing to be contacted to learn about participation in assessment and treatment? ☐ Yes ☐ No

Coparent's Name: ______________________________

Coparent's Phone Number: ______________________________

Additional information for the clinical team about contact with the coparent (e.g., safety concerns, best times to reach them):

Please email this form to clinician listed above. Thank you.

FORM 6.1 Assessment and Treatment Agreement

Please read the guidelines below carefully, list several goals you have for yourself, and sign the bottom of the form.

1. I understand that I will be asked to complete assessment tools and questionnaires.
2. I agree that I will be asked to submit to random urine and Breathalyzer screens during my assessment and treatment.
3. I understand that this treatment will be 4 to 6 months in duration, and I agree to participate for this length of time.
4. I agree to attend the sessions and to be ***prompt!***
5. I understand that this treatment is intended for people who want to remain abstinent from alcohol or drugs, to manage their anger, to be violence-free, and focus on their roles as parents and coparents.
6. I understand that I must participate and practice the exercises to be most effective.
7. I understand that I *may* be asked to attend sessions with my coparent and/or children as part of the treatment.
8. I understand that my coparent and/or child may participate in sessions where I am not present.
9. I agree to work on the following goals during the program:

   a. ______________________________

   b. ______________________________

   c. ______________________________

______________________	______________________	______________
Client Name Printed	Client Signature	Date
______________________	______________________	______________
Clinician Name Printed	Clinician Signature	Date

HANDOUT 6.1 Impact of Exposure to Parental Violence and Substance Misuse on Children

Parents' use of aggression or violence (both physical and verbal) and substance misuse affect children beginning in pregnancy and infancy. The more exposure over a longer period, the more likely children will have difficulties. Some specific symptoms you may see in children at different ages are as follows:

Ages Birth to 5	Ages 6 to 11	Ages 12 to 18
• Sleep trouble • Disruptions in eating (too much or too little) • Withdrawal/lack of responsiveness • Intense separation anxiety (cannot be separated from caregivers) • Inconsolable crying/ unable to be soothed when distressed • Loss of acquired skills (toileting, talking, etc.) • Intense anxiety, worries, and/or new fears • Aggression/hyperactivity • Impulsive behavior • Failure to thrive	• Sleep trouble/nightmares • Aggression and difficulty with peer relationships • Difficulty with concentration • Withdrawal and/or emotional numbing • School avoidance and/or truancy • Hyperactivity–impulsivity • Change in grades/school performance • Poor self-esteem • Anxiety • Hypervigilance • Oppositional behaviors • Irritability	• Sleep trouble • Nightmares • Difficulty in peer relationships • Poor grades/school failure • Impulsive and/or reckless behavior • School truancy • Substance use • Running away • Involvement in violent or abusive dating relationships • Depression • Irritability/anger • Anxiety/hypervigilance • Withdrawal

WORKSHEET 6.1 How Healthy Is My Relationship?

Review the list below and check the behaviors or characteristics that describe your relationship. Total the number of checked items per column. Which one is higher?

Healthy Characteristics

Check off if you and your partner . . .

- ☐ Have fun together more often than not
- ☐ Each enjoy spending time separately, with your own friends, as well as with each other's friends
- ☐ Always feel safe with each other
- ☐ Trust each other
- ☐ Are faithful to each other
- ☐ Support each other's individual goals in life such as educational or career goals
- ☐ Respect each other's opinions
- ☐ Solve conflicts without putting each other down, cursing or making threats
- ☐ Both accept responsibility for your actions
- ☐ Both apologize when you're wrong
- ☐ Have equal decision-making power about what you do in your relationship
- ☐ Have equal decision-making power
- ☐ Are proud to be with each other
- ☐ Have some privacy; your texts, journal, personal phone calls, are respected as your own
- ☐ Have close friends and family who like your partner
- ☐ Never feel like you're being pressured for sex
- ☐ Communicate about sex if your relationship is sexual
- ☐ Allow each other "space" when you need it
- ☐ Always treat each other with respect

Total # Healthy Checked _____

Unhealthy Characteristics

Check off if you and your partner . . .

- ☐ Get extremely jealous or accuse the other of cheating
- ☐ Put the other down by name-calling, swearing, or making the other feel bad about themselves
- ☐ Yell at and treat the other like a child
- ☐ Don't take the other person or things that are important to them seriously
- ☐ Don't listen when the other talks
- ☐ Frequently criticize the other's friends or family
- ☐ Pressure the other for sex or make sex hurt or feel humiliating
- ☐ Has ever threatened to hurt the other or to commit suicide if they leave
- ☐ Cheat or threaten to cheat
- ☐ Tell the other how to dress
- ☐ Has ever grapped, pushed, hit, or used other violence
- ☐ Blame the other for their own behavior ("If you hadn't made me mad, I wouldn't have . . .")
- ☐ Embarrass or humiliate the other
- ☐ Smash, throw, or destroy things
- ☐ Try to keep the other person from having a job or furthering their education
- ☐ Make all the decisions about what the two of you do
- ☐ Try to make the other feel crazy or play mind games
- ☐ Go back on promises
- ☐ Act controlling or possessive
- ☐ Use alcohol or drugs as an excuse for hurtful behavior
- ☐ Ignore or withhold affection to punish the other
- ☐ Completely depend on the other to meet social emotional needs

Total # Unhealthy Checked _____

HANDOUT 6.2 Good Role-Modeling Tips for Dads

Fathers are models for their children. You are an example to your children about what fathers and men should be like. You teach many lessons about life, relationships, and responsibility.

Here are some important things to remember:

1. You never stop being a role model even if you are not around: Research shows that when dads are not in the picture, kids wonder why and often think they did something wrong or that they are not good enough for their dad.
2. Actions speak more loudly than words: If you say one thing but do another, your child will remember your action, NOT your words.
3. Most mistakes are not forever: Most of the time, if you acknowledge your mistake, take responsibility, and change your behavior, you can regain trust and respect.

WHAT ARE SOME ESSENTIALS OF A GOOD ROLE MODEL?

Treat others with respect, especially your coparent:

- If you can be positive, respectful, and work out conflicts and disagreements in good ways, you model how men should treat women and respect for adults in general. You are teaching your sons how to treat women and teaching your daughters how they can expect to be treated by men.
- Harsh criticism, showing contempt, stonewalling, and defensiveness can hurt children emotionally.
- Using force with the children's other parent can cause fear and lasting hurt to your child.
- If you use aggression and violence when you are angry, you are teaching your children that is how to solve problems.
- If you want to have your rules respected, you must follow them yourself. For example, if you hold back your temper when you're mad, it shows that you value self-control and teaches responsible behavior.
- If you are polite to people in general (e.g., in stores, while driving, and when someone is rude to you), you highlight the importance of respect.

(continued)

Contribute at home:

- Doing chores at home or outdoors and making other contributions, either alone or with the kids, teaches responsibility and shows you care about your household and family life.

Spend time together:

- How you spend your time shows your commitment. Spending time with your family and doing things with them illustrates that you care and want to be with them.

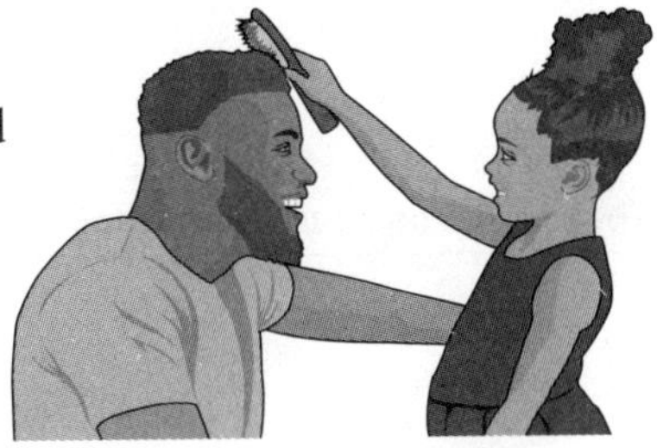

REMEMBER THAT YOU NEVER STOP BEING A ROLE MODEL.

FORM 6.2 Change Plan

I understand that verbal and physical aggression, yelling, screaming, and controlling behaviors are unhealthy for my family.

Why is it important to make changes now?

What will successful change look like?

What resources and strengths do I have that can help me reach these goals?

What barriers stand in my way?

What are specific ways I can ensure there is no physical aggression, yelling, screaming, and controlling behaviors in my family? How can I plan for high-risk situations?

Client Signature

Date

WORKSHEET 7.1 Functional Analysis of Behaviors

Fill in the boxes below to examine what led up to behaviors you'd like to change (e.g., yelling, lashing out, aggression).

What and Where	• Where was I? • What was happening? • Who was with me?
Thoughts	• What was I thinking?
Feelings Sensations	• What were my feelings? • What sensations did I have in my body?
Behaviors	• What did I do?
Consequences	• What happened right after? • How did other people react? • How did I feel? • Any other consequences?

HANDOUT 7.1 Shame versus Guilt: How Are They Different?

Shame

Shame is feeling bad about yourself as a person.

"I am a bad father."

"I am a terrible person."

"I am worthless."

Shame says:
I AM BAD

What do we do when we feel Shame?

- Get defensive.
- Deny responsibility.
- Blame others.
- Avoid the issue.

What can we do to move out of Shame?

- Recognize the feeling.
- Have empathy for yourself because we all make mistakes.
- Seek healthy connections with others.
- Talk to a therapist.

Guilt

Guilt is feeling bad about something we did.

"I should not have yelled at my daughter like that."

"I should not have acted that way."

Guilt says:
I DID SOMETHING WRONG

What do we do when we feel Guilt?

- Reflect on our behaviors.
- Take responsibility.
- Apologize or seek to make amends.

What can we do when we feel Guilty?

- Acknowledge what we did was wrong.
- Apologize and seek forgiveness.
- Be open to learning alternative ways to handle situations.
- Work to change our behaviors.

WORKSHEET 7.2 Emotion Triggers

Fill in the boxes below to examine situations where you got emotionally triggered (e.g., yelled, got angry, reacted in a way you did not like afterward). See example below.

Trigger situation (what, when, where, who)	What do you feel? (try to name more than one)	Unhelpful: angry, anxious, or substance-craving thought	Does this trigger remind you of anything from the past?	What might be the other person's experience of the situation?
Came home from work and the kitchen was a mess.	*Annoyed/angry*	*She just sits around all day on social media and doesn't do anything. She doesn't care about keeping our house nice.*	*My parents were always very worried about the way our house looked and what other people would think. What if someone showed up unexpected? What would they think of us if our house was a mess?*	*Maybe she was busy with the kids and couldn't get to the dishes.*

WORKSHEET 7.3 Emotion and Substance Misuse Thermometer

List types of anger or other emotion (e.g., anxiety) next to levels from 1 to 10 (with 10 being the highest level) on one side of the thermometer, along with substance use craving levels from 1 to 10 (with 10 being the highest level). Include physiological body sensations at each level on the thermometer.

Physiological Sensations **Descriptive Word** **Craving Thoughts?**

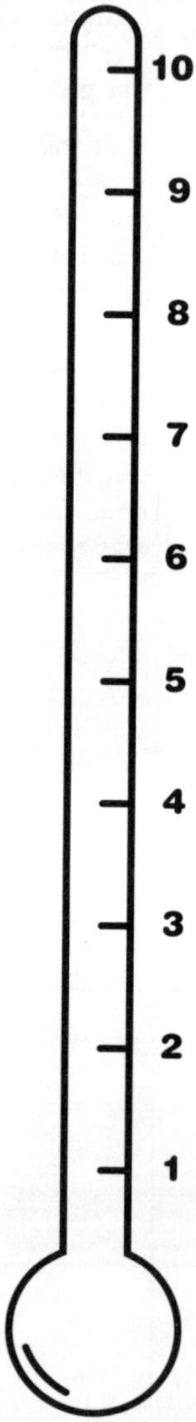

HANDOUT 7.2 Impact of High Emotion/Stress on Brain Functioning

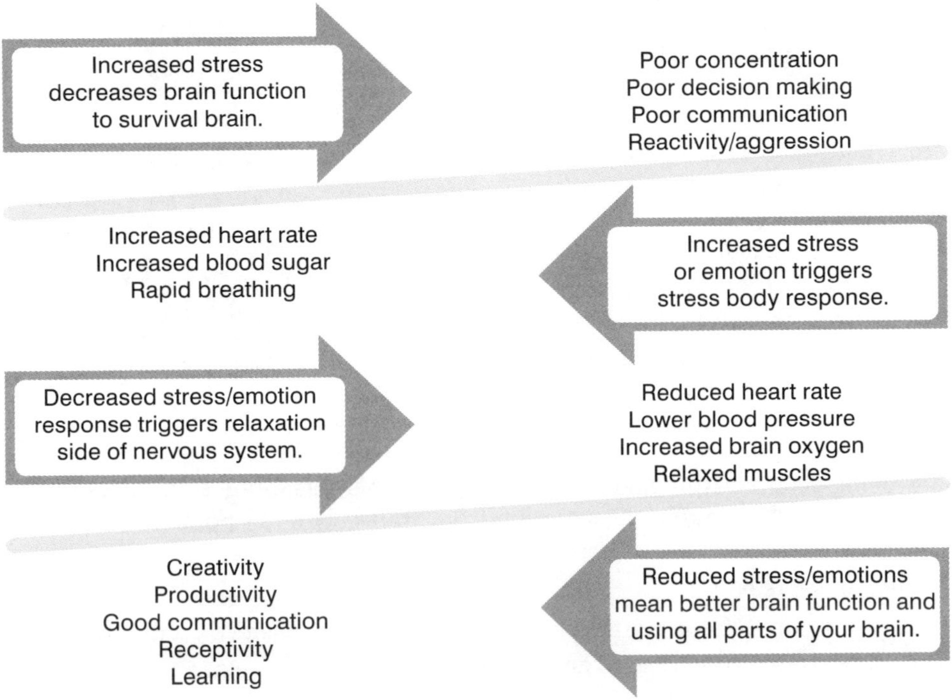

When our stress response system turns on, the greater the stress, the fewer the parts of our brain that are functioning. At the highest levels of stress, only our survival brain is responding. The other two parts, our emotional brain and our thinking brain, are not being used. All signals to our brain are going only through the survival brain, making us react without thought.

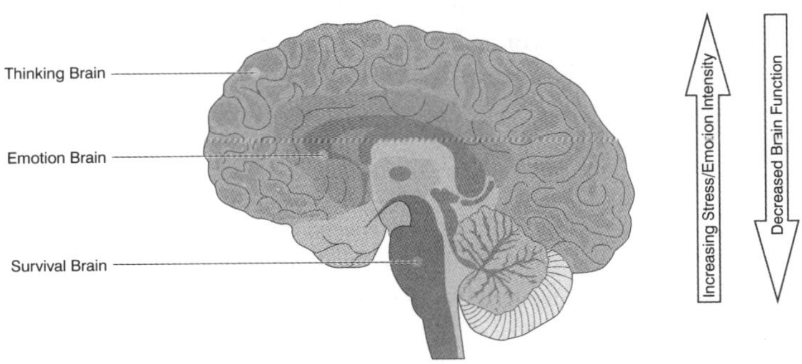

HANDOUT 7.3 Steps to Taking Space

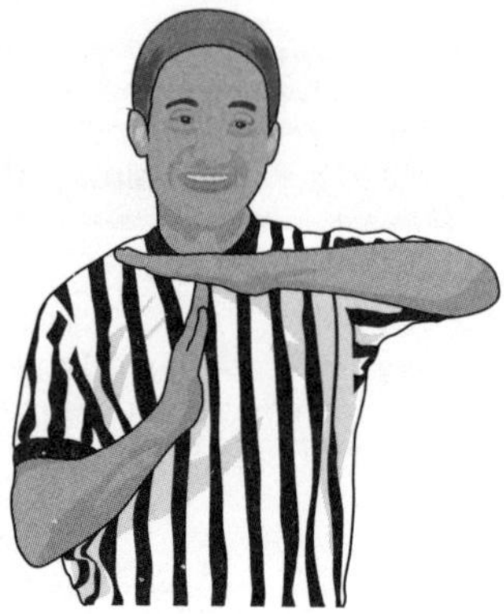

- Explain to your coparent what you are doing quickly and calmly. This should include the following:
  - where you are going
  - what time you will return
- State that you will return to the topic later, when you are both calm.
- Sample language: *"I'm going to go for a walk to calm down. I'll be back within 1 hour. We can talk about this more then."*
- Exit the room quickly and use the time to calm down, using health coping strategies such as the following:
  - taking a walk
  - doing deep breathing, guided imagery, or other relaxation techniques
  - trying to think about the situation from your coparent's point of view

Taking Space Is NOT:

- storming out without saying where you are going or when you will return.
- an opportunity or excuse to go out with friends, go drinking, and so forth.
- staying out for many hours.
- using the time to come up with a list of complaints/attacks against your partner.
- returning and ignoring the problem/acting as if nothing happened.

Coparent Support of Taking Space

- Always grant taking space, if requested, so the coparent can calm down.
- Expect to return to the conversation later. Use the time to calm down yourself and think through what is important to say when they return.
- Take deep breaths; try to think about the situation from your coparent's perspective.
- Do not:
  - stand in the way of the person trying to take a time out.
  - follow them, trying to continue the conversation.
  - make threats of what you will do if they take a take space.
  - use the time to compile a list of complaints/attacks to use when they return.

WORKSHEET 7.4 Cognitive Triangle Exercise

Choose a triggering event and write it on the lines below the arrow for "trigger event." Then, fill in the thought, feeling, and action that followed that event on the first line provided at each corner of the triangle. Next, try to change the initial unhelpful thought to a more helpful thought, and see how this new thought changes your feelings and the actions you might take. Record those feelings and actions on the second line at each corresponding corner.

THOUGHT 1. ____________________________

____

2. ____________________________

____

TRIGGER EVENT

____

____

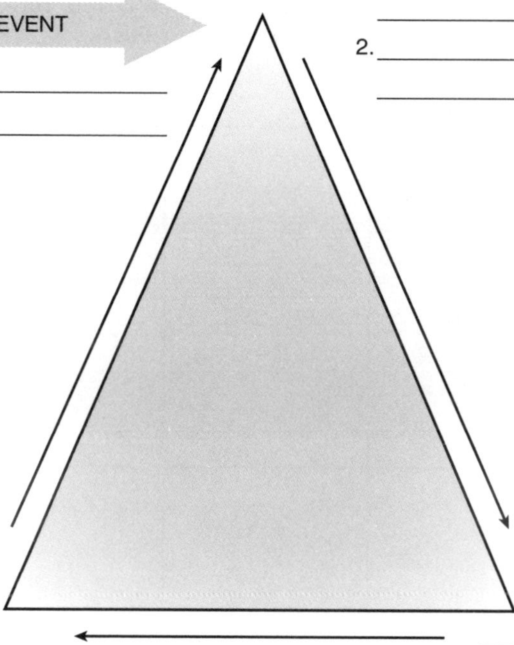

ACTION

1. ____________________________

____

2. ____________________________

____

FEELING

1. ____________________________

____

2. ____________________________

____

WORKSHEET 7.5 Changing Your Unhelpful Thoughts

When you experience a strong emotion such as anger or anxiety over the week, write down the situation that triggered the emotion. Then write what thoughts you have after the event. Are there alternative, more helpful, thoughts that you could have, and what feeling follows those more helpful thoughts? See example below.

Trigger (what, when, where, who)	Emotion/ feeling?	Unhelpful thought?	Alternative helpful thought?	Feeling?
My partner didn't answer my text right away.	*Agitated.*	*She's ignoring me. She's out with someone else.*	*She's busy right now or her phone died.*	*Concerned but not agitated.*

HANDOUT 8.1 Coparenting Session Rules

- One person talks at a time.

- When it is not your turn to talk, listen to understand what the other person is saying.

- Stay on session topic.

- The clinician will interrupt to help provide feedback, correct, teach a skill, or redirect a conversation as needed.

- Yelling, interrupting, or demeaning your coparent or the clinician is not allowed.

- Topics for discussion are focused on coparenting and raising your children together, and not talking through ways your partner has hurt you in the past.

- Stick to the goals of the coparenting sessions:
  - Decrease conflict/aggression/violence in the relationship.
  - Improve communication related to coparenting.

- If needed, the session will be stopped and the clinician will meet with each partner separately.

- Phones should be silenced and put away.

- ______________________________

- ______________________________

______________________________ ______________________________

Parent 1 Signature Parent 2 Signature

WORKSHEET 8.1 Catch Your Coparent Doing Something You Appreciate

A satisfying coparenting relationship is based on feeling good about your coparent's behavior toward your child. Sometimes we don't notice all the positive, helpful, important things, big or small, that our coparents do to take care of and parent our children or support us as coparents. Write down the things you notice your coparent doing as a parent that you appreciate. See example below.

Date	Time of Day	Behavior	Why do you appreciate this tbehavior?
January 5	*Morning*	*You fixed the kids' favorite breakfast.*	*It made the kids feel special and started the day off well.*

HANDOUT 8.2 Steps for Active Listening

1. **<u>LISTEN</u> to the other person.**
   - Listen to understand. If you focus only on winning or getting your own point across, then you do not hear the other person or understand them.
   - Listen carefully so you can repeat what you just heard the other person say.
   - Listen with your full attention by making eye contact and facing the person. Sit in an open position (don't fold your arms or be distracted by your phone or other things).
   - *Do NOT interrupt.*
   - Do not judge or criticize what the other person said.
2. **<u>REPEAT</u> what the other person just said. This shows you really heard them correctly.**
   - When the person finishes speaking, say "Let me be sure I heard you correctly."
   - Repeat what you heard.
   - After you say what you think you heard, ask the other person if you have heard correctly.
   - Be prepared that you might have gotten something wrong. We often misunderstand when we are communicating, especially if we are emotionally triggered. That is OK, and asking for clarification will help you understand what the other person was trying to say.
3. **<u>ASK</u> questions to clarify and to continue the conversation.**
   - Don't assume you know what the other person means or is thinking. Ask, "Do you mean . . . ?"
   - Ask open-ended questions such as the following:
     - "What do you think we should do about this situation?"
     - "What do you think are our options?"
   - Make sure your tone is calm and sincere. Watch out for use of sarcastic or hostile tones of voice, or use of nonverbal communication such as eye rolling, sighing, turning away from the person.
4. **<u>ACCEPT</u> the other's feelings, thoughts, or ideas by putting yourself in their shoes.**
   - This does *not* mean you have to agree with the other person.
   - This does *not* mean you have to "give in" to the other person.

It means you are trying to solve a problem, and not just be right or get your way. Each of you is entitled to your own feelings. Feelings are not wrong.

HANDOUT 8.3 How to Make an "I" Statement

"I" statements are an important way to communicate. Let's practice.

1. Say "I" (instead of "you" or "they").
2. Say what you feel (e.g., worried, annoyed, upset, scared, sad, angry).
3. Say the event/situation that provoked your feelings.
4. Say what it is about the behavior or its consequences that you do not like.
5. Say what you would like or prefer to happen (alternative to the behavior).

This becomes a sentence:

#1 I feel ______ **#2** ______ when ______ **#3** ______

because ______ **#4** ______.

I'd appreciate it if ______ **#5** ______.

Examples:

1. I feel **worried** when **you get home late and don't let me know** because **I think something has happened to you.** I'd appreciate it if **you sent me a text when you are running late so I know you are OK.**
2. I feel **frustrated** when **you sit downstairs while I get the kids ready for bed,** because **I think you want me to do all the parenting work alone.** I'd appreciate it **if you could help me by getting them in their pajamas and seeing that they brush their teeth. It would make the evening go more smoothly.**

Tips:

- Avoid inserting words such as *that* and *like,* because they are often about an opinion or judgment.
- Don't use lines like "I feel like you . . ." or "I feel that you . . ."
- Don't start with the word *you,* because the *you* sounds like blaming.

Now you try writing one:

I feel ______________________ when ______________________

because ____.

I'd appreciate it if ___________________________________.

HANDOUT 8.4 Areas of Coparenting

Below is a list of areas of coparenting. Review the list and identify which aspects of coparenting are the most challenging for you.

1. **Opinions about how to raise your child**
   - How to discipline your child
   - What moral values to teach your child
   - How to teach good behavior
   - How to identify and respond to your child's emotional needs
   - What education is important for your child?
   - What is safe for your child?
   - What is allowable in terms of friends or peer relationships?

2. **Division of labor: Who does what when it comes to parenting of the kids?**
   - How do each of you contribute to caring for and parenting your child?

3. **Support: How do you balance each other?**
   - How do you support the parenting of your child's other parent?
   - How does your child's other parent support you?
   - When one parent falls behind, does the other pick up the slack?

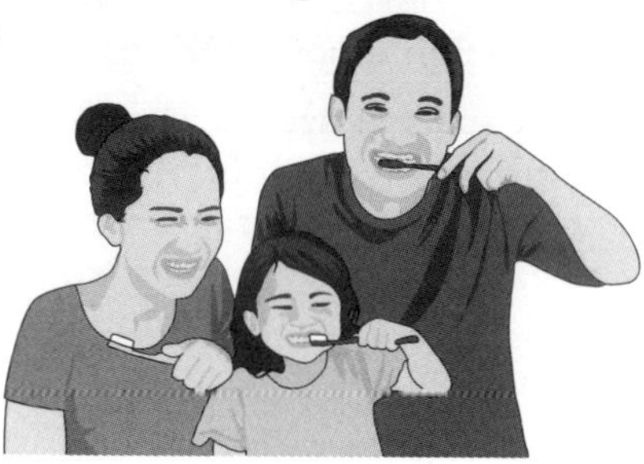

4. **Family management**
   - Managing the household
   - Finances
   - Transportation

HANDOUT 8.5 Rules for Healthy Problem-Solving Discussions

✓ **Talk about one thing at a time.** It is not helpful to bring up a long list of complaints during an argument. This turns a conversation about an area of disagreement into a war of complaints. There's no winning this kind of argument. Stay focused on one issue and resolve it before bringing up anything else. Try starting the conversation with an "I" statement focused on one thing only.

✓ **Listen.** Use your new active listening skills to try to really listen and understand your partner and their point of view. It does not mean you have to agree with them, but you can acknowledge their point of view and understand them better.

✓ **Do not bring up the other person's family members or best friends.** Blaming things on the other person's parents, family, best friend, or childhood history is one of the worst things you could do. Criticizing other people the person cares about or making them feel shame for their family or childhood will only cause them to get defensive or shut down.

✓ **Do not yell, threaten, name-call, or use physical aggression.** People often think that if they yell, their partner will hear them better. They do not. When people are yelled at, they stop listening and often start yelling, too. Physical aggression is never OK.

✓ **Take space if needed.** When people get flooded with feelings, they cannot think clearly, and they make bad decisions. When one or both of you become flooded, it's important to take some space from each other and the discussion to calm down. Don't just storm out. Calmly say something like "I need to take some space. I'm going to go for a walk, and I'll be back in half an hour." When you come back, ask, "Can we try again to talk?"

✓ **Acknowledge your part.** Ask yourself, "What did I do to contribute to this problem?" If one person is willing to admit their part in a conflict, sometimes the other person's anger softens. Admitting your mistakes lets you address the only behaviors you really have any control over—your own. **No behavior of the other person excuses your use of physical or verbal aggression toward them. You are in control of your own behavior.**

✓ **Apologize when you are wrong.** Be sincere when you say, "I'm sorry." An apology is a powerful way to soothe hurt feeling and get a discussion back on track.

Based on *Figuring It Out for the Child* (McHale et al., 2022).

WORKSHEET 8.2 Rules for Healthy Problem Solving

Answer the questions below related to how often you break the healthy problem-solving rules.

1. Talk about one issue at a time.

   I break this rule: ____ a lot ____ sometimes ____ never

2. Use "I" statements.

   I break this rule: ____ a lot ____ sometimes ____ never

3. Listen to my partner rather than preparing my own side of the argument.

   I break this rule: ____ a lot ____ sometimes ____ never

4. No yelling, threatening, intimidating, name-calling, or use of physical aggression.

   I break this rule: ____ a lot ____ sometimes ____ never

5. No bringing up the other person's family members or best friends.

   I break this rule: ____ a lot ____ sometimes ____ never

6. No dredging up the past; focus on the current issue only.

   I break this rule: ____ a lot ____ sometimes ____ never

7. Take space when things get heated; walk away and allow time to cool off.

   I break this rule: ____ a lot ____ sometimes ____ never

8. Acknowledge my part or contribution to the problem rather than blaming my partner for my actions.

   I break this rule: ____ a lot ____ sometimes ____ never

9. Apologize when I am wrong.

   I break this rule: ____ a lot ____ sometimes ____ never

The rules I break the most are: ____

____

The one I most want to work on is: ____

____

WORKSHEET 8.3 Planning for Disagreements

Disagreements in relationships are going to happen. It is OK to disagree. It is never OK to yell, scream, or use manipulation/control or physical aggression to win a disagreement. Solving problems rather than winning arguments is your goal as coparents. Answer the questions below to prepare for future disagreements.

1. What are ways you can be supportive to your coparent at times of stress?
2. What are ways you can remember that your goal as coparents is to work out any problems/conflicts for the good of your children?
3. What is a way you can signal your coparent to stop arguing if you are in front of your children and need or want to take space?
4. What is your "Taking Space" plan (what will you say to your partner and where will you go to take your space and for how long)?
5. If you can't solve a problem yourselves, where could you go for impartial support?

FORM 8.1 Healthy Problem-Solving Contract

1. I agree not to use yelling, screaming, threatening, manipulation, or physical aggression during disagreements.
2. I agree to calmly solve problems in the best interests of our children.
3. I will apologize when I am wrong.
4. I will not bring up my coparent's family, best friends, or old history when trying to solve a problem.
5. I will recognize my part in the problem and not blame my partner for my own actions.
6. I agree to use the following strategies to have good communication with my coparent:
   a. Listen to my coparent and try to think about things from their point of view.
   b. Accept their feelings even if I do not agree with them.
   c. Use "I" statements to express my feelings and bring up issues for discussion.
   d. If I am overwhelmed or too angry to talk, I will tell my coparent I am taking space and set a time we can discuss the topic later.

____________________________________ ______________

Coparent 1 Signature Date

____________________________________ ______________

Coparent 2 Signature Date

WORKSHEET 8.4 Daily Routines

Write down the typical daily routine during the week. Start with wake up and end when children are asleep at night. Who does what? Highlight areas that are a struggle or that go especially well.

5:00 A.M. ____________________

5:30 A.M. ____________________

6:00 A.M. ____________________

6:30 A.M. ____________________

7:00 A.M. ____________________

7:30 A.M. ____________________

8:00 A.M. ____________________

8:30 A.M. ____________________

9:00 A.M. ____________________

9:30 A.M. ____________________

10:00 A.M. ____________________

10:30 A.M. ____________________

11:00 A.M. ____________________

11:30 A.M. ____________________

12:00 P.M. ____________________

12:30 P.M. ____________________

1:00 P.M. ____________________

1:30 P.M. ____________________

2:00 P.M. ____________________

2:30 P.M. ____________________

3:00 P.M. ____________________

3:30 P.M. ____________________

4:00 P.M. ____________________

4:30 P.M. ____________________

5:00 P.M. ____________________

5:30 P.M. ____________________

6:00 P.M. ____________________

6:30 P.M. ____________________

7:00 P.M. ____________________

7:30 P.M. ____________________

8:00 P.M. ____________________

8:30 P.M. ____________________

9:00 P.M. ____________________

9:30 P.M. ____________________

10:00 P.M. ____________________

10:30 P.M. ____________________

11:00 P.M. ____________________

11:30 P.M. ____________________

12:00 A.M. ____________________

12:30 A.M. ____________________

1:00 A.M. ____________________

1:30 A.M. ____________________

2:00 A.M. ____________________

2:30 A.M. ____________________

3:00 A.M. ____________________

3:30 A.M. ____________________

4:00 A.M. ____________________

4:30 A.M. ____________________

WORKSHEET 9.1 Catch Your Child Doing Something You Appreciate

A satisfying parenting relationship is based on feeling good about your child. Sometimes we don't notice all of our childrens' positive behaviors. Each day, notice at least one positive or helpful thing that your child does and write it on the chart below. It is ALWAYS POSSIBLE to notice at least one behavior you appreciate. See example below.

Date	Child's behavior	Praise given	Child's response
September 5th	*Picked up toys when asked*	*"I like the way you put your toys away when you were done."*	*Smiled*

HANDOUT 9.1 What Is Time In?

Time ins can be used when your child is having a temper tantrum, when there's a power struggle, or when your child is being aggressive, or noncooperative. Time in can be used instead of Time out to provide a supportive space for emotion coaching.

1. **RESIST BEING REACTIVE IN RESPONSE TO THE MISBEHAVIOR:** This is often the hardest part for parents. When you react to a child's misbehavior with your own anger, it can make the situation worse rather than better. If your child is hitting or being destructive, you need to stop the behavior immediately. If they're not destructive or aggressive, take three deep breaths before you address the situation, or take a few minutes to gather yourself if you are really upset or angry. Before responding:
   a. Remind yourself that a child's aggressive or oppositional behaviors are common following exposure to family conflict and domestic violence.
   b. Think about what your child's needs might be or how they may be experiencing the situation.
2. **REMOVE YOURSELF AND YOUR CHILD TO A NEUTRAL LOCATION:** Whether you pick them up or just ask them to join you, it's a good idea to move to a different location from where the behavior took place. You can say, "Let's meet on the couch," or "Let's go sit out on the porch."
3. **LOOK FOR THE UNDERLYING UNMET NEED OR FEELING:** Usually, kids misbehave to get their needs met or express/release strong emotions. Looking for the hidden cause can help problem-solve how the child can ask for what they need appropriately next time.
4. **ACKNOWLEDGE FEELINGS AND NEEDS:** This is a great time to use the emotion coaching skill of identifying feelings. Help your child identify what they felt. "I know that you are angry that it is time to come inside and you really want to keep playing now."
5. **DISCUSS WHY THE BEHAVIOR IS A PROBLEM:** When your child has visibly calmed down is the time to talk about their behavior. Invite your child to talk about what happened. "I can see you're feeling calmer now. Can we talk now about what happened?"
   - Talk about why the child's behavior was a problem. "The problem is that it's not OK to hit or yell at others, even when you are upset or angry."
   - Keep the focus on how the child can improve next time—reinforcing their responsibility for their own behavior. "What could you do next time instead of hitting when you are angry?" or "How could you avoid this from happening again?"
   - Discuss the feelings of other people who were affected to help the child develop empathy for others and see how their behavior impacts others. "I was really upset when you hit me."
6. **DISCUSS RESTITUTION AND RECONCILIATION:** Ask something like "What can you do to make this situation better?" When a child comes up with their own solutions, they are more genuine, and the child is more likely to feel control over the situation. Forcing your child to say "sorry" will not have the same impact as their coming up with solutions themselves.

HANDOUT 9.2 What Is Time Out?

Time out is a safe and very effective form of discipline, but it is also a way for children to calm down when they are overstimulated or distressed. When kids are given a time out, they do not get parental attention and they are not allowed to do anything fun or interesting.

What kinds of behaviors should I use time out for?

- Threatening people
- Loud, hostile arguing
- Being mean to people or animals
- Breaking or throwing things
- Swearing
- Hitting
- Dangerous behavior

Prepare for time out in advance

- Identify a place in the house to do time out with your child (a specific chair, etc.).
- Identify a timer to keep accurate time (a watch, your phone, a timer on the stove).
- Identify specific behaviors you will use time out for with your child(ren).*

Implement time out

- Use a calm, firm voice, state what the child did wrong and the consequence: "Hitting your sister is not OK. You will need to take a time out. Let's go to the time out chair. I will set the timer for 4 minutes, and you need to sit in this chair until you hear the beep. When the timer rings, we can talk about what happened."
- Set the timer for the number of minutes equal to the child's age (4-year-old = 4 minutes).
- During time out, the parent should not engage with the child. Ignore the child unless they are hurting themselves or in danger.
- Once the timer sounds, the parent can talk with the child about what happened and how they could better manage their emotions or get their needs met. This is the time to use emotion coaching skills.

*DO NOT use time out for every little offense, but for more serious behaviors only.

HANDOUT 9.3 Why Not Spanking?

- Studies show spanking children is NOT an effective way to control behavior long term. Spanking doesn't work because:
  - it does not teach children self-control or what to do instead.
  - it becomes less effective over time.
  - it has long-term, harmful side effects.
  - it tends to increase negative behavior rather than decrease it.
  - it encourages children to hide their misbehavior or mistakes.

- Parents typically spank when they are angry.

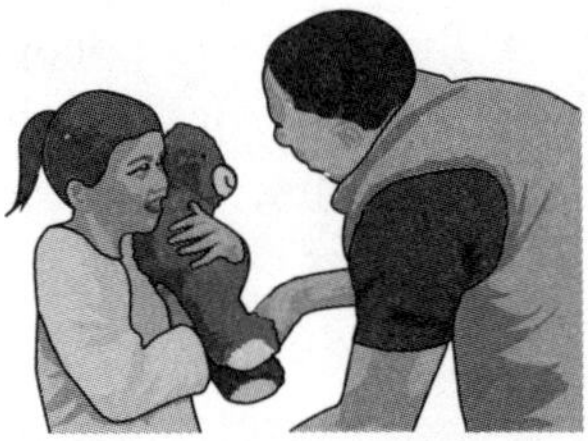

- Spanking provokes anger in both the parent and the child. Children may then misbehave even more.

- Spanking also creates a distance in the relationship between a parent and a child.

- Children who have been repeatedly spanked or threatened to be hit/spanked may:
  - develop low self-esteem.
  - fear adults so they will not ask them for help when they need it.
  - feel unloved and unwanted.
  - exhibit a high degree of anxiety.
  - struggle with feelings of helplessness.
  - seek revenge against others.
  - destroy property and break things belonging to others.
  - tend to be more aggressive.
  - learn hitting is a way to deal with anger and frustration.

HANDOUT 9.4 Talking with Your Kids about Your Addiction and Treatment

Many parents in recovery agonize over what to tell their children about things that happened when they were using drugs or alcohol.

Don't lie or sugarcoat your addiction.

It can be tempting to think that you don't need to tell a child (especially a young child) the truth about why you are not living together. But it is far better to tell them in words they can understand given their age and development stage. They know that something is wrong, and they usually blame themselves for whatever they imagine that "something" is. You can strengthen your current relationship with your children and set the stage for better future relationships by telling the truth.

Teach your children about addiction, recovery, and relapse.

1. Let them know how using drugs made you do things you would not normally do, such as hurting them or leaving them alone.
2. You can explain that drugs cause people who are dependent on them to make using drugs (or alcohol) come ahead of everything else, even their children. This was not your choice, but the drugs have effects on your body and mind.
3. Teach them about recovery and relapse. They should know that people do recover from drug addiction, but that it is really hard work and parents in recovery need help. Sometimes parents who have stopped using—even for a long time—relapse. This does not mean failure. It means that your treatment plan must be adjusted.
4. Don't make the promise that you will never use again.
5. Reassure them that you are working on your recovery, and that you will keep working on it every day from now on.

Reassure your child.

Children whose parents misuse substances often believe that their parents' problems are their fault, and that they should be able to do something to change the parent. Teach them the following:

1. **Cause:** Your children did not cause your alcohol or drug problem.
2. **Control:** Your children cannot control your alcohol/drug problem—by behaving perfectly, getting straight A's in school, or throwing out your liquor/drugs.
3. **Cure:** Your child cannot cure your addiction. You are responsible for your recovery.

(continued)

The most important thing is that they understand that your addiction is not their fault.

Other key concepts for you to share with your child include the following:

- You never stopped loving your child, even when the drugs or alcohol were making you put using ahead of your child's needs. Your child deserves love.
- Many children have parents with drug or alcohol problems, and they grow up to be strong, healthy, and happy adults.
- Children whose parents misuse substances are at especially high risk for their own substance misuse. Their bodies respond differently to alcohol and other drugs than the bodies of their friends, so they need to be especially careful about avoiding drugs or alcohol in the first place. This is something to talk about with children who are school age and older, but not young children who are fearful of illnesses.

It is usually very difficult for parents in recovery to talk with their children about their own addiction, recovery, and relapse. It brings up feelings of shame and guilt, and parents often worry that they will lose their children's respect. You may be afraid that once you start to talk about it, you will have to face your children's questions and feelings, such as disappointment and anger, about your past actions. And you will. But the good news is that this is all part of the family's healing process. Being honest about your addiction and letting your child know it is OK to talk about it is one of the best ways to earn back your child's trust. It's necessary and healthy to have these conversations and, over time, you will feel more and more comfortable talking about it.

Sample Language about Addiction:

"I have a kind of sickness called addiction. It isn't a sickness you can catch. It means that I take drugs [or drink alcohol], and it is very hard for me to stop. I am getting help for my addiction. My counselor is helping me with my sickness, and I am getting better. My addiction sickness is not your fault. Nothing you did made me use drugs. There is nothing you can do to make me stop. I need to stop myself, and I am working very hard, with the help of my counselor. I love you and I'm sorry that I cannot be with you all the time, because I need to be in treatment for my sickness now. Do you have any questions?"

WORKSHEET 9.2 Guidelines for Making Amends Session Letter

1. What have your children experienced/witnessed that you need to acknowledge or for what behaviors do you need to take responsibility? ______________________

2. In what ways have these experiences or your behaviors impacted your children? _____

3. What are you trying to do differently now so your children do not have these experiences again? What skills have you learned, or what behaviors are you changing?

4. Write a statement in developmentally appropriate language for your children that includes an acknowledgment of what they experienced, an apology for your behavior, and how you are trying to change:

HANDOUT 9.5 Child-Directed Play Guidelines

- Encourage your child's curiosity to explore objects and activities.
- Follow your child's lead—let them be in charge of the play.
- Be attentive, patient, and enthusiastic.
- Don't focus on the "correct" way or specific rules for a game—let your child play how they choose.
- Model cooperation by doing what your child asks you to do.
- Observe and respond to your child's requests or bids for your attention and try not to ask questions.
- Praise and encourage your child.
- Avoid criticism.
- Engage in pretend and make-believe play with your child.
- Curb your desire to give too much help—give just enough support to avoid frustration but not so much you take over.
- Laugh and have fun.

REMEMBER TO CATCH YOUR CHILD DOING SOMETHING YOU APPRECIATE AND PRAISE THIS BEHAVIOR AT LEAST ONCE PER DAY—OR MORE, IF POSSIBLE!

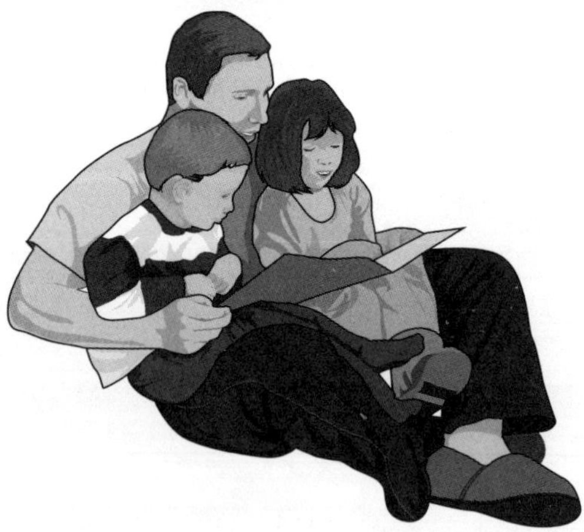

APPENDIX B

Suggested Readings and Resources

MINDFULNESS RESOURCES

Mindful
www.mindful.org

YouTube: Trauma-Sensitive Mindfulness Series with David Treleaven
www.youtube.com/playlist?list=plskhqn-oiolbkjp1amwjftbn_kilfgydj

PsychologyTools.com
www.psychologytools.com/resource/progressive-muscle-relaxation

Urge surfing
www.therapistaid.com/worksheets/urge-surfing-handout

SMARTPHONE APPS

Ten Percent Happier
Calm
Headspace

CHILD DEVELOPMENT RESOURCES

Geffner, R., Igelman, R. S., & Zellner, J. (2014). *The effects of intimate partner violence on children*. Routledge.

Jaffe, P. G., Wolfe, D. A., & Campbell, M. (2011). *Growing up with domestic violence* (vol. 23). Hogrefe Publishing.
Lieberman, A. F. (2017). *The emotional life of the toddler*. Simon & Schuster.
Miller, K. (2012). *Ages and stages revised*. Teleshare.

Centers for Disease Control and Prevention Developmental Milestones
www.cdc.gov/ncbddd/actearly/milestones/index.html

ZERO TO THREE Early Development
www.zerotothree.org/issue-areas/early-development

CHILDREN'S BOOKS

Calvin, G. (2019). *Addie's mom isn't home anymore: Addiction is scary—especially when you don't know what it is*. Independently Published.
Curtis, J. L. (1998). *Today I feel silly and other moods that make my day*. HarperCollins.
Ghosh Ippen, C. (2017). *Once I was very very scared*. Pilpo Productions.
Ghosh Ippen, C. (2019). *Holdin Pott*. Pilpo Productions.
Ghosh Ippen, C. (2019). *You weren't with me*. Pilpo Publications.
Holmes, M. A. (2000). *A terrible thing happened*. Magination Press.
Kraulis, J. (2013). *Whimsy's heavy things*. Tundra Books.
Wilgocki, J. (2002). *Maybe days: A book for children in foster care*. American Psychological Association.

FURTHER READING TO INFORM FATHERS FOR CHANGE THERAPY PRACTICE

Akbar, M. (2017). *Urban trauma: A legacy of racism*. Publish Your Purpose Press.
Dana, D. (2020). *Polyvagal exercises for safety and connection: 50 client-centered practices*. Norton.
Dana, D. (2021). *Anchored: How to befriend your nervous system using polyvagal theory*. Sounds True.
Dimeff, L. A., Rizvi, S. L., & Koerner, K. (Eds.). (2021). *Dialectical behavior therapy in clinical practice* (2nd ed.). Guilford Press.
Hamby, S., & Clark, S. (2012). The VIGOR: The Victim Inventory of Goals, Options and Risks: A safety planning tool to help survivors of violence assess their risk and decide how to cope. Retrieved November, 6, 2022, from *www.ywcayork.org/wp-content/uploads/sites/51/website-safety-plan.pdf*.
Kendi, I. X. (2019). *How to be an antiracist*. One World.
Levine, P. (1997). *Waking the tiger: Healing trauma*. North Atlantic Books.

Lieberman, A. F., Ippen, C. G., & Van Horn, P. (2015). *"Don't hit my mommy!": A manual for child–parent psychotherapy with young children exposed to violence and other trauma.* ZERO TO THREE.

McHale, J. P., & Lindahl, K. M. (2011). *Coparenting: A conceptual and clinical examination of family systems.* American Psychological Association.

Miller, W. R., & Rollnick, S. (2023). *Motivational interviewing: Helping people change and grow* (4th ed.). Guilford Press.

Powell, B., Cooper, G., Hoffman, K., & Marvin, B. (2013). *The circle of security intervention: Enhancing attachment in early parent–child relationships.* Guilford Press.

Schwartz, R. C. (2021). *No bad parts: Healing trauma and restoring wholeness with the internal family systems model.* Sounds True.

Schwartz, R. C. (2021). *You are the one you've been waiting for: Bringing courageous love to intimate relationships.* Author.

Schwartz, R. C., & Sweezy, M. (2019). *Internal family systems* therapy (2nd ed.). Guilford Press.

Treleaven, D. A. (2018). *Trauma-sensitive mindfulness: Practices for safe and transformative healing.* Norton.

GENERAL RESOURCE WEBSITES

Brené Brown: *https://brenebrown.com*—Materials and resources related to shame versus guilt.

National Child Traumatic Stress Network: *www.nctsn.org*—Materials, trainings, and handouts on domestic violence. Of particular interest is this handout on talking to children about domestic violence: *www.nctsn.org/resources/children-and-domestic-violence-listening-and-talking-your-child-about-domestic-violence.*

Therapist Aid: *www.therapistaid.com/therapy-worksheets*—Worksheets and scripts that can be used for general techniques discussed in this book (e.g., urge surfing).

Yale School of Medicine, Child Study Center: *https://medicine.yale.edu/childstudy/education-and-training/professional-development/fathers-for-change*—Information and updates about Fathers for Change Research and Training.

References

Abidin, R. R., & Brunner, J. F. (1995). Development of a parenting alliance inventory. *Journal of Clinical Child Psychology, 24*(1), 31–40.

Achenbach, T. M., & Rescorla, L. A. (2001). *Manual for the ASEBA school-age forms and profiles.* Research Centre for Children, Youth, and Families, University of Vermont.

Adhia, A., & Jeong, J. (2019). Fathers' perpetration of intimate partner violence and parenting during early childhood: Results from the Fragile Families and Child Wellbeing Study. *Child Abuse and Neglect, 96*, Article 104103.

Ahmadabadi, Z., Najman, J. M., Williams, G. M., Clavarino, A. M., d'Abbs, P., & Abajobir, A. A. (2018). Maternal intimate partner violence victimization and child maltreatment. *Child Abuse and Neglect, 82*, 23–33.

Aldao, A., Nolen-Hoeksema, S., & Schweizer, S. (2010). Emotion-regulation strategies across psychopathology: A meta-analytic review. *Clinical Psychology Review, 30*(2), 217–237.

Amodia-Bidakowska, A., Laverty, C., & Ramchandani, P. G. (2020). Father–child play: A systematic review of its frequency, characteristics and potential impact on children's development. *Developmental Review, 57*, Article 100924.

Antunes-Alves, S., & Stefano, J. (2014). Intimate partner violence: Making the case for joint couple treatment. *Family Journal, 22*(1), 62–68.

Arias, E., Arce, R., & Vilariño, M. (2013). Batterer intervention programmes: A meta-analytic review of effectiveness. *Psychosocial Intervention, 22*(2), 153–160.

Armenti, N. A., & Babcock, J. C. (2016). Conjoint treatment for intimate partner violence: A systematic review and implications. *Couple and Family Psychology: Research and Practice, 5*(2), 109–123.

Arnsten, A. F. T. (2015). Stress weakens prefrontal networks: Molecular insults to higher cognition. *Nature Neuroscience, 18*(10), 1376–1385.

Arroyo, K., Lundahl, B., Butters, R., Vanderloo, M., & Wood, D. S. (2017).

Short-term interventions for survivors of intimate partner violence: A systematic review and meta-analysis. *Trauma, Violence, and Abuse, 18*(2), 155–171.

Asen, E., & Fonagy, P. (2017). Mentalizing family violence: Part 1. Conceptual framework. *Family Process, 56*(1), 6–21.

Babcock, J. C., Green, C. E., & Robie, C. (2004). Does batterers' treatment work?: A meta-analytic review of domestic violence treatment. *Clinical Psychology Review, 23*(8), 1023–1053.

Babcock, J. C., Green, C. E., & Webb, S. (2008). Decoding deficits of different types of batterers during presentation of facial affect slides. *Journal of Family Violence, 23*(5), 295–302.

Babcock, J. C., Green, C. E., Webb, S. A., & Graham, K. H. (2004). A second failure to replicate the Gottman et al. (1995) typology of men who abuse intimate partners . . . and possible reasons why. *Journal of Family Psychology, 18*(2), 396–400.

Baldwin, D. V. (2013). Primitive mechanisms of trauma response: An evolutionary perspective on trauma-related disorders. *Neuroscience and Biobehavioral Reviews, 37*(8), 1549–1566.

Bancroft, L., Silverman, J., & Ritchie, D. (2012). *The batterer as parent: Addressing the impact of domestic violence on family dynamics* (2nd ed.). SAGE.

Bavolek, S. J. (1984). *Handbook for the Adult–Adolescent Parenting Inventory (AAPI).* Family Development Associates.

Bayarri Fernandez, E., Ezpeleta, L., Granero, R., de la Osa, N., & Domènech, J. M. (2011). Degree of exposure to domestic violence, psychopathology, and functional impairment in children and adolescents. *Journal of Interpersonal Violence, 26*(6), 1215–1231.

Bearss, K. E., & Eyberg, S. (1998). A test of the parenting alliance theory. *Early Education and Development, 9*(2), 179–185.

Beck, A. T., Steer, R. A., & Brown, G. K. (1987). *Beck Depression Inventory.* Harcourt Brace Jovanovich.

Beck, R., & Fernandez, E. (1998). Cognitive-behavioral therapy in the treatment of anger: A meta-analysis. *Cognitive Therapy and Research, 22*(1), 63–74.

Beebe, R., Clough, M., Bernstein, B., Grasso, D., & Stover, C. S. (submitted for publication). *Reducing family violence through child welfare intervention: A propensity score matched study of Fathers for Change.* Unpublished manuscript.

Berking, M., Wupperman, P., Reichardt, A., Pejic, T., Dippel, A., & Znoj, H. (2008). Emotion-regulation skills as a treatment target in psychotherapy. *Behaviour Research and Therapy, 46*(11), 1230–1237.

Birkley, E. L., & Eckhardt, C. I. (2015). Anger, hostility, internalizing negative emotions, and intimate partner violence perpetration: A meta-analytic review. *Clinical Psychology Review, 37,* 40–56.

Brady, K. T., & Backs, S. E. (2012). Childhood stress, posttraumatic stress disorder, and alcohol dependence. *Alcohol Research: Current Reviews, 34,* 408–413.

Braga, T., Gonçalves, L. C., Basto-Pereira, M., & Maia, A. (2017). Unraveling the link between maltreatment and juvenile antisocial behavior: A meta-analysis of prospective longitudinal studies. *Aggression and Violent Behavior, 33,* 37–50.

Brown, P. D., & O'Leary, K. D. (2000). Therapeutic alliance: Predicting continuance and success in group treatment for spouse abuse. *Journal of Consulting and Clinical Psychology, 68*(2), 340–345.

Burelomova, A. S., Gulina, M. A., & Tikhomandritskaya, O. A. (2018). Intimate partner violence: An overview of the existing theories, conceptual frameworks, and definitions. *Psychology in Russia: State of Art, 11*(3), 128–144.

Cabrera, N. J., Hofferth, S. L., & Chae, S. (2011). Patterns and predictors of father–infant engagement across race/ethnic groups. *Early Childhood Research Quarterly, 26*(3), 365–375.

Camara, K. A., & Resnick, G. (1989). Styles of conflict resolution and cooperation between divorced parents: Effects on child behavior and adjustment. *American Journal of Orthopsychiatry, 59*(4), 560–575.

Campbell, J. C., Webster, D. W., & Glass, N. (2009). The danger assessment: Validation of a lethality risk assessment instrument for intimate partner femicide. *Journal of Interpersonal Violence, 24*(4), 653–674.

Cano, T., Perales, F., & Baxter, J. (2019). A matter of time: Father involvement and child cognitive outcomes. *Journal of Marriage and Family, 81*(1), 164–184.

Caprara, G. V., Paciello, M., Gergino, M., & Cugini, C. (2007). Individual differences conducive to aggression and violence: Trajectories and correlates of irritability and hostile rumination through adolescence. *Aggressive Behavior, 33*, 359–374.

Carter, A. S., & Briggs-Gowan, M. J. (2006). *The Infant–Toddler Social and Emotional Assessment (ITSEA) manual*. Harcourt Assessment.

Centers for Disease Control and Prevention. (2015). Intimate partner violence surveillance: Uniform definitions and recommended data elements. Version 2.0. Retrieved from *www.cdc.gov/violenceprevention/pdf/ipv/intimatepartnerviolence.pdf*.

Chan, Y. C., & Yeung, J. W. K. (2009). Children living with violence within the family and its sequel: A meta-analysis from 1995–2006. *Aggression and Violent Behavior, 14*(5), 313–322.

Chemtob, C. M., Novaco, R. W., Hamada, R. S., Gross, D. M., & Smith, G. (1997). Anger regulation deficits in combat-related posttraumatic stress disorder. *Journal of Traumatic Stress, 10*(1), 17–36.

Cheng, S. Y., Davis, M., Jonson-Reid, M., & Yaeger, L. (2021). Compared to what? A meta-analysis of batterer intervention studies using nontreated controls or comparisons. *Trauma, Violence, & Abuse, 22*(3), 496–511.

Choenni, V., Hammink, A., & van de Mheen, D. (2017). Association between substance use and the perpetration of family violence in industrialized countries: A systematic review. *Trauma, Violence, and Abuse, 18*(1), 37–50.

Choi, J., Jeong, B., Polcari, A., Rohan, M. L., & Teicher, M. H. (2012). Reduced fractional anisotropy in the visual limbic pathway of young adults witnessing domestic violence in childhood. *NeuroImage, 59*(2), 1071–1079.

Ciesinski, N. K., Sorgi-Wilson, K. M., Cheung, J. C., Chen, E. Y., & McCloskey, M. S. (2022). The effect of dialectical behavior therapy on anger and aggressive behavior: A systematic review with meta-analysis. *Behaviour Research and Therapy, 154*, Article 104122.

Connell, R. W., & Messerschmidt, J. W. (2005). Hegemonic masculinity: Rethinking the concept. *Gender & Society, 19*(6), 829–859.

Costa, D., & Babcock, J. (2008). Articulated thoughts of intimate partner abusive men during anger arousal: Correlates with personality disorder features. *Journal of Family Violence, 23*(6), 395–402.

Cox, E. D., Smith, M. A., Brown, R. L., & Fitzpatrick, M. A. (2007). Effect of gender and visit length on participation in pediatric visits. *Patient Education and Counseling, 65*, 320–328.

Cunradi, C. B., Todd, M., Mair, C., & Remer, L. (2013). Intimate partner violence among California couples: Multilevel analysis of environmental and partner risk factors. *Partner Abuse, 4*(4), 419–443.

Daniels, J. W., & Murphy, C. M. (1997). Stages and processes of change in batterers' treatment. *Cognitive and Behavioral Practice, 4*(1), 123–145.

Dankoski, M., Keiley, M., Thomas, V., Choice, P., Lloyd, S., & Seery, B. (2006). Affect regulation and the cycle of violence against women: New directions for understanding the process. *Journal of Family Violence, 21*(5), 327–339.

Denson, T. F., Capper, M. M., Oaten, M., Friese, M., & Schofield, T. P. (2011). Self-control training decreases aggression in response to provocation in aggressive individuals. *Journal of Research in Personality, 45*(2), 252–256.

Derogatis, L. R., & Melisaratos, N. (1983). The Brief Symptom Inventory: An introductory report. *Psychological Medicine, 13*(3), 595–605.

Diemer, K., Humphreys, C., Fogden, L., Gallant, D., Spiteri-Staines, A., Bornemisza, A., & Vercoe, E. (2020). *Caring Dads program: Helping fathers value their children*. University of Melbourne.

Dimeff, L. A., Rizvi, S. L., & Koerner, K. (Eds.). (2021). *Dialectical behavior therapy in clinical practice* (2nd ed.). Guilford Press.

Dobash, R. E., & Dobash, R. P. (1979). *Violence against wives: A case against the patriarchy*. Free Press.

Dubowitz, H. (2014). The safe environment for every kid model: Promotion of children's health, development, and safety, and prevention of child neglect. *Pediatric Annals, 43*(11), e271–e277.

Duffy, K. A., Mclaughlin, K. A., & Green, P. A. (2018). Early life adversity and health-risk behaviors: Proposed psychological and neural mechanisms. *Annals of the New York Academy of Sciences, 1428*(1), 151–169.

Easton, C. J., Crane, C. A., & Mandel, D. (2018). A randomized controlled trial assessing the efficacy of cognitive behavioral therapy for substance-dependent domestic violence offenders: An integrated substance abuse–domestic violence treatment approach (SADV). *Journal of Marital and Family Therapy, 44*(3), 483–498.

Easton, C. J., Mandel, D. L., Hunkele, K. A., Nich, C., Rounsaville, B. J., & Carroll, K. M. (2007). A cognitive behavioral therapy for alcohol-dependent domestic violence offenders: An integrated substance abuse–domestic violence treatment approach (SADV). *American Journal on Addictions, 16*(1), 24–31.

Eckhardt, C., Holtzworth-Munroe, A., Norlander, B., Sibley, A., & Cahill, M. (2008). Readiness to change, partner violence subtypes, and treatment outcomes among men in treatment for partner assault. *Violence and Victims, 23*(4), 446–475.

Eckhardt, C. I., Samper, R. E., & Murphy, C. M. (2008). Anger disturbances among perpetrators of intimate partner violence: Clinical characteristics and outcomes of court-mandated treatment. *Journal of Interpersonal Violence, 23*(11), 1600–1617.

Edwards, A., Shipman, K., & Brown, A. (2005). The socialization of emotional understanding: A comparison of neglectful and nonneglectful mothers and their children. *Child Maltreatment, 10*(3), 293–304.

Evans, S. E., Davies, C., & DiLillo, D. (2008). Exposure to domestic violence: A meta-analysis of child and adolescent outcomes. *Aggression and Violent Behavior, 13*(2), 131–140.

Fainsilber, K. L., & Low, S. M. (2004). Marital violence, co-parenting, and family-level processes in relation to children's adjustment. *Journal of Family Psychology, 18*(2), 372–382.

Feinberg, M. E. (2003). The internal structure and ecological context of coparenting: A framework for research and intervention. *Parenting, 3*(2), 95–131.

Feldman, R. (1998). *Coding of interactive behavior.* Unpublished manual, Department of Psychology, Bar Ilan University, Israel.

Finkel, E. J. (2007). Impelling and inhibiting forces in the perpetration of intimate partner violence. *Review of General Psychology, 11*(2), 193–207.

Finkel, E. J., DeWall, C. N., Slotter, E. B., Oaten, M., & Foshee, V. A. (2009). Self-regulatory failure and intimate partner violence perpetration. *Journal of Personality and Social Psychology, 97*(3), 483–499.

First, M. B., Williams, J. B., Karg, R. S., & Spitzer, R. L. (2016). *User's guide for the SCID-5-CV Structured Clinical Interview for DSM-5® disorders: Clinical version.* American Psychiatric Publishing.

Foa, E. B., Asnaani, A., Zang, Y., Capaldi, S., & Yeh, R. (2018). Psychometrics of the Child PTSD Symptom Scale for DSM-5 for trauma-exposed children and adolescents. *Journal of Clinical Child and Adolescent Psychology, 47*(1), 38–46.

Fonagy, P. (2003). The developmental roots of violence in the failure of mentalization. In F. Pfäfflin & G. Adshead (Eds.), *A matter of security: The application of attachment theory to forensic psychiatry and psychotherapy* (pp. 13–56). Jessica Kingsley.

Fonagy, P., & Bateman, A. W. (2016). Adversity, attachment, and mentalizing. *Comprehensive Psychiatry, 64*, 59–66.

Fonagy, P., Steele, M., Steele, H., Moran, G. S., & Higgitt, A. C. (1991). The capacity for understanding mental states: The reflective self in parent and child and its significance for security of attachment. *Infant Mental Health Journal, 12*(3), 201–218.

Forssell, A. M., & Cater, Å. (2015). Patterns in child–father contact after parental separation in a sample of child witnesses to intimate partner violence. *Journal of Family Violence, 30*(3), 339–349.

Fossati, A., Acquarini, E., Feeney, J. A., Borroni, S., Grazioli, F., Giarolli, L. E., . . . Maffei, C. (2009). Alexithymia and attachment insecurities in impulsive aggression. *Attachment and Human Development, 11*(2), 165–182.

Fox, G. L., & Benson, M. L. (2004). Violent men, bad dads?: Fathering profiles of men involved in intimate partner violence. In R. D. Day & M. E. Lamb (Eds.), *Conceptualizing and measuring father involvement* (pp. 359–384). Erlbaum.

Fox, G. L., Sayers, J., & Bruce, C. (2002). Beyond bravado: Redemption and rehabilitation in the fathering accounts of men who batter. *Marriage and Family Review, 32*(3–4), 137–163.

Franklin, C. A., & Kercher, G. A. (2012). The intergenerational transmission of intimate partner violence: Differentiating correlates in a random community sample. *Journal of Family Violence, 27*(3), 187–199.

Fuller-Thomson, E., Roane, J. L., & Brennenstuhl, S. (2016). Three types of adverse childhood experiences, and alcohol and drug dependence among adults: An investigation using population-based data. *Substance Use and Misuse, 51*(11), 1451–1461.

Gerhardt, M., Feng, X., Wu, Q., Hooper, E., Ku, S., & Chan, M. (2020). A naturalistic study of parental emotion socialization. *Journal of Family Psychology, 34*(2), 204–214.

Germine, L., Dunn, E. C., McLaughlin, K. A., & Smoller, J. W. (2015). Childhood adversity is associated with adult theory of mind and social affiliation, but not face processing. *PLOS One, 10*(6), e0129612.

Gerson, R., & McGoldrick, M. (1985). The computerized genogram. *Primary Care, 12*(3), 535–545.

Gillette, M. T., & Gudmunson, C. G. (2014). Processes linking father absence to educational attainment among African American females. *Journal of Research on Adolescence, 24*(2), 309–321.

Goodman, R. (2002). Strengths and Difficulties Questionnaire. In *Mental Health National Outcomes and Casemix Collection: Overview of Clinician-Rated and Consumer Self-Report Measures V1.50*. Mental Health and Suicide Prevention Branch, Department of Health and Ageing, Australia.

Gordon, D. M., Oliveros, A., Hawes, S. W., Iwamoto, D. K., & Rayford, B. S. (2012). Engaging fathers in child protection services: A review of factors and strategies across ecological systems. *Children and Youth Services Review, 34*(8), 1399–1417.

Gottman, J. M., & DeClaire, J. (2001). *The relationship cure: A five-step guide to strengthening your marriage, family, and friendships*. Harmony.

Gottman, J. M., Jacobson, N. S., Rushe, R. H., Shortt, J. W., Babcock, J., La Taillade, J. J., & Waltz, J. (1995). The relationship between heart rate reactivity, emotionally aggressive behaviour, and general violence in batterers. *Journal of Family Psychology, 9*(2), 227–248.

Graham-Bermann, S. A., Castor, L. E., Miller, L. E., & Howell, K. H. (2012). The impact of intimate partner violence and additional traumatic events on trauma symptoms and PTSD in preschool-aged children. *Journal of Traumatic Stress, 25*, 393–400.

Grasso, D. J., Felton, J. W., & Reid-Quinoñes, K. (2015). *Structured Trauma-Related Experiences and Symptoms Screener (STRESS)*. Unpublished measure.

Gratz, K. L., & Roemer, L. (2004). Multidimensional assessment of emotion regulation and dysregulation: Development, factor structure, and initial validation of the difficulties in emotion regulation scale. *Journal of Psychopathology and Behavioral Assessment, 26*, 41–54.

Greif, G. L., & Hegar, R. L. (1993). *Perspectives on parents who abduct their children: Windows on a limited sample* (OJJDP Juvenile Justice Bulletin, No. NCJ 157159). U.S. Department of Justice, Office of Justice Programs, Office of Juvenile Justice and Delinquency Prevention.

Grych, J. H., Jouriles, E. N., Swank, P. R., McDonald, R., & Norwood, W. D. (2000). Patterns of adjustment among children of battered women. *Journal of Consulting and Clinical Psychology, 68*(1), 84.

Halpern, S. C., Schuch, F. B., Scherer, J. N., Sordi, A. O., Pachado, M., Dalbosco, C., . . . Von Diemen, L. (2018). Child maltreatment and illicit substance abuse: A systematic review and meta-analysis of longitudinal studies. *Child Abuse Review, 27*(5), 344–360.

Hamby, S. (2013). *Battered women's protective strategies: Stronger than you know.* Oxford University Press.

Hamby, S., & Clark, S. (2012). The VIGOR: The Victim Inventory of Goals, Options and Risks: A safety planning tool to help survivors of violence assess their risk and decide how to cope. Retrieved November 6, 2022, from *www.ywcayork.org/wp-content/uploads/sites/51/website-safety-plan.pdf.*

Hamby, S., Finkelhor, D., Turner, H., & Ormrod, R. (2010). The overlap of witnessing partner violence with child maltreatment and other victimizations in a nationally representative survey of youth. *Child Abuse and Neglect, 34*(10), 734–741.

Hardesty, J. L., Crossman, K. A., Khaw, L., & Raffaelli, M. (2016). Marital violence and coparenting quality after separation. *Journal of Family Psychology, 30*(3), 320–330.

Hardesty, J. L., Khaw, L., Chung, G. H., & Martin, J. M. (2008). Coparenting relationships after divorce: Variations by type of marital violence and fathers' role differentiation. *Family Relations, 57*(4), 479–491.

Hardesty, J. L., Ogolsky, B. G., Raffaelli, M., Whittaker, A., Crossman, K. A., Haselschwerdt, M. L., . . . Khaw, L. (2017). Coparenting relationship trajectories: Marital violence linked to change and variability after separation. *Journal of Family Psychology, 31*(7), 844–854.

Hare, R. D. (2003). *The Psychopathy Checklist–Revised, second edition.* Multi-Health Systems.

Harper, C. C., & McLanahan, S. S. (2004). Father absence and youth incarceration. *Journal of Research on Adolescence, 14*(3), 369–397.

Hayes, S. C., Strosahl, K. D., & Wilson, K. G. (2009). *Acceptance and commitment therapy.* American Psychological Association.

Heatherton, T. F., & Wagner, D. D. (2011). Cognitive neuroscience of self-regulation failure. *Trends in Cognitive Sciences, 15*(3), 132–139.

Hein, T. C., & Monk, C. S. (2017). Research Review: Neural response to threat in children, adolescents, and adults after child maltreatment—A quantitative meta-analysis. *Journal of Child Psychology and Psychiatry, 58*(3), 222–230.

Henry, J. B., Julion, W. A., Bounds, D. T., & Sumo, J. N. (2020). Fatherhood matters: An integrative review of fatherhood intervention research. *Journal of School Nursing, 36*(1), 19–32.

Hohman, M. (2021). *Motivational interviewing in social work practice* (2nd ed.). Guilford Press.

Holtzworth-Munroe, A., & Hutchinson, G. (1993). Attributing negative intent to wife behavior: The attributions of maritally violent versus nonviolent men. *Journal of Abnormal Psychology, 102*(2), 206–211.

Holtzworth-Munroe, A., Meehan, J. C., Herron, K., Rehman, U., & Stuart, G. L. (2000). Testing the Holtzworth-Munroe and Stuart (1994) batterer typology. *Journal of Consulting and Clinical Psychology, 68*, 1000–1019.

Hooper, L. M., Stockton, P., Krupnick, J. L., & Green, B. L. (2011). Development, use, and psychometric properties of the Trauma History Questionnaire. *Journal of Loss and Trauma, 16*(3), 258–283.

Howell, K. H., Barnes, S. E., Miller, L. E., & Graham-Bermann, S. A. (2016). Developmental variations in the impact of intimate partner violence exposure during childhood. *Journal of Injury and Violence Research, 8*(1), 1–15.

Hunter, E. C., & Graham-Bermann, S. A. (2013). Intimate partner violence and child adjustment: Moderation by father contact? *Journal of Family Violence, 28*(5), 435–444.

Israel, E., & Stover, C. (2009). Intimate partner violence: The role of the relationship between perpetrators and children who witness violence. *Journal of Interpersonal Violence, 24*(10), 1755–1764.

Iwaoka-Scott, A. Y., & Lieberman, A. F. (2015). Moving from dyads to triads: Implementation of child–parent psychotherapy with fathers. *ZERO TO THREE, 35*(5), 18–24.

Iwata, B. A., Dorsey, M. F., Slifer, K. J., Bauman, K. E., & Richman, G. S. (1994). Toward a functional analysis of self-injury. *Journal of Applied Behavior Analysis, 27*(2), 197–209.

Jacobson, N. S., Gottman, J. M., & Shortt, J. W. (1995). The distinction between Type 1 and Type 2 batterers: Further considerations: Reply to Ornduff et al. (1995), Margolin et al. (1995), and Walker (1995). *Journal of Family Psychology, 9*(3), 272–279.

Jarvis, K. L., Gordon, E. E., & Novaco, R. W. (2005). Psychological distress of children and mothers in domestic violence emergency shelters. *Journal of Family Violence, 20*(6), 389–402.

Johnson, M. P. (2010). *A typology of domestic violence: Intimate terrorism, violent resistance, and situational couple violence.* University Press of New England.

Johnston, J. R., & Girdner, L. K. (2001, January). *Family abductors: Descriptive profiles and preventive interventions* (Juvenile Justice Bulletin, No. NCJ 182788). U.S. Department of Justice, Office of Justice Programs, Office of Juvenile Justice and Delinquency Prevention.

Jouriles, E. N., & McDonald, R. (2014). Intimate partner violence, coercive control, and child adjustment problems. *Journal of Interpersonal Violence, 30*(3), 459–474.

Jouriles, E. N., Rosenfield, D., McDonald, R., Vu, N. L., Rancher, C., & Mueller, V. (2018). Children exposed to intimate partner violence: Conduct problems, interventions, and partner contact with the child. *Journal of Clinical Child and Adolescent Psychology, 47*(3), 397–409.

Karakurt, G., Koç, E., Çetinsaya, E. E., Ayluçtarhan, Z., & Bolen, S. (2019). Meta-analysis and systematic review for the treatment of perpetrators of intimate partner violence. *Neuroscience and Biobehavioral Reviews, 105*, 220–230.

Kaufman, E. A., Xia, M., Fosco, G., Yaptangco, M., Skidmore, C. R., & Crowell, S. E. (2016). The Difficulties in Emotion Regulation Scale Short Form (DERS-SF): Validation and replication in adolescent and adult samples. *Journal of Psychopathology and Behavioral Assessment, 38*, 443–455.

Kelly, J. B., & Lamb, M. E. (2000). Using child development research to make appropriate custody and access decisions for young children. *Family Court Review, 38*(3), 297–311.

Kennedy, H., Landor, M., & Todd, L. (2011). *Video interaction guidance.* Jessica Kingsley.

Kiesel, L. R., Piescher, K. N., & Edleson, J. L. (2016). The relationship between child maltreatment, intimate partner violence exposure, and academic performance. *Journal of Public Child Welfare, 10*(4), 434–456.

Kistenmacher, B. R., & Weiss, R. L. (2008). Motivational interviewing as a mechanism for change in men who batter: A randomized controlled trial. *Violence and Victims, 23*(5), 558–570.

Kitzmann, K. M., Gaylord, N. K., Holt, A. R., & Kenny, E. D. (2003). Child witnesses to domestic violence: A meta-analytic review. *Journal of Consulting and Clinical Psychology, 71*(2), 339.

Kolko, D. J. (1996). Individual cognitive behavioral treatment and family therapy for physically abused children and their offending parents: A comparison of clinical outcomes. *Child Maltreatment, 1*(4), 322–342.

Kolko, D. J., Baumann, B. L., Herschell, A. D., Hart, J. A., Holden, E. A., & Wisniewski, S. R. (2012). Implementation of AF-CBT by community practitioners serving child welfare and mental health: A randomized trial. *Child Maltreatment, 17*(1), 32–46.

Kolko, D. J., Herschell, A. D., Baumann, B. L., Hart, J. A., & Wisniewski, S. R. (2018). AF-CBT for families experiencing physical aggression or abuse served by the mental health or child welfare system: An effectiveness trial. *Child Maltreatment, 23*(4), 319–333.

Kugler, K. C., Guastaferro, K., Shenk, C. E., Beal, S. J., Zadzora, K. M., & Noll, J. G. (2019). The effect of substantiated and unsubstantiated investigations of child maltreatment and subsequent adolescent health. *Child Abuse and Neglect, 87*, 112–119.

Labarre, M., Bourassa, C., Holden, G. W., Turcotte, P., & Letourneau, N. (2016). Intervening with fathers in the context of intimate partner violence: An analysis of ten programs and suggestions for a research agenda. *Journal of Child Custody, 13*(1), 1–29.

Lamb, K., Humphreys, C., & Hegarty, K. (2018). "Your behaviour has consequences": Children and young people's perspectives on reparation with their fathers after domestic violence. *Children and Youth Services Review, 88*, 164–169.

Langhinrichsen-Rohling, J., Misra, T. A., Selwyn, C., & Rohling, M. L. (2012). Rates of bidirectional versus unidirectional intimate partner violence across samples, sexual orientations, and race/ethnicities: A comprehensive review. *Partner Abuse, 3*(2), 199–230.

Lanier, P., Jonson-Reid, M., Stahlschmidt, M. J., Drake, B., & Constantino, J. (2010). Child maltreatment and pediatric health outcomes: A longitudinal study of low-income children. *Journal of Pediatric Psychology, 35*(5), 511–522.

Lawrence, E., Langer Zarling, A., & Orengo-Aguayo, R. (2014). *Achieving change through value-based behavior (ACTV)*. University of Iowa Foundation.

Lawrence, S. K., Watson, J., & Stepteau-Watson, D. (2013). President Obama and the fatherhood initiative. *Race, Gender & Class, 20*(3–4), 98–113.

Lerner, C. F., & Kennedy, L. T. (2000). Stay–leave decision making in battered women: Trauma, coping and self-efficacy. *Cognitive Therapy and Research, 24*, 215–232.

Lieberman, A. F., Ippen, C. G., & Van Horn, P. (2006). Child-parent psychotherapy: 6-month follow-up of a randomized controlled trial. *Journal of the American Academy of Child and Adolescent Psychiatry, 45*(8), 913–918.

Lieberman, A. F., Ippen, C. G., & Van Horn, P. (2015). *"Don't hit my mommy!":*

A manual for child–parent psychotherapy with young children exposed to violence and other trauma. ZERO TO THREE.

Lieberman, A. F., & Van Horn, P. (2011). *Psychotherapy with infants and young children: Repairing the effects of stress and trauma on early attachment.* Guilford Press.

Lieberman, A. F., Van Horn, P., & Ghosh Ippen, C. (2005). Toward evidence-based treatment: Child–parent psychotherapy with preschoolers exposed to marital violence. *Journal of the American Academy of Child and Adolescent Psychiatry, 44*(12), 1241–1248.

Linehan, M. M. (2020). *Dialectical behavior therapy in clinical practice.* Guilford Press.

Liston, C., McEwen, B. S., & Casey, B. J. (2009). Psychosocial stress reversibly disrupts prefrontal processing and attentional control. *Proceedings of the National Academy of Sciences of the USA, 106*(3), 912–917.

Lupien, S. J., Parent, S., Evans, A. C., Tremblay, R. E., Zelazo, P. D., Corbo, V., . . . Séguin, J. R. (2011). Larger amygdala but no change in hippocampal volume in 10-year-old children exposed to maternal depressive symptomatology since birth. *Proceedings of the National Academy of Sciences of the USA, 108*(34), 14324–14329.

Luyten, P., Mayes, L. C., Nijssens, L., & Fonagy, P. (2017). The Parental Reflective Functioning Questionnaire: Development and preliminary validation. *PLOS One, 12*(5), e0176218.

Madigan, S., Cyr, C., Eirich, R., Fearon, R. P., Ly, A., Rash, C., . . . Alink, L. R. (2019). Testing the cycle of maltreatment hypothesis: Meta-analytic evidence of the intergenerational transmission of child maltreatment. *Development and Psychopathology, 31*(1), 23–51.

Maiuro, R. D., & Murphy, C. (Eds.). (2009). *Motivational interviewing and stages of change in intimate partner violence.* Springer.

Maldonado, A. I., & Murphy, C. M. (2021). Readiness to change as a predictor of treatment engagement and outcome for partner violent men. *Journal of Interpersonal Violence, 36*(7–8), 3041–3064.

Maliken, A. C., & Fainsilber Katz, L. (2013). Fathers' emotional awareness and children's empathy and externalizing problems: The role of intimate partner violence. *Journal of Interpersonal Violence, 28*(4), 718–734.

Maneta, E. K., White, M., & Mezzacappa, E. (2017). Parent–child aggression, adult–partner violence, and child outcomes: A prospective, population-based study. *Child Abuse and Neglect, 68*, 1–10.

Martin, A. J., Berenson, K. R., Griffing, S., Sage, R. E., Madry, L., Bingham, L. E., & Primm, B. J. (2000). The process of leaving an abusive relationship: The role of risk assessments and decision-certainty. *Journal of Family Violence, 15*, 109.

Mathews, B., & Kenny, M. C. (2008). Mandatory reporting legislation in the United States, Canada, and Australia: A cross-jurisdictional review of key features, differences, and issues. *Child Maltreatment, 13*(1), 50–63.

Mathwasa, J., & Okeke, C. I. O. (2016). Barriers educators face in involving fathers in the education of their children at the foundation phase. *Journal of Social Sciences, 46*(3), 229–240.

Maxwell, N., Scourfield, J., Featherstone, B., Holland, S., & Tolman, R. M.

(2012). Engaging fathers in child welfare services: A narrative review of recent research evidence. *Child and Family Social Work, 17*(2), 160–169.

McHale, J. P., Stover, C. S., Dubé, C., Sirotkin, Y. S., Lewis, S., & McKay, K. (2022). A culturally grounded prenatal coparenting intervention: Results of a randomized controlled trial with unmarried Black parents. *Journal of Family Psychology, 36*(4), 479.

McLanahan, S., Tach, L., & Schneider, D. (2013). The causal effects of father absence. *Annual Review of Sociology, 39*, 399–427.

McLellan, T. A., Kushner, H., Metzger, D., Peters, R., Smith, I., Grissom, G., . . . Argeriou, M. (1992). Addiction Severity Index—fifth edition. *Journal of Substance Abuse Treatment, 9*(3), 199–213.

McNeil, C. B., & Hembree-Kigin, T. L. (2011). *Parent–child interaction therapy* (2nd ed.). Springer.

McTavish, J. R., MacGregor, J. C. D., Wathen, C. N., & MacMillan, H. L. (2016). Children's exposure to intimate partner violence: An overview. *International Review of Psychiatry, 28*(5), 504–518.

Meehan, J. C., Holtzworth-Munroe, A., & Herron, K. (2001). Maritally violent men's heart rate reactivity to marital interactions: A failure to replicate the Gottman et al. (1995) typology. *Journal of Family Psychology, 15*(3), 394–408.

Miller, W. R., & Rollnick, S. (2023). *Motivational interviewing: Helping people change and grow* (4th ed.). Guilford Press.

Mohaupt, H., & Duckert, F. (2016). Parental reflective functioning in fathers who use intimate partner violence: Findings from a Norwegian clinical sample. *Nordic Psychology, 68*(4), 272–286.

Mohaupt, H., Duckert, F., & Askeland, I. R. (2021). How do memories of having been parented relate to the parenting-experience of fathers in treatment for intimate partner violence?: A phenomenological analysis. *Journal of Family Violence, 36*(4), 467–480.

Mueller, I., & Tronick, E. (2019). Early life exposure to violence: Developmental consequences on brain and behavior. *Frontiers in Behavioral Neuroscience, 13*, Article 156.

Nielsen, S. K., Hardesty, J. L., & Raffaelli, M. (2016). Exploring variations within situational couple violence and comparisons with coercive controlling violence and no violence/no control. *Violence Against Women, 22*(2), 206–224.

O'Farrell, T. J., & Fals-Stewart, W. (2000). Behavioral couples therapy for alcoholism and drug abuse. *Journal of Substance Abuse Treatment, 18*(1), 51–54.

O'Farrell, T. J., & Fals-Stewart, W. (2012). *Behavioral couples therapy for alcoholism and drug abuse*. Guilford Press.

O'Leary, K. D., Van Hasselt, V. B., Morrison, R. L., Bellack, A. S., & Hersen, M. (1988). Physical aggression between spouses: A social learning theory perspective. In V. B. Van Hasselt, R. L. Morrison, A. S. Bellack, & M. Hersen (Eds.), *Handbook of family violence* (pp. 31–55). Plenum Press.

Osofsky, J. D. (2003). Prevalence of children's exposure to domestic violence and child maltreatment: Implications for prevention and intervention. *Clinical Child and Family Psychology Review, 6*(3), 161–170.

Owen, A. E., Thompson, M. P., Shaffer, A., Jackson, E. B., & Kaslow, N. J. (2009). Family variables that mediate the relation between intimate partner violence (IPV) and child adjustment. *Journal of Family Violence, 24*, 433–445.

Paymar, M., & Barnes, G. (2007). *Countering confusion about the Duluth Model.* Domestic Abuse Intervention Programs.

Pence, E., & Paymar, M. (1993). *Education groups for men who batter: The Duluth Model.* Springer.

Perel, G., & Peled, E. (2008). The fathering of violent men: Constriction and yearning. *Violence Against Women, 14*(4), 457–482.

Poole, G. M., & Murphy, C. M. (2019). Fatherhood status as a predictor of intimate partner violence (IPV) treatment engagement. *Psychology of Violence, 9*(3), 340.

Porter, T. (n.d.). A call to men (TED talk). Retrieved January 9, 2022, from *www.ted.com/talks/tony_porter_a_call_to_men.*

Reynolds, C. R., & Kamphaus, R. W. (2002). *The clinician's guide to the Behavior Assessment System for Children (BASC).* Guilford Press.

Rohner, R. P., Khaleque, A., & Cournoyer, D. E. (2005). Parental acceptance–rejection: Theory, methods, cross-cultural evidence, and implications. *Ethos, 33*(3), 299–334.

Rollè, L., Gullotta, G., Trombetta, T., Curti, L., Gerino, E., Brustia, P., & Caldarera, A. M. (2019). Father involvement and cognitive development in early and middle childhood: A systematic review. *Frontiers in Psychology, 10*, Article 2405.

Rothenberg, B. (2003). "We don't have time for social change": Cultural compromise and the battered woman syndrome. *Gender and Society, 17*(5), 771–787.

Rothman, E. F., Mandel, D. G., & Silverman, J. G. (2007). Abusers' perceptions of the effect of their intimate partner violence on children. *Violence Against Women, 13*(11), 1179–1191.

Salisbury, E. J., Henning, K., & Holdford, R. (2009). Fathering by partner-abusive men: Attitudes on children's exposure to interparental conflict and risk factors for child abuse. *Child Maltreatment, 14*(3), 232–242.

Saunders, D. G. (1996). Feminist-cognitive-behavioral and process-psychodynamic treatments for men who batter: Interaction of abuser traits and treatment models. *Violence and Victims, 11*(4), 393–414.

Saunders, J. B., & Babor, T. F. (1993). AUDIT questionnaire. *Addiction, 88*, 791–804.

Scheeringa, M. S. (2019). Development of a brief screen for symptoms of posttraumatic stress disorder in young children: The Young Child PTSD Screen (YCPS). *Journal of Developmental and Behavioral Pediatrics, 40*(2), 105–111.

Scher, C. D., Stein, M. B., Asmundson, G. J., McCreary, D. R., & Forde, D. R. (2001). The childhood trauma questionnaire in a community sample: Psychometric properties and normative data. *Journal of Traumatic Stress, 14*(4), 843–857.

Scott, K. L., & Crooks, C. V. (2007). Preliminary evaluation of an intervention program for maltreating fathers. *Brief Treatment and Crisis Intervention, 7*(3), 224.

Scott, K., Francis, K., Crooks, C., & Kelly, T. (2006). *Caring dads: Helping fathers value their children.* Trafford.

Scott, K. L., & Lishak, V. (2012). Intervention for maltreating fathers: Statistically and clinically significant change. *Child Abuse and Neglect, 36*(9), 680–684.

Scott, K. L., & Wolfe, D. A. (2003). Readiness to change as a predictor of outcome in batterer treatment. *Journal of Consulting and Clinical Psychology, 71*(5), 879.

Semiatin, J. N., Murphy, C. M., & Elliott, J. D. (2013). Observed behavior during group treatment for partner-violent men: Acceptance of responsibility and promotion of change. *Psychology of Violence, 3*(2), 126–139.

Shepard, M. F., & Campbell, J. A. (1992). The Abusive Behavior Inventory: A measure of psychological and physical abuse. *Journal of Interpersonal Violence, 7*(3), 291–305.

Shipman, K. L., & Zeman, J. (1999). Emotional understanding: A comparison of physically maltreating and nonmaltreating mother–child dyads. *Journal of Clinical Child Psychology, 28*(3), 407–417.

Siegel, J. M. (1986). The Multidimensional Anger Inventory. *Journal of Personality and Social Psychology, 51*(1), 191.

Siegel, J. P. (2013). Breaking the links in intergenerational violence: An emotional regulation perspective. *Family Process, 52*(2), 163–178.

Silove, D. (1998). Is posttraumatic stress disorder an overlearned survival response?: An evolutionary-learning hypothesis. *Psychiatry, 61*(2), 181–190.

Simmons, C., Steinberg, L., Frick, P. J., & Cauffman, E. (2018). The differential influence of absent and harsh fathers on juvenile delinquency. *Journal of Adolescence, 62*, 9–17.

Singh, A., Yeh, C. J., & Blanchard, S. B. (2017). Ages and Stages Questionnaire: A global screening scale. *Boletín Médico del Hospital Infantil de México* (English Edition), *74*(1), 5–12.

Skinner, H. (1982). The Drug Abuse Screening Test. *Addictive Behaviour, 7*, 363–371.

Slade, A. (2005). Parental reflective functioning: An introduction. *Attachment and Human Development, 7*(3), 269–281.

Slade, A., Aber, J. L., Bresgi, I., Berger, B., & Kaplan, M. (2004). *The Parent Development Interview—Revised*. Unpublished protocol, The City University of New York, New York, New York.

Snyder, D. K., Klein, M. A., Gdowski, C. L., Faulstich, C., & LaCombe, J. (1988). Generalized dysfunction in clinic and nonclinic families: A comparative analysis. *Journal of Abnormal Child Psychology, 16*(1), 97–109.

Spilsbury, J. C., Kahana, S., Drotar, D., Creeden, R., Flannery, D. J., & Friedman, S. (2008). Profiles of behavioral problems in children who witness domestic violence. *Violence and Victims, 23*(1), 3–17.

Stith, S. M., McCollum, E. E., & Rosen, K. H. (2011). *Couples therapy for domestic violence: Finding safe solutions*. American Psychological Association.

Stith, S. M., Rosen, K. H., Middleton, K. A., Busch, A. L., Lundeberg, K., & Carlton, R. P. (2000). The intergenerational transmission of spouse abuse: A meta-analysis. *Journal of Marriage and Family, 62*(3), 640–654.

Stover, C. S. (2013). Fathers for change: A new approach to working with fathers who perpetrate intimate partner violence. *Journal of the American Academy of Psychiatry and the Law, 41*(1), 65.

Stover, C. S. (2015a). Fathers for Change for substance use and intimate partner violence: Initial Community Pilot. *Family Process, 54*(4), 600–609.

Stover, C. S. (2015b). Throw-away dads?: Promoting healthy father–child attachment in families affected by intimate partner violence. *ZERO TO THREE, 35*(5), 36–42.

Stover, C. S., Beebe, R., Clough, M., DiVietro, S., Madigan, L., & Grasso, D. J. (2022). Evaluation of a statewide implementation of Fathers for Change: A fathering intervention for families impacted by partner violence. *Journal of Family Violence, 37*, 449–459.

Stover, C. S., Carlson, M., & Patel, S. (2017). Integrating intimate partner violence and parenting intervention into residential substance use disorder treatment for fathers. *Journal of Substance Abuse Treatment, 81*, 35–43.

Stover, C. S., Carlson, M., Patel, S., & Manalich, R. (2018). Where's Dad?: The importance of integrating fatherhood and parenting programming into substance use treatment for men.*Child Abuse Review, 27*(4), 280–300.

Stover, C. S., Easton, C. J., & McMahon, T. J. (2013). Parenting of men with co-occurring intimate partner violence and substance abuse. *Journal of Interpersonal Violence, 28*(11), 2290–2314.

Stover, C. S., Ippen, C. G., Liang, L. J., Briggs, E. C., & Berkowitz, S. J. (2019). An examination of partner violence, polyexposure, and mental health functioning in a sample of clinically referred youth. *Psychology of Violence, 9*(3), 359–369.

Stover, C. S., & Kahn, M. (2013). Family of origin influences on the parenting of men with co-occurring substance abuse and intimate partner violence. *Advances in Dual Diagnosis, 6*(2), 84–94.

Stover, C. S., & Kiselica, A. J. (2014). An initial examination of the association of reflective functioning to parenting of fathers. *Infant Mental Health Journal, 35*(5), 452–461.

Stover, C. S., & Lent, K. (2014). Training and certification for domestic violence service providers: The need for a national standard curriculum and training approach. *Psychology of Violence, 4*(2), 117–127.

Stover, C. S., McMahon, T. J., & Moore, K. (2019). A randomized pilot trial of two parenting interventions for fathers in residential substance use disorder treatment. *Journal of Substance Abuse Treatment, 104*, 116–127.

Stover, C. S., Meadows, A. L., & Kaufman, J. (2009). Interventions for intimate partner violence: Review and implications for evidence-based practice. *Professional Psychology: Research and Practice, 40*(3), 223–233.

Stover, C., & Spink, A. (2012). Affective awareness in parenting of fathers with co-occurring substance abuse and intimate partner violence. *Advances in Dual Diagnosis, 5*(2), 74–85.

Stover, C. S., Van Horn, P., & Lieberman, A. F. (2006). Parental representations in the play of preschool aged witnesses of marital violence. *Journal of Family Violence, 21*, 417–424.

Stover, C. S., Van Horn, P., Turner, R., Cooper, B., & Lieberman, A. F. (2003). The effects of father visitation on preschool-aged witnesses of domestic violence. *Journal of Interpersonal Violence, 18*(10), 1149–1166.

Taft, C. T., Macdonald, A., Monson, C. M., Walling, S. M., Resick, P. A., & Murphy, C. M. (2013). "Strength at Home" group intervention for military populations engaging in intimate partner violence: Pilot findings. *Journal of Family Violence, 28*(3), 225–231.

Taft, C. T., Murphy, C. M., King, D. W., Musser, P. H., & DeDeyn, J. M. (2003).

Process and treatment adherence factors in group cognitive-behavioral therapy for partner violent men. *Journal of Consulting and Clinical Psychology, 71*(4), 812–820.

Taft, C. T., Vogt, D. S., Marshall, A. D., Panuzio, J., & Niles, B. L. (2007). Aggression among combat veterans: Relationships with combat exposure and symptoms of posttraumatic stress disorder, dysphoria, and anxiety. *Journal of Traumatic Stress, 20*(2), 135–145.

Taubner, S., White, L. O., Zimmermann, J., Fonagy, P., & Nolte, T. (2013). Attachment-related mentalization moderates the relationship between psychopathic traits and proactive aggression in adolescence. *Journal of Abnormal Child Psychology, 41*(6), 929–938.

Teicher, M. H., Anderson, C. M., Ohashi, K., Khan, A., McGreenery, C. E., Bolger, E. A., . . . Vitaliano, G. D. (2018). Differential effects of childhood neglect and abuse during sensitive exposure periods on male and female hippocampus. *NeuroImage, 169*, 443–452.

Teicher, M. H., Dumont, N. L., Ito, Y., Vaituzis, C., Giedd, J. N., & Andersen, S. L. (2004). Childhood neglect is associated with reduced corpus callosum area. *Biological Psychiatry, 56*(2), 80–85.

Teubert, D., & Pinquart, M. (2010). The association between coparenting and child adjustment: A meta-analysis. *Parenting: Science and Practice, 10*(4), 286–307.

Thibodeau, M.-E., Lavoie, F., Hébert, M., & Blais, M. (2017). Childhood maltreatment and adolescent sexual risk behaviors: Unique, cumulative and interactive effects. *Child Abuse and Neglect, 72*, 411–420.

Thompson-Walsh, C. A., Scott, K. L., Dyson, A., & Lishak, V. (2018). Are we in this together?: Post-separation co-parenting of fathers with and without a history of domestic violence. *Child Abuse Review, 27*(2), 137–149.

Toth, S. L., Maughan, A., Manly, J. T., Spagnola, M., & Cicchetti, D. (2002). The relative efficacy of two interventions in altering maltreated preschool children's representational models: Implications for attachment theory. *Development and Psychopathology, 14*(4), 877–908.

Treleaven, D. A. (2018). *Trauma-sensitive mindfulness: Practices for safe and transformative healing.* Norton.

Turner, H. A., Finkelhor, D., & Ormrod, R. (2010). Poly-victimization in a national sample of children and youth. *American Journal of Preventive Medicine, 38*(3), 323–330.

Velotti, P., Rogier, G., Beomonte Zobel, S., Chirumbolo, A., & Zavattini, G. C. (2022). The relation of anxiety and avoidance dimensions of attachment to intimate partner violence: A meta-analysis about perpetrators. *Trauma, Violence, and Abuse, 23*(1), 196–212.

Voith, L. A., Logan-Greene, P., Strodthoff, T., & Bender, A. E. (2020). A paradigm shift in batterer intervention programming: A need to address unresolved trauma. *Trauma, Violence, and Abuse, 21*(4), 691–705.

Waterman, E. A., & Lefkowitz, E. S. (2017). Are mothers' and fathers' parenting characteristics associated with emerging adults' academic engagement? *Journal of Family Issues, 38*(9), 1239–1261.

Weathers, F. W., Litz, B. T., Herman, D. S., Huska, J. A., & Keane, T. M. (1993, October). *The PTSD Checklist (PCL): Reliability, validity, and diagnostic utility*. Paper presented at the ninth annual convention of the International Society for Traumatic Stress Studies, San Antonio, Texas.

Wei, M. F., Russell, D. W., Mallinckrodt, B., & Vogel, D. L. (2007). The experiences in Close Relationship Scale (ECR)–Short form: Reliability, validity, and factor structure. *Journal of Personality Assessment, 88*(2), 187–204.

Whitaker, D. J., Haileyesus, T., Swahn, M., & Saltzman, L. S. (2007). Differences in frequency of violence and reported injury between relationships with reciprocal and nonreciprocal intimate partner violence. *American Journal of Public Health, 97*(5), 941–947.

White, R. J., & Gondolf, E. W. (2000). Implications of personality profiles for batterer treatment. *Journal of Interpersonal Violence, 15*(5), 467–488.

Whittle, S., Dennison, M., Vijayakumar, N., Simmons, J. G., Yücel, M., Lubman, D. I., . . . Allen, N. B. (2013). Childhood maltreatment and psychopathology affect brain development during adolescence. *Journal of the American Academy of Child and Adolescent Psychiatry, 52*(9), 940–952.

Wilson, H. W., Stover, C. S., & Berkowitz, S. J. (2009). Research Review: The relationship between childhood violence exposure and juvenile antisocial behavior: A meta-analytic review. *Journal of Child Psychology and Psychiatry, 50*(7), 769–779.

Winters, K. C., Botzet, A. M., Fahnhorst, T., Baumel, L., & Lee, S. (2008). Impulsivity and its relationship to risky sexual behaviors and drug abuse. *Journal of Child and Adolescent Substance Abuse, 18*(1), 43–56.

Witkiewitz, K., & Villarroel, N. A. (2009). Dynamic association between negative affect and alcohol lapses following alcohol treatment. *Journal of Consulting and Clinical Psychology, 77*, 633–644.

Wood, S. L., & Sommers, M. S. (2011). Consequences of intimate partner violence on child witnesses: A systematic review of the literature. *Journal of Child and Adolescent Psychiatric Nursing, 24*(4), 223–236.

Wride, A. (2020). *Classifying intimate partner violence: A functional typology*. Unpublished thesis, Victoria University of Wellington.

Yoman, J. (2008). A primer on functional analysis. *Cognitive and Behavioral Practice, 15*(3), 325–340.

Zarling, A., Bannon, S., & Berta, M. (2019). Evaluation of acceptance and commitment therapy for domestic violence offenders. *Psychology of Violence, 9*(3), 257–266.

Zinzow, H. M., Ruggiero, K. J., Resnick, H., Hanson, R., Smith, D., Saunders, B., & Kilpatrick, D. (2009). Prevalence and mental health correlates of witnessed parental and community violence in a national sample of adolescents. *Journal of Child Psychology and Psychiatry, 50*(4), 441–450.

Zisser, A., & Eyberg, S. M. (2010). Parent–child interaction therapy and the treatment of disruptive behavior disorders. In J. R. Weisz & A. E. Kazdin (Eds.), *Evidence-based psychotherapies for children and adolescents* (pp. 179–193). Guilford Press.

Zvara, B. J., & Mills-Koonce, R. (2021). Intimate partner violence, parenting, and children's representations of caregivers. *Journal of Interpersonal Violence, 36*(21–22), NP11756–NP11779.

Index

Note. f or *t* after a page number indicates a figure or a table.

Prof. József Verhás, D.Sc. (1939–2020)

The present Special Issue is dedicated to the memory of our beloved, respected friend, colleague and teacher, the late Professor József Verhas.

Prof. Verhás played a pioneering role in establishing and strengthening the Hungarian tradition of thermodynamics.

He was active both scientifically and socially, having membership in the Roland Eötvös Physical Society, the János Bolyai Mathematical Society, the International Society for the Interaction of Mechanics and Mathematics, and in the Editorial Advisory Board of *Journal of Non-Equilibrium Thermodynamics*. He was also a member of the Accademia Peloritana dei Pericolanti.

Prof. Verhás was a master of irreversible thermodynamics with extremely broad interests and knowledge. He contributed to the progress of the variational principles of irreversible thermodynamics and wave theory of thermodynamics, and introduced the concept of dynamic degrees of freedom and developed the nonequilibrium thermodynamic theory of liquid crystals.
He also worked on the theory of cellular division, turbulence, plasticity, and in many other applications and areas of irreversible thermodynamics.

The Kluitenberg-Verhás body and the rheological Verhás element bear his name, in honor of his work in elaborating the thermodynamic basis of rheology.

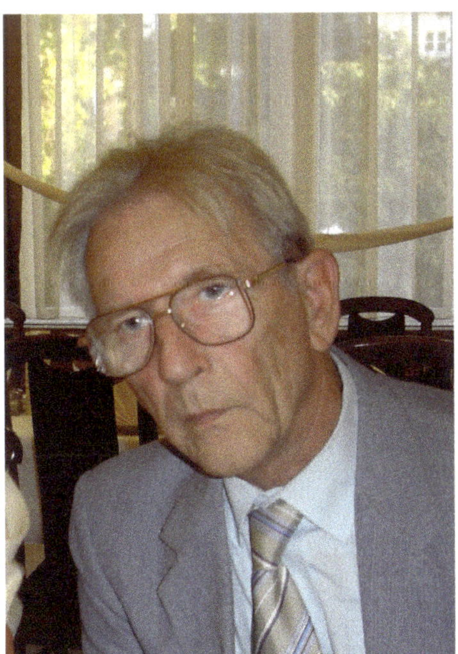

Contents

About the Special Issue Editors

Róbert Kovács graduated with a degree in Mechanical Engineering in 2015 before attaining his Ph.D. in 2017 from Budapest University of Technology and Economics (BME) in collaboration with the Hungarian Academy of Sciences. He is currently working on continuum thermodynamics, both experimental and theoretical problems, including the development of numerical schemes, analytical solutions of evolution equations, and other mathematical aspects. He has been a Visiting Researcher at Northeastern University, MA, USA; Messina University, Sicily, Italy; and Université du Québec à Chicoutimi, Québec, Canada.

Antonio M. Scarfone is a theoretical physics researcher working mainly in the field of statistical mechanics. He graduated from University of Torino in 1996 and completed his Ph.D. in Physics at Politecnico of Torino in 2000. He has been a Postdoctoral Researcher at INFM (2000–2002) and received a Research Fellowship at the University of Cagliari in 2003. Since 2004, he has carried out research activities at CNR-ISC based in Politecnico of Torino. To date, he has authored approximately 100 scientific papers published in international journals on the topics of statistical mechanics, kinetic theory, geometry information, nonlinear classical and quantum dynamics, and noncommutative algebras. He is Editor-in-Chief of the Section Statistical Physics of *Entropy*, a member of the Editorial Board of *Advances in Mathematical Physics*, and belongs to the advisory panel of *Journal of Physics A*. Finally, he is one of the organizers of the SigmaPhi international conference series that has been held every three years starting from 2005.

Sumiyoshi Abe has recently been serving as Full Professor at Mie University in Japan until March 2020. Currently, he is a Visiting Professor at Huaqiao University in China, Kazan Federal University in Russia, Turin Polytechnic University in Tashkent in Uzbekistan, and ESIEA in France.

entropy

MDPI

Editorial

Entropy and Non-Equilibrium Statistical Mechanics

Róbert Kovács [1,2,3,*], Antonio M. Scarfone [4] and Sumiyoshi Abe [5,6,7,8]

1 Department of Energy Engineering, Faculty of Mechanical Engineering, Budapest University of Technology and Economics, 1111 Budapest, Hungary
2 Department of Theoretical Physics, Wigner Research Centre for Physics, Konkoly-Thege M. 29-33, 1121 Budapest, Hungary
3 Montavid Thermodynamic Research Group, 1112 Budapest, Hungary
4 Istituto dei Sistemi Complessi, Consiglio Nazionale delle Ricerche (ISC-CNR), c/o, Politecnico di Torino, Corso Duca degli Abruzzi 24, I-10129 Torino, Italy; antonio.scarfone@polito.it
5 Physics Division, College of Information Science and Engineering, Huaqiao University, Xiamen 361021, China; suabe@sf6.so-net.ne.jp
6 Institute of Physics, Kazan Federal University, 420008 Kazan, Russia
7 Department of Natural and Mathematical Sciences, Turin Polytechnic University in Tashkent, Tashkent 100095, Uzbekistan
8 ESIEA, 9 Rue Vesale, 75005 Paris, France
* Correspondence: kovacs.robert@wigner.mta.hu

Received: 24 April 2020; Accepted: 27 April 2020; Published: 29 April 2020

Keywords: non-equilibrium phenomena; kinetic theory; second law of thermodynamics; statistical distributions; stochastic processes

---

The present Special Issue, 'Entropy and Non-Equilibrium Statistical Mechanics', consists of seven original research papers. Although the issue has a long history, still it remains as one of the most fundamental subjects in physics. These seven papers actually cover various latest relevant topics, ranging from gravity as an entropic force to exotic statistics, including conservation laws, dynamics generated by entropy production, quantum measurements and the limits on the constitutive laws in classical gaseous systems.

We hope that the Special Issue will be able to play a role in further progress to come in the future.

In this paper, 'Classical Model of Quons', by G. Kaniadakis and A. M Scarfone [1] by using a kinetic interaction principle an evolution equation describing quons statistics is proposed by properly generalizing the inclusion/exclusion principle of standard boson and fermion statistics. In this way, a nonlinear Fokker-Planck equation for quons particles of type I and type II is introduced and the corresponding steady distribution is derived.

The paper 'Statistics of the Bifurcation in Quantum Measurement', by K.-E. Eriksson and K. Lindgren [2], deals with a quantum measurement of a two-level system improving the already known methods, basing the analysis of the interaction with the measurement device on the quantum field theory. In this way, a microscopic details of the measurement apparatus affect the process so that it takes the eigenstates of the measured observable by recording the corresponding measurement result.

The paper written by R. Kovács [3] deals with the experiments on rarefied gases. The generalized system of Navier-Stokes-Fourier equations is presented, which is required to model the ballistic effects appearing in gases at low pressures. The experimental evaluation consists of the investigation of scaling properties of models originating from the kinetic theory and continuum thermodynamics, especially emphasizing the importance of mass density dependence of material properties.

In the paper 'A Note on the Entropy Force in Kinetic Theory and Black Holes' by R. A. Treumann and W. Baumjohann [4] is derived a kinetic equations of a large system of particles including a collective integral term to the Klimontovich equation for the evolution of the signle-particle distribution function. The integral character of this equation transforms the basic signle particle kinetics into an integro-differential equation showing that not only the microscopic forces but the hole system gets its probability distribution in a holistic way.

In their paper [5], motivated by the contact geometric structure in thermodynamics, V. Klika, M. Pavelka, P. Vágner, and M. Grmela present an approach to multilevel modeling based on the recognition that the state variables and their conjugate variables are independent. That procedure is called Dynamic MaxEnt, and demonstrated on various examples from continuum physics such as hyperbolic heat conduction and magnetohydrodynamics.

In the paper 'A Fourth Order Entropy Stable Scheme for Hyperbolic Conservation Laws' [6], Xiaohan Cheng presents the development of a numerical procedure with fourth order accuracy in order to solve hyperbolic system of partial differential equations of conservative form, for one-dimensional situations. Here, the novelty is to endow great importance for the entropy balance equation in updating the state variables, thus the numerical compatibility with the second law of thermodynamics is ensured. Its efficiency is demonstrated on several examples, e.g., on shock tubes and on the nonlinear Burgers equation.

In the paper [7], Ou, Yokoi and Abe note a possible diversity of baths in quantum thermodynamics. They discuss the isoenergetic processes in terms of the concept of weak invariants, where the time-dependent Hamiltonian is a weak invariant associated with a relevant master equation. In particular, they analyze as an explicit example the finite-time isoenergetic process of the nonequilibrium dissipative system of the Pauli spin in a varying external magnetic field based on the Lindblad master equation.

Acknowledgments: We would like to express our gratitude to the Editorial Board of Entropy for they helpful attitude and also to the Authors who made this Special Issue successful.

Conflicts of Interest: The authors declare no conflict of interest.

References

1. Kaniadakis, G.; Scarfone, A.M. Classical Model of Quons. *Entropy* **2019**, *21*, 841. [CrossRef]
2. Eriksson, K.-E.; Lindgren, K. Statistics of the Bifurcation in Quantum Measurement. *Entropy* **2019**, *21*, 834. [CrossRef]
3. Kovács, R. On the Rarefied Gas Experiments. *Entropy* **2019**, *21*, 718. [CrossRef]
4. Treumann, R.A.; Baumjohann, W. A Note on the Entropy Force in Kinetic Theory and Black Holes. *Entropy* **2019**, *21*, 716. [CrossRef]
5. Klika, V.; Pavelka, M.; Vágner, P.; Grmela, M. Dynamic Maximum Entropy Reduction. *Entropy* **2019**, *21*, 715. [CrossRef]
6. Cheng, X. A Fourth Order Entropy Stable Scheme for Hyperbolic Conservation Laws. *Entropy* **2019**, *21*, 508. [CrossRef]
7. Ou, C.; Yokoi, Y.; Abe, S. Spin Isoenergetic Process and the Lindblad Equation. *Entropy* **2019**, *21*, 503. [CrossRef]

entropy

MDPI

Article

Classical Model of Quons

Giorgio Kaniadakis [1,*] and Antonio M. Scarfone [2]

1 Dipartimento di Scienza Applicata e Tecnologia, Politecnico di Torino, Corso Duca degli Abruzzi 24, 10129 Torino, Italy
2 Istituto dei Sistemi Complessi, Consiglio Nazionale delle Ricerche (ISC-CNR), c/o Politecnico di Torino, Corso Duca degli Abruzzi 24, 10129 Torino, Italy
* Correspondence: giorgio.kaniadakis@polito.it; Tel.: +39-011-090-7331

Received: 29 July 2019; Accepted: 24 August 2019; Published: 27 August 2019

Abstract: By using the kinetic interaction principle, the quons statistics in the framework of kinetic theory is introduced. This is done by properly generalizing the inclusion/exclusion principle of standard boson and fermion statistics within a nonlinear classical model. The related nonlinear Fokker-Planck equation is introduced and the corresponding steady distribution describing quons statistics of type I and type II is derived.

Keywords: classical model of boson and fermion statistics; inclusion/exclusion principle; nonlinear Fokker-Planck equation; type I quon statistics; type II quon statistics

---

1. Introduction

As is well known, one of the most fundamental theorems in quantum field theory and in quantum statistical mechanics, at the basis of many physical and chemical phenomena, is the spin-statistics theorem stated by Pauli [1,2].

This theorem fixes the statistical behavior of a many-body quantum system according to its spin. Bosons are integer spin particles whose creation and annihilation operators obey bilinear commutation relations. Their many-body wave function is symmetrical and the occupation number of particle in a given state is unlimited. On the opposite side, fermions are half-integer spin particles whose creation and annihilation operators obey bilinear anti-commutation relations. Their many-body wave function is anti-symmetric and the occupation number of the particle in a given state can never exceed the unity.

Experimental tests [3–5] have placed a straight limit to the possible violations of this theorem so that, today, it is widely accepted that elementary particles can be only bosons or fermions.

However, statistical deviations from bosons or fermions can be observed in quasi-particle excitations that occur in various condensed matter systems. Therefore, the study of physical systems that obey non-conventional statistics is one of the pillars of contemporary statistical physics [6–12]. Their interest spans from the theoretical foundation of generalized statistical mechanics [13,14], Fermi gas superfluid [15], high-temperature gas [16] and high-T_c superconductivity [17], Laughlin particle with fractional charge related to fractional quantum Hall effect [18,19], Josephson junctions [20] and applications to quantum computation [21,22].

Basically, there are two different approaches to introduce non-conventional statistics. The first one is by modifying the bilinear algebraic relation between creation and annihilation operators and therefore the exchange factor between permuted particles. The second is by modifying the number of possible ways to put particles in a collection of single-particles state.

Within the first method we find: parastatistics [23], obtained by generalizing, respectively, the bilinear commutative and anti-commutative relation of creation annihilation operators in trilinear relation for para-Boson and para-Fermion; quons statistics of type I [24,25], with asymmetric q-numbers and type II [26,27], with symmetric q-numbers, obtained in the framework of q-deformed harmonic oscillator based on q-calculus [28]; fractional statistics of anyons [29–31] that are topological bi-dimensional quasi-particles derived in the framework of quantum groups arising from the study of quantum integrable systems and Yang-Baxter equation; Majorana fermions quasiparticles [32]; and Gentilionic statistics [33], obtained by using the permutation group theory with the indistinguishability principle of identical particles in the framework of non relativistic quantum mechanics.

Differently, within the second approaches we find: Haldane-Wu statistics [34,35], including semion [36], obtained by generalizing Pauli exclusion principle; intermediate statistics by Gentile [37], derived in a thermodynamical context by assuming that the maximum occupation particle number of an energy level is between one (standard fermions) and infinity (standard bosons); and more recently the interpolating boson-fermion statistics [38–42], used to study non relativistic quantum systems that obey to a generalized inclusion/exclusion principle, obtained by modifying the dependency of the transition probability from the occupation particle number of the starting and the arriving site [43,44].

In this paper, we propose an algebraic approach to introduce non-conventional statistics within a semiclassical kinetic framework. Following the kinetic interaction principle proposed in [43], which fixes the form of the transition probability $\pi(t, \mathbf{v}_i \to \mathbf{v}_{i+1})$ in such a way to take into account its dependence on the particle population of the starting site $a(f_i)$ and of the arrive site $b(f_{i+1})$, we obtain a nonlinear Fokker-Planck equation describing the particle evolution.

In standard boson and fermion statistics, the inclusion/exclusion principle is taken into account by the relation

$$b(f) \mp a(f) = 1 \,. \tag{1}$$

In fact, when, $a(f) = f$ is fixed, it follows $b(f) = 1 \pm f$, and the Bose (+) and Fermi (-) factors are obtained.

The relation (1) can be generalized in

$$b(f) \bigoplus a(f) = 1 \,, \tag{2}$$

where $x \bigoplus y$ is a deformed composition law, depending on a deformation parameter ξ, and is reduced to the standard sum and subtraction in a suitable limit $\xi \to \xi_0$. Equation (2) defines the functional dependence between $a(f)$ and $b(f)$, and fixes the steady particle distribution. The relationship between the generalized composition law $x \bigoplus y$ and the induced statistics is the main goal of this work.

The plane of the paper is as follows. In the next Section 2, we briefly recall the kinetic interaction principle used to introduce the nonlinear Fokker-Planck equation governing the time evolution of the particles system toward the equilibrium. Section 3 contains our main result. Non-conventional statistics are introduced by means of a generalized composition law between the functions $a(f)$ and $b(f)$, which introduces nonlinear terms in the Fokker-Planck equation and then modifies substantially its steady state solution. Several well known statistics can be easily derived within this algebraic approach and new statistics can be obtained through the introduction of suitable composition laws. This is discussed in the subsequent Sections 4 and 5, which introduce, within the present formalism, type II quons statistics and type I quons statistics, respectively. In the last Section 6 we report our conclusions.

2. The Exclusion-Inclusion Principle

Let us consider a classical stochastic Markovian process in the n-dimensional velocity space. It is described by the distribution function $f \equiv f(t, \mathbf{v})$ which obeys the Pauli master equation

$$\frac{\partial f}{\partial t} = \int \Big[\pi(t, \mathbf{v}' \to \mathbf{v}) - \pi(t, \mathbf{v} \to \mathbf{v}')\Big] \, d^n \mathbf{v}' \,. \tag{3}$$

According to the kinetic interaction principle the transition probability $\pi(t,\, \boldsymbol{v} \to \boldsymbol{v}')$, from the site $\boldsymbol{v}$ to the site $\boldsymbol{v}'$, can be written in

$$\pi(t,\, \boldsymbol{v} \to \boldsymbol{v}') = W(t;\, \boldsymbol{v},\, \boldsymbol{v}')\, a(f(\boldsymbol{v}))\, b(f(\boldsymbol{v}')) \,. \tag{4}$$

This quantity defines a special interaction between the particles of the system that involve, separately and/or together, the two-particle bunches entertained at the start and arrival sites. It is factorized into the product of three terms. The first term $W(t;\, \boldsymbol{v},\, \boldsymbol{v}')$ is the transition rate that depends on the nature of the interaction between the particles and the bath, and is a velocity function of the starting $\boldsymbol{v}$ and arrival $\boldsymbol{v}'$ sites. The second factor $a(f) \equiv a(f(\boldsymbol{v}))$ is an arbitrary function of the particle population of the starting site and satisfies the condition $a(0) = 0$ because, if the initial site is empty, the transition probability is equal to zero. Without loss of generality, we can always impose on $a(f)$ the further condition $a(1) = 1$ by re-scaling the function $a(f)$ and opportunely redefining the quantity $W(t;\, \boldsymbol{v},\, \boldsymbol{v}')$. The last factor $b(f) \equiv b(f(\boldsymbol{v}))$ is an arbitrary function of the arrival site population and satisfies the condition $b(0) = 1$ since the transition probability does not depend on the arrival site if, in it, particles are absent. The expression of the function $b(f)$ plays a very important role as it allows us to introduce a sort of inclusion/exclusion effect in the system stimulating or inhibiting the transition to the arrival site, as a consequence of the interactions originated from collective effects.

Accounting for Equation (4), by using the Kramer-Moyal expansion, the Pauli master equation can be transformed in the following Fokker-Planck equation

$$\frac{\partial f}{\partial t} = \boldsymbol{\nabla} \cdot \left[D\, a(f)\, b(f)\, \boldsymbol{\nabla} \left(\beta\, U + \ln \frac{a(f)}{b(f)} \right) \right] , \tag{5}$$

where $\boldsymbol{\nabla} \equiv (\partial/\partial v_1,\, \dots,\, \partial/\partial v_n)$ is the gradient operator in the velocity space, D is the diffusion coefficient, $\beta = 1/k_{\rm B}\, T$ the inverse temperature and $U = \frac{1}{2}\, m\, v^2$ is the single particle kinetic energy.

Equation (5) can be rewritten in

$$\frac{\partial f}{\partial t} = \boldsymbol{\nabla} \cdot \Big(D\, m\, \beta\, \gamma(f)\, \boldsymbol{v} + D\, \Omega(f)\, \boldsymbol{\nabla} f \Big) , \tag{6}$$

where

$$\gamma(f) = a(f)\, b(f) \,, \tag{7}$$

affects the drift current $j_{\rm drift} = D\, m\, \beta\, \gamma(f)\, \boldsymbol{v}$, while

$$\Omega(f) = b(f)\, \frac{\partial\, a(f)}{\partial f} - a(f)\, \frac{\partial\, b(f)}{\partial f} \,, \tag{8}$$

models the diffusion current $j_{\rm diff} = D\, \Omega(f)\, \boldsymbol{\nabla} f$. The functions $\gamma(f)$ and $\Omega(f)$ are scalar quantities depending only on $f(t,\, \boldsymbol{v})$. In this way, both drift and diffusion current depend, in a nonlinear manner, on the distribution function through the population of the starting and arrival site.

The stationary distribution of the system described by Equation (5) follows from the condition

$$\frac{\partial f}{\partial t} = 0 \,, \tag{9}$$

that, without loss of generality, implies the reletion

$$\beta\, U + \ln \frac{a(f)}{b(f)} = \beta\, \mu \,, \tag{10}$$

where μ is a constant. This last, can be rewritten in

$$\frac{a(f)}{b(f)} = e^{-\epsilon} \,. \tag{11}$$

which defines implicitly the statistical distribution of the steady state of the system, where $\epsilon = \beta\,(U-\mu)$, with μ the chemical potential fixed by the normalization of the distribution function.

As well known, Fokker-Planck equation (5) is strictly related to a generalized entropic form, as discussed in [43], so that the steady state obtained from Equation (11) can also be obtained starting from an optimizing program performed to the corresponding entropic form.

3. Generalized Exclusion-Inclusion Principle

The kinetics of already known statistics can be derived from ansatz (4) by choosing opportunely the functions $a(f)$ and $b(f)$. For instance, the bosons and fermions statistics follow, in the quasi-classical picture, by posing

$$a(f) = f \,, \tag{12}$$

$$b(f) = 1 \pm f \,. \tag{13}$$

The corresponding Fokker-Planck equation for quasi-classical Bose and Fermi particles reads

$$\frac{\partial f}{\partial t} = \boldsymbol{\nabla}\cdot\Big(D\,m\,\beta\,f\,(1\pm f)\,v + D\,\boldsymbol{\nabla} f\Big)\,, \tag{14}$$

that describes a drift-diffusion process with a constant diffusive current, being $\Omega(f) = 1$, and a nonlinear drift term. The corresponding steady state

$$f(\epsilon) = \frac{1}{e^{\epsilon} \mp 1}\,, \tag{15}$$

follows by solving Equation (11) with the position (12) and (13).

To go one step further and introduce more general statistics, let us observe that Equation (13) actually may be rewritten in the two equivalent forms

$$b(f) = 1 \pm a(f)\,, \tag{16}$$

or, alternatively

$$b(f) = a(1 \pm f)\,. \tag{17}$$

However, it is easy to see that, although both of these formulations are equivalent for $a(f) = f$, for another choice of $a(f)$ different from the identity, Equations (16) and (17) in general do not coincide.

To overcome this problem and have a consistent relationship between the functions $a(f)$ and $b(f)$, we introduce a generalized operation $x \oplus y$ to denote a new composition law between real numbers, hereinafter named deformed sum. It depends on a deformation parameter ξ such that the generalized sum $\oplus$ reduces to the ordinary sum $+$ in a suitable limit $\xi \to \xi_0$, that is $x \oplus y \to x + y$.

Reasonably, a deformed sum $x \oplus y$ should preserve the main proprieties of standard sum like commutativity, $x \oplus y = y \oplus x$; associativity $x \oplus (y \oplus z) = (x \oplus y) \oplus z$; the existence of neutral element $x \oplus 0^* = 0^* \oplus x = x$; the opposite $x \oplus \overline{x} = \overline{x} \oplus x = 0^*$, where, in general, $0^* \neq 0$ and $\overline{x} \neq -x$. Equipped with these properties, the algebraic structure $\mathcal{A} \equiv (\oplus : \Re \times \Re \to \Re)$ forms an Abelian group.

In this way, a deformed subtraction can be introduced as the inverse operation of the deformed sum, that is $x \ominus y \equiv x \oplus \overline{y}$.

Within the algebra $\mathcal{A}$, we can generalize Equations (16) and (17) in

$$b(f) = 1 \bigoplus a(f)\,, \tag{18}$$

$$b(f) = a(c \pm f)\,, \tag{19}$$

where c is a constant depending on the deformation parameter that must reduce to the identity in the $\xi \to \xi_0$ limit.

Consistently, by requiring that both Equations (18) and (19) define the same function $b(f)$ for any choice of $a(f)$, we obtain the following functional equation

$$1 \bigoplus a(f) = a(c \pm f)\,. \tag{20}$$

Thus, the generalized composition $\bigoplus$ fixes univocally the function $a(f)$. In fact, by posing

$$x \bigoplus y = a\left(a^{-1}(x) \pm a^{-1}(y)\right)\,, \tag{21}$$

we easily realize that Equations (18) and (19) coincide each to the other whenever we choose $c = a^{-1}(1)$.

According to definition (21), the neutral element is given by $0^* \equiv a(0)$ while the opposite is $\overline{x} \equiv a(-a^{-1}(x))$.

Clearly, Equation (20) imposes $a(f)$, and then $b(f)$, to depend on the deformation parameter too so that, as expected in the $\xi \to \xi_0$ limit, these functions behave like $a(f) \to f$ and $b(f) \to 1 \pm f$, respectively.

Notice also that ansatz (21) requires that $a(x)$ be a monotonic, and then invertible, function at least in the range $[0, 1]$ of a distribution function.

Based on the algebra $\mathcal{A}$, we can introduce several relevant generalized functions. Among them, the generalized exponential $E(x) \in \Re^+$, defined in

$$E(x) = \exp\left(a^{-1}(x)\right)\,, \tag{22}$$

that satisfies the relation

$$E(x \oplus y) = E(x)\,E(y)\,, \tag{23}$$

as well as its inverse function, the generalized logarithm $L(x)$ for $x \in \Re^+$, with $L(E(x)) = E(L(x)) = x$, defined in

$$L(x) = a\left(\ln(x)\right)\,, \tag{24}$$

that satisfies the dual relation

$$L(x\,y) = L(x) \oplus L(y)\,. \tag{25}$$

In the $\xi \to \xi_0$ limit, in which $\oplus$ reduces to the standard sum, both the functions $E(x)$ and $L(x)$ reduce to the standard exponential and logarithm, respectively and Equations (23) and (25) reproduce the well know algebraic relation of standard exponential and logarithm functions.

4. Type II Quons

Within the formalism introduced above, let us now derive some statistics starting from deformed algebras already proposed in literature.

To start with, let us consider the κ-sum [43] defined in

$$x \oplus y = x\,\sqrt{1+\kappa^2\,y^2} + y\,\sqrt{1+\kappa^2\,x^2}\,, \tag{26}$$

whose deformation parameter $\xi \equiv \kappa$ is limited to $|\kappa| \leq 1$ and the κ-sum recovers the standard sum in the $\kappa \to 0$ limit.

The above κ-sum is the momenta relativistic additivity law of special relativity and plays a central role in the construction of κ-statistical mechanics [45].

According to Equation (21), the function $a(x)$ should be determined from the relation

$$a^{-1}(x \oplus y) = a^{-1}(x) + a^{-1}(y) \,. \tag{27}$$

In order to solve this functional equation we use the following identity

$$x = \frac{1}{\kappa} \sinh\left(\mathrm{arcsinh}\,(\kappa\, x)\right) \,, \tag{28}$$

in the r.h.s. of Equation (26) that becomes

$$\begin{aligned} x \oplus y &= \frac{1}{\kappa} \sinh\Big(\mathrm{arcsinh}\,(\kappa\, x)\Big) \sqrt{1 + \Big(\sinh\Big(\mathrm{arcsinh}\,(\kappa\, y)\Big)\Big)^2} \\ &\quad + \frac{1}{\kappa} \sinh\Big(\mathrm{arcsinh}\,(\kappa\, y)\Big) \sqrt{1 + \Big(\sinh\Big(\mathrm{arcsinh}\,(\kappa\, x)\Big)\Big)^2} \\ &= \frac{1}{\kappa} \sinh\Big(\mathrm{arcsinh}\,(\kappa\, x)\Big) \cosh\Big(\mathrm{arcsinh}\,(\kappa\, y)\Big) + \frac{1}{\kappa} \sinh\Big(\mathrm{arcsinh}\,(\kappa\, y)\Big) \cosh\Big(\mathrm{arcsinh}\,(\kappa\, x)\Big) \\ &= \frac{1}{\kappa} \sinh\Big(\mathrm{arcsinh}\,(\kappa\, x) + \mathrm{arcsinh}\,(\kappa\, y)\Big) \,. \end{aligned} \tag{29}$$

This means that

$$\mathrm{arcsinh}\,(\kappa(x \oplus y)) = \mathrm{arcsinh}\,(\kappa\, x) + \mathrm{arcsinh}\,(\kappa\, y) \,. \tag{30}$$

which forces us to define

$$a^{-1}(x) = \frac{1}{\kappa} \mathrm{arcsinh}\,(\kappa\, x) \quad \Rightarrow \quad a(x) = \frac{\sinh(\kappa\, x)}{\kappa} \,. \tag{31}$$

It is worth observing that function $a(x)$, derived in our approach within the κ-algebra, has already been studied in literature starting from [26,27] where quon statistics of type II has been introduced from a Hermitian version of the q-oscillator algebra of creation and annihilation operators.

In fact, recalling that algebra of type II quons is based on the symmetric q-numbers

$$[x] = \frac{q^x - q^{-x}}{q - q^{-1}} \,, \tag{32}$$

which are invariant under the exchange $q \to 1/q$; it is easy to verify as definition (32) is related to function (31) according to

$$[x] = \frac{a(x)}{a(1)} \,. \tag{33}$$

with $\kappa = \ln q$.

Within the κ-algebra the generalized exponential reads $E(x) \equiv \exp_\kappa(x)$ and analogously the generalized logarithm reads $L(x) \equiv \ln_\kappa(x)$, where

$$\exp_\kappa(x) = \left(\sqrt{1 + \kappa^2\, x^2} + \kappa\, x\right)^{1/\kappa} \,, \tag{34}$$

$$\ln_\kappa(x) = \frac{x^\kappa - x^{-\kappa}}{2\,\kappa} \,, \tag{35}$$

and fulfill relations (23) and (25), respectively, with the κ-sum given in (26).

The deformed-subtraction is given in

$$x \ominus y \equiv x\sqrt{1+\kappa^2 y^2} - y\sqrt{1+\kappa^2 x^2}\,, \tag{36}$$

being, in this case, $0^* \equiv 0$ and $\overline{x} \equiv -x$.

The function $a(f)$ given in Equation (31) defines univocally the function $b(f)$ throughout Equations (18) or (19) with $c = \text{arcsinh}(\kappa)/\kappa$.

Therefore, the nonlinear kinetic underling type II quons statistics is depicted by a linear Fick diffusive current

$$j_{\text{diff}} = D\,\nabla f\,, \tag{37}$$

with a constant diffusive coefficient. In fact, it is straightforward to verify from Equation (8) that in this case $\Omega = 1$ [46]. Thus, like standard bosons and fermions, type II quons also undergo classical diffusive process governed by a linear diffusion current.

The corresponding nonlinear Fokker-Planck equation becomes

$$\frac{\partial f}{\partial t} = \nabla\Big(D\,m\,\beta\,\gamma(f)\,v + D\,\nabla f\Big)\,, \tag{38}$$

where

$$\gamma(f) = \gamma_+\,e^{2\kappa f} + \gamma_-\,e^{-2\kappa f} + \gamma_0\,, \tag{39}$$

with

$$\gamma_+ = \frac{\pm\sqrt{1+\kappa^2}+\kappa}{4\kappa^2}\,, \qquad \gamma_- = \frac{\pm\sqrt{1+\kappa^2}-\kappa}{4\kappa^2}\,, \qquad \gamma_0 = -\gamma_+ - \gamma_-\,. \tag{40}$$

The steady state follows from Equation (11), that in this case reads

$$\frac{\sinh(\kappa f)}{\sinh(\text{arcsinh}(\kappa) \pm \kappa f)} = c^{-\epsilon}\,, \tag{41}$$

that solved for $f(\epsilon)$ gives

$$f(\epsilon) = \frac{1}{\kappa}\,\text{arctanh}\left(\frac{\kappa}{e^{\epsilon} \mp \sqrt{1+\kappa^2}}\right)\,. \tag{42}$$

As easy check, in the $\kappa \to 0$ limit, functions $a(f)$ and $b(f)$ reduce to the one of standard bosons and fermions (12) and (13), as well as the nonlinear Fokker-Planck equation (38) reduces to Equation (14) and, in the same limit, the steady state (42) reproduces distribution (15).

5. Type I Quons

As known, type I quons firstly studied in [23], are based on the asymmetric version of q-numbers

$$[x]_q = \frac{q^x - 1}{q - 1}\,, \tag{43}$$

that is strictly related to the q-calculus introduced by Jackson [28]. In the present context, type I quons can be derived starting from the following deformed sum

$$x \oplus y = x + y + (q-1)\,x\,y\,, \tag{44}$$

emerging also in the context of generalized statistical mechanics [47]. The deformation parameter $\xi \equiv q$, is restricted to $q \geq 0$ and the q-sum recovers the standard sum in the $q \to 1$ limit.

Equation (44) can be rewritten in

$$x \oplus y = \frac{[1 + (q-1)\,x]\,[1 + (q-1)\,y] - 1}{q-1}\,, \tag{45}$$

so that

$$1 + (q-1)\,(x \oplus y) = [1 + (q-1)\,x]\,[1 + (q-1)\,y]\,, \tag{46}$$

which forces us to define the quantity

$$a^{-1}(x) = \frac{1}{\ln q}\,\ln(1 + (q-1)\,x)\,, \tag{47}$$

and its inverse $a(x)$ coincides with function defined in Equation (43), that is

$$a(x) \equiv [x]_q\,. \tag{48}$$

Asymmetric q-numbers have been employed in [23–25] to introduce quon statistics of type I starting from the q-generalization of the quantum oscillator algebras of creation and annihilation operators, like for the type II.

However, the algebra of asymmetric q numbers differs from those of the symmetric one since

$$\overline{[x]}_q = -q^{-x}\,[x]_q\,, \tag{49}$$

being, in general $0^* = 0$ and

$$\overline{x} = -\frac{x}{1 + (q-1)\,x}\,, \tag{50}$$

that is, the opposite in $\mathcal{A} \equiv (\oplus_q,\,\Re)$ does not coincides with the opposite of the ordinary algebras in $\Re$ like in the symmetric case.

Within the q-algebra the generalized exponential reads $E(x) \equiv \exp_q(x)$ and analogously the generalized logarithm reads $L(x) \equiv \ln_q(x)$ where

$$\exp_q(x) = (1 + (q-1)\,x)^{1/\ln q}\,, \tag{51}$$

$$\ln_q(x) = \frac{q^{\ln x} - 1}{q-1}\,, \tag{52}$$

that are strictly related to the q-exponential and q-logarithm introduced in the generalized statistical mechanics [47] and fulfill relations (23) and (25), respectively, with the q-sum given in (44).

The function $a(f)$ given in Equation (48) defines univocally the function $b(f)$ throughout Equations (18) or (19) with $c = 1$. However, in this case due to relation (49), we must separate the case of boson-like quons, with

$$b(f) = 1 + q\,[f]_q\,, \tag{53}$$

from the case of fermion-like quons, with

$$b(f) = 1 - q^{1-f}\,[f]_q\,. \tag{54}$$

5.1. Bosons-Like Quons

The kinetic of boson-like quons is depicted by the nonlinear Fokker-Planck equation

$$\frac{\partial f}{\partial t} = \boldsymbol{\nabla}\Big(D\, m\, \beta\, \gamma_{\rm Bose}(f)\, \boldsymbol{v} + D\, \Omega_{\rm Bose}(f)\, \boldsymbol{\nabla} f\Big)\,, \tag{55}$$

with a nonlinear drift term

$$\gamma_{\rm Bose}(f) = \gamma_2\, q^{2f} + \gamma_1\, q^f + \gamma_0\,, \tag{56}$$

where

$$\gamma_2 = \frac{q}{(q-1)^2}\,, \qquad \gamma_1 = -\frac{1+q}{(q-1)^2}\,, \qquad \gamma_0 = -\gamma_2 - \gamma_1\,, \tag{57}$$

and a nonlinear diffusive term

$$\Omega_{\rm Bose}(f) = \frac{\ln q}{q-1}\, q^f\,, \tag{58}$$

that reduces to a constant $\Omega_{\rm Bose}(f) \to 1$ in the $q \to 1$ limit. Therefore, differently from the symmetric case, Boson-like type I quons undergo classical diffusive process governed by a nonlinear diffusion current.

The steady state classical Boson-like quons follows from Equation (11) that in this case reads

$$\frac{q^f - 1}{q^{1+f} - 1} = e^{-\epsilon}\,, \tag{59}$$

that solved for $f(\epsilon)$ gives

$$f_{\rm Bose}(\epsilon) = \frac{1}{\ln q}\, \ln \frac{e^\epsilon - 1}{e^\epsilon - q}\,. \tag{60}$$

As expected, in the $q \to 1$ limit, the steady state of the Boson-like quons (60) reduces to the stationary distribution of bosons.

5.2. Fermions-Like Quons

The kinetic of fermion-like quons is depicted by the nonlinear Fokker-Planck equation

$$\frac{\partial f}{\partial t} = \boldsymbol{\nabla}\Big(D\, m\, \beta\, \gamma_{\rm Fermi}(f)\, \boldsymbol{v} + D\, \Omega_{\rm Fermi}(f)\, \boldsymbol{\nabla} f\Big)\,, \tag{61}$$

with a nonlinear drift term

$$\gamma_{\rm Fermi}(f) = \gamma_+\, q^f + \gamma_-\, q^{-f} + \gamma_0\,, \tag{62}$$

where

$$\gamma_+ = -\frac{1}{(q-1)^2}\,, \qquad \gamma_- = -\frac{q}{(q-1)^2}\,, \qquad \gamma_0 = -\gamma_+ - \gamma_-\,, \tag{63}$$

and a nonlinear diffusive term

$$\Omega_{\rm Fermi}(f) = \omega_0 + \omega_+\, q^f + \omega_-\, q^{-f}\,, \tag{64}$$

where

$$\omega_0 = \frac{2q\ln q}{(q-1)^2}, \qquad \omega_+ = -\frac{\ln q}{(q-1)^2}, \qquad \omega_- = -\frac{q\ln q}{(q-1)^2}. \tag{65}$$

and reduces to a constant $\Omega_{\text{Fermi}}(f) \to 1$ in the $q \to 1$ limit. Again, type I quons undergo classical diffusive process governed by a nonlinear diffusion current.

The steady state now follows from relation

$$\frac{q^f - 1}{q^{1-f} - 1} = e^{-\epsilon}, \tag{66}$$

that solved for $f(\epsilon)$ gives

$$f_{\text{Fermi}}(\epsilon) = \frac{1}{\ln q}\ln\left(\frac{1-e^{-\epsilon}}{2} + \sqrt{\left(\frac{1-e^{-\epsilon}}{2}\right)^2 + q\,e^{-\epsilon}}\right). \tag{67}$$

and reduces to the stationary distribution of fermion particles in the $q \to 1$ limit.

6. Conclusions

In this paper we have proposed an algebraic approach to study many body particle systems obeying a non-conventional statistics, in the semiclassical picture. A nonlinear Fokker-Planck equation, describing the kinetic of collectively interacting particles, has been obtained according to a kinetic interaction principle. The particle current is fixed by the two functions $a(f)$ and $b(f)$ that regulate the transition probability from the departing site to the arrival site in a way that depends only on the population of the initial and final sites, respectively. In this formalism, bosons-like and fermions-like particles follow from a very easy assumption on the function $a(f)$ and $b(f)$ by means of a generalized version of the inclusion/exclusion principle given by $b(f) \bigoplus a(f) = 1$, with $b(f) = a(c \pm f)$ for a generalized composition law that fixes the form of the functions $a(f)$, and then $b(f)$, and consequently fixes the steady particle distribution.

Following this approach, we have studied boson-like and fermion like quons of type II [26], whose underling algebra is related with the generalized sum (26), as well as boson-like and fermion like quons of type I [13], whose underlying algebra is defined by the generalized sum (44). It has been shown that the kinetic of type II quons is described by a nonlinear Fokker-Planck equation with a nonlinear drift current and a linear diffusive current like in the case of standard Bose and Fermi particles; otherwise, the kinetic of type I quons is described by a nonlinear Fokker-Planck equation with a nonlinear drift current and a nonlinear diffusive current.

Finally, let us remark that, following the same approach described in this work, several non conventional statistics in the classical picture can be obtained employing different composition laws. For instance, in addition to the κ-sum and the q-sum studied in this paper, other examples can be found in the framework of the generalized statistical mechanics [48,49].

Author Contributions: The authors have equally contributed to the manuscript. They all have read and approved its final version.

Funding: This research received no external funding.

Conflicts of Interest: The authors declare no conflict of interest.

References

1. Pauli, W. The connection between spin and statistics. *Phys. Rev.* **1940**, *58*, 716–722. [CrossRef]
2. Luders, G.; Zumino, B. Connection between spin and statistics. *Phys. Rev.* **1958**, *110*, 1450–1453. [CrossRef]

3. Reines, F.; Sobel, H.W. Test of the Pauli exclusion principle for atomic electrons. *Phys. Rev. Lett.* **1974**, *32*, 954. [CrossRef]
4. Modugno, G.; Inguscio, M.; Tino, G.M. Search for small violations of the symmetrization postulate for spin-0 particles. *Phys. Rev. Lett.* **1998**, *81*, 4790–4793. [CrossRef]
5. VIP Collaboration. New experimental limit on the Pauli exclusion principle violation by electrons. *Phys. Lett. B* **2006**, *641*, 18–22. [CrossRef]
6. Campagnano, G.; Zilberberg, O.; Gornyi, I.V.; Feldman, D.E.; Potter, A.C.; Gefen, Y. Hanbury Brown–Twiss interference of anyons. *Phys. Rev. Lett.* **2012**, *109*, 106802. [CrossRef]
7. Shen, Y.; Ai, Q.; Long, G.L. The relation between properties of Gentile statistics and fractional statistics of anyon. *Physica A* **2010**, *389*, 1565–1570. [CrossRef]
8. Lavagno, A.; Swamy, P.N. Thermostatistics of deformed bosons and fermions. *Found. Phys.* **2009**, *40*, 814–828. [CrossRef]
9. Bagarello, F. Quons, coherent states and intertwining operators. *Phys. Lett. A* **2009**, *373*, 2637–2642. [CrossRef]
10. Kibler, M.R. Miscellaneous applications of quons. *SIGMA* **2007**, *3*, 092. [CrossRef]
11. El Baz, M.; Hassouni, Y. Deformed exterior algebra, quons and their coherent states. *Int. J. Mod. Phys. A* **2003**, *18*, 3015–3040. [CrossRef]
12. Greenberg, O.W.; Delgado, J.D. Construction of bosons and fermions out of quons. *Phys. Lett. A* **2001**, *288*, 139–144. [CrossRef]
13. Greenberg, O.W. Particles with small violations of Fermi or Bose statistics. *Phys. Rev. D* **1991**, *43*, 4111–4120. [CrossRef]
14. Acharya, R.; Swamy, P.N. Statistical mechanics of anyons. *J. Phys. A*, **1994**, *27*, 7247–7263. [CrossRef]
15. Truscott, A.G.; Strecker, K.E.; McAlexander, W.I.; Partridge, G.B.; Hulet R.G. Observation of Fermi pressure in a gas of trapped atoms. *Science* **2001**, *291*, 2570–2572. [CrossRef]
16. Algin, A.; Senay, M. High-temperature behavior of a deformed Fermi gas obeying interpolating statistics. *Phys. Rev. E* **2012**, *85*, 041123. [CrossRef]
17. Wilczek, F. (Ed.) *Fractional Statistics and Anyon Superconductivity*; World Scientific: Singapore, 1990.
18. Camino, F.E.; Zhou, W.; Goldman, V.J. Realization of a Laughlin quasiparticle interferometer: Observation of fractional statistics. *Phys. Rev. B* **2005**, *72*, 075342. [CrossRef]
19. Stern, A. Anyons and the quantum Hall effect—A pedagogical review. *Ann. Phys.* **2008**, *323*, 204–249. [CrossRef]
20. Ezawa, Z.F.; Iwazaki, A. Quantum Hall liquid, Josephson effect, and hierarchy in a double-layer electron system. *Phys. Rev. B* **1993**, *47*, 7295–7311. [CrossRef]
21. Kitaev, A.Y. Fault-tolerant quantum computation by anyons. *Ann. Phys.* **2003**, *303*, 2–30. [CrossRef]
22. Das Sarma, S.; Freedman S.M.; Nayak, C. Topologically protected qubits from a possible non-abelian fractional quantum Hall state. *Phys. Rev. Lett.* **2005** *94*, 166802. [CrossRef]
23. Green, H.S. A Generalized Method of Field Quantization. *Phys. Rev.* **1953**, *90*, 270–273. [CrossRef]
24. Greenberg, O.W. Example of infinite statistics. *Phys. Rev. Lett.* **1990**, *64*, 705–708. [CrossRef]
25. Chaturvedi, S.; Kapoor, A.K.; Sandhya, R.; Srinivasan, V.; Simon, R. Generalized commutation relations for a single-mode oscillator. *Phys. Rev. A* **1991**, *43*, 4555–4557. [CrossRef]
26. Biedenharn, L.C. The quantum group $SU_q(2)$ and a q-analogue of the boson operators. *J. Phys. A* **1989**, *22*, L873–L878. [CrossRef]
27. Macfarlane, A.J. On q-analogues of the quantum harmonic oscillator and the quantum group $SU_q(2)$. *J. Phys. A* **1989**, *22*, 4581–4588. [CrossRef]
28. Jackson, F. q-Form of Taylor's theorem. *Mess. Math.* **1909**, *38*, 57–61.
29. Leinaas, J.M.; Myrheim, J. On the theory of identical particles. *Il Nuovo Cim. B* **1977**, *37*, 1–23. [CrossRef]
30. Wilczek, F. Magnetic flux, angular momentum, and statistics. *Phys. Rev. Lett.* **1982**, *48*, 1144–1146. [CrossRef]
31. Lerda, A. *Anyons: Quantum Mechanics of Particles with Fractional Statistics*; Springer: Berlin/Heidelberg, Germany, 1992.
32. Carollo, A.; Spagnolo, B.; Valenti, D. Uhlmann curvature in dissipative phase transitions, *Sc. Rep. Nat.* **2018**, *8*, 9852.
33. Cattani M.; Fernandes, N.C. Baryon states as colorspinors in gentilionic statistics. *Phys. Lett. A* **1987**, *124*, 229–232. [CrossRef]

34. Haldane, F.D.M. "Spinon gas" description of the $S = 1/2$ Heisenberg chain with inverse-square exchange: Exact spectrum and thermodynamics. *Phys. Rev. Lett.* **1991**, *66*, 1529–1532. [CrossRef]
35. Wu, Y.S. Statistical distribution for generalized ideal gas of fractional-statistics particles. *Phys. Rev. Lett.* **1994**, *73*, 922–925. [CrossRef] [PubMed]
36. Chaturvedi, S.; Srinivasan, V. Microscopic interpretation of Haldane's semion statistics. *Phys. Rev. Lett.* **1997**, *78*, 4316–4319. [CrossRef]
37. Gentile, G., Jr. Osservazioni sopra le statistiche intermedie. *Nuovo Cim.* **1940**, *17*, 493–497 [CrossRef]
38. Kaniadakis, G.; Quarati, P. Classical model of bosons and fermions. *Phys. Rev. E* **1994**, *49*, 5103–5110. [CrossRef] [PubMed]
39. Toscani, G. Finite time blow up in Kaniadakis-Quarati model of Bose Einstein particles. *Commun. Part. Differ. Equ.* **2011**, *37*, 77–87. [CrossRef]
40. Carrillo, J.A.; Hopf, K.; Wolfran, M-T. Numerical study of Bose-Einstein condensation in the Kaniadakis-Quarati model for bosons. *arXiv* **2019**, arXiv:1902.06266.
41. Carrillo, J.A.; Hopf, K.; Rodrigo, J.L. On the singularity formation and relaxation to equilibrium in 1D Fokker-Planck model with superlinear drift. *arXiv* **2019**, arXiv:1901.11098.
42. Kaniadakis, G.; Hristopulos, D.T. Nonlinear kinetics on lattices based on the kinetic interaction principle. *Entropy* **2018**, *20*, 426. [CrossRef]
43. Kaniadakis, G. Non-linear kinetics underlying generalized statistics. *Physica A* **2001**, *296*, 405–425. [CrossRef]
44. Kaniadakis, G.; Quarati, P.; Scarfone, A.M. Kinetical foundations of non-conventional statistics. *Physica A* **2001**, *305*, 76–83. [CrossRef]
45. Kaniadakis, G. Relativistic entropy and related Boltzmann kinetics. *Eur. Phys. J. A* **2009**, *40*, 275–287. [CrossRef]
46. Kaniadakis, G.; Lavagno, A.; Quarati, P. Kinetic model for q-deformed bosons and fermions. *Phys. Lett. A* **1997**, *227*, 227–231. [CrossRef]
47. Tsallis, C. *Introduction to Nonexstensive Statistical Mechanics*; Springer: New York, NY, USA, 2009.
48. El Kaabouchi, A.; Nivanen, L.; Wang, Q.A.; Badiali, J.P.; Le Méhauté, A. A mathematical structure for the generalization of conventional algebra. *Cent. Eur. J. Phys.* **2009**, *7*, 549–554. [CrossRef]
49. Scarfone, A.M. Entropic forms and related algebras. *Entropy* **2013**, *15*, 624–649. [CrossRef]

entropy

MDPI

Article

Statistics of the Bifurcation in Quantum Measurement

Karl-Erik Eriksson and Kristian Lindgren *

Complex Systems Group, Department of Space, Earth and Environment, Chalmers University of Technology, SE-412 96 Gothenburg, Sweden
* Correspondence: kristian.lindgren@chalmers.se

Received: 29 June 2019; Accepted: 24 August 2019; Published: 26 August 2019

Abstract: We model quantum measurement of a two-level system μ. Previous obstacles for understanding the measurement process are removed by basing the analysis of the interaction between μ and the measurement device on quantum field theory. This formulation shows how inverse processes take part in the interaction and introduce a non-linearity, necessary for the bifurcation of quantum measurement. A statistical analysis of the ensemble of initial states of the measurement device shows how microscopic details can influence the transition to a final state. We find that initial states that are efficient in leading to a transition to a final state result in either of the expected eigenstates for μ, with ensemble averages that are identical to the probabilities of the Born rule. Thus, the proposed scheme serves as a candidate mechanism for the quantum measurement process.

Keywords: quantum measurement; scattering theory; statistics; Born's rule

1. Introduction

Quantum mechanics is at the basis of all modern physics and fundamental for the understanding of the world that we live in. As a general theory, quantum mechanics should apply also to the measurement process. From the general experience of non-destructive measurements, we draw conclusions about the interaction between the observed system and the measurement apparatus and how this can be described within quantum mechanics.

We thus consider a quantum system μ, interacting with a measurement device. For simplicity we assume that μ is a two-level system that is not destroyed in the process. Then after the measurement, μ ends up in one of the eigenstates of the measured observable. If μ is prepared in one of these eigenstates, it remains in that state after the measurement. If μ is initially in a superposition of the two eigenstates, it still ends up in one of the eigenstates and the measurement result is the corresponding eigenvalue. The probability for a certain outcome is the squared modulus of the corresponding state component in the superposition (Born's rule).

An essential question is whether the probabilistic nature of quantum measurement with Born's rule is an inherent feature of quantum mechanics or whether it can be shown to hold as a result of a quantum-mechanical treatment of the measurement process combined with a statistical analysis. In the latter case, a single measurement would be a quantum-mechanical process in which the state of the measurement apparatus (possibly including its surroundings) determines the result. Born's rule would then emerge from the statistics of the ensemble that describes the measurement apparatus in interaction with the system subject to measurement.

The requirement that μ, if initially in an eigenstate of the observable, remains in that eigenstate after interacting with the apparatus, is usually considered to lead to a well-known dilemma: If applying the (linear) quantum mechanics of the 1930s to μ in an initial superposition of those eigenstates, the result of the process appears to be a superposition of the two possible resulting states for μ and the apparatus without any change in the proportions between the channels. This has been referred to as von Neumann's dilemma [1], and it has led to paradoxical conclusions such as Schrödinger's cat.

Attempts to get around this problem include Everett's relative-state formulation [2] and its continuation in DeWitt's many-worlds interpretation [3] as well as non-linear modifications of quantum mechanics [4–8]. In the non-linear modifications, one gets the bifurcation of the measurement process but the non-linear character of the basic theory introduces new conceptual difficulties. Mathematically our treatment can be seen to be very close to quantum diffusion [5]; we have chosen to follow the same conventions in handling the statistics of stochastic variables as in Ref. [5]. The ambition to understand quantum measurement as a deterministic process we share with the De Broglie-Bohm theory [9], with the difference that we look for how details in the measurement device influence the process.

Bell pointed out that the Everett-DeWitt theory does not properly reflect the fact that the presence of inverse processes and interference are inherent features of quantum mechanics [10]:

> Thus, DeWitt seems to share our idea that the fundamental concepts of the theory should be meaningful on a microscopic level and not only on some ill-defined macroscopic level. However, at the microscopic level there is no such asymmetry in time as would be indicated by the existence of branching and the non-existence of debranching. [...] [I]t even seems reasonable to regard the coalescence of previously different branches, and the resulting interference phenomena, as the characteristic feature of quantum mechanics. In this respect an accurate picture, which does not have any tree-like character, is the 'sum over all possible paths' of Feynman.

Therefore, as suggested by Bell, we investigate work of Feynman for a correct theory. We choose the scattering theory of quantum field theory, including Feynman diagrams, as a basis for our description of the measurement process. This theory contains inverse processes that result in a non-linear dependence on the initial state which removes the von Neumann dilemma.

In the field of investigation of the measurement process, a strong belief has been established that microscopic details of the measurement interaction cannot lead to the bifurcation determining the result of measurement (see, e.g., [11,12]). This belief is based on von Neumann's way of handling linear quantum mechanics. In this situation, many have abandoned the ambition to understand the mechanism of a single measurement and concentrated on the full ensemble of measurements. There one has studied the irreversible decoherence process that takes the initial ensemble, with μ in a pure state, into a mixed state for the final ensemble after measurement. Since 1970, the year of DeWitt's many-worlds theory [3] and Zeh's paper on decoherence [11], a new tradition has developed that includes different views on how to interpret quantum mechanics, see for instance Refs. [13,14]. Epistemological aspects play an important role in these interpretations.

Our idea is that the microscopic details of the measurement apparatus affect the process so that it takes μ into either of the eigenstates of the measured observable and initiates a recording of the corresponding measurement result. This is possible to see in a more developed form of linear deterministic quantum mechanics, namely the scattering theory of quantum field theory.

The development of relativistic quantum mechanics led to quantum field theory. For a situation where a quantum system μ meets a part A of a measurement device, interacts with it and then leaves it, scattering theory can be an adequate description. As we have pointed out already, the scattering theory of quantum field theory has the reversibility that was requested by Bell. These are our reasons for the choice of studying measurement in the scattering theory of quantum field theory.

In our approach, measurement is part of the physics studied, rather than a subject for epistemological analysis. We show how non-linearities can be generated within quantum theory. Our statistical study of measurement processes then shows that those states of the apparatus which are competitive in leading to a final state, also take μ into *one* of the eigenstates of the measured observable. Moreover, this bifurcation, leading to one of the two possible final states for μ, occurs with the frequencies given by Born's rule.

In the following sections, we shall first give our scattering theory description and then make all possible processes subject to a statistical analysis.

2. The Initial Phase of Measurement as A Scattering Process

Here we study the interaction between the small system μ and a larger system A with a large number of degrees of freedom. The larger system is assumed to be characterized by an ensemble of possible *initial* microstates of A. We consider this interaction to be the first part of a measurement process.

Since we are dealing with a two-level system μ, the Pauli matrices provide a suitable formalism with $\sigma_3 = \left(\begin{smallmatrix} 1 & 0 \\ 0 & -1 \end{smallmatrix}\right)$ representing the observable to be measured, with eigenstates $|+\rangle_\mu = \left(\begin{smallmatrix} 1 \\ 0 \end{smallmatrix}\right)$ and $|-\rangle_\mu = \left(\begin{smallmatrix} 0 \\ 1 \end{smallmatrix}\right)$.

Let us investigate the characteristics of the interaction between μ and A in scattering theory for the case with A in a state with (unknown) microscopic details that are summarized in a variable α. We then denote the normalized initial state of A by $|0,\alpha\rangle_A$ (with 0 indicating a state of preparedness). This means that we assume α to represent one microstate in an ensemble of possible initial states.

A basic requirement is that if μ is initially in the state $|j\rangle_\mu$ ($j = +$ or $-$), after the interaction with A, its state remains the same. In this process A changes from the initial state $|0,\alpha\rangle_A$ to a final state $|j,\beta_j(\alpha)\rangle_A$, also normalized. The first j here indicates that A has been marked by the state $|j\rangle_\mu$ of μ. All other characteristics of the final state of A are collected in $\beta_j(\alpha)$. The interaction thus transforms the system A from an initial state of readiness, characterized by α, to a final state, marked by $|j\rangle_\mu$ and characterized by $\beta_j(\alpha)$.

For a general normalized state of μ, $|\psi\rangle_\mu = \psi_+ |+\rangle_\mu + \psi_- |-\rangle_\mu$ (with $|\psi_+|^2 + |\psi_-|^2 = 1$), the combined initial state of $\mu \cup A$ is

$$|\psi\rangle_\mu \otimes |0,\alpha\rangle_A = \left(\psi_+ |+\rangle_\mu + \psi_- |-\rangle_\mu\right) \otimes |0,\alpha\rangle_A \, . \tag{1}$$

A measurement of σ_3 on μ leads to a certain result. Since two different results are possible, the μA-interaction should in general result in a transition to one of the following states,

$$|+\rangle_\mu \otimes |+,\beta_+(\alpha)\rangle_A \qquad \text{or} \qquad |-\rangle_\mu \otimes |-,\beta_-(\alpha)\rangle_A \, . \tag{2}$$

The conclusion is then that the outcome must depend on the initial state of A, i.e., on α.

In scattering theory, the interaction between μ and A is characterized by a transition operator M, and this leads to the (non-normalized) final state (see Figure 1),

$$M\,|\psi\rangle_\mu \otimes |0,\alpha\rangle_A = b_+(\alpha)\psi_+ |+\rangle_\mu \otimes |+,\beta_+(\alpha)\rangle_A + b_-(\alpha)\psi_- |-\rangle_\mu \otimes |-,\beta_-(\alpha)\rangle_A \, . \tag{3}$$

In general, the amplitudes, $b_+(\alpha)$ and $b_-(\alpha)$, are not equal and therefore the proportions between $+$ and $-$ can change in a way that depends on the initial state $|0,\alpha\rangle_A$ of A. (Please note that M must not to be confused with the unitary scattering operator S, see Appendix A).

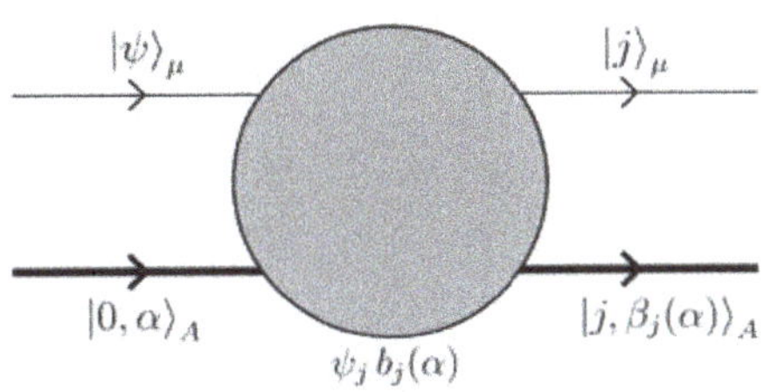

Figure 1. Schematic Feynman diagram for a transition from the initial state $|\psi\rangle_\mu \otimes |0,\alpha\rangle_A$ to the final state $|j\rangle_\mu \otimes |j,\beta_j(\alpha)\rangle_A$, $j = \pm$. The transition amplitude $\psi_j b_j(\alpha)$ depends on the microscopic details of the initial state $|0,\alpha\rangle_A$ of the larger system A and on the initial state $|\psi\rangle_\mu$ of μ.

The requirement of a statistically unbiased measurement means that $\langle\langle |b_+|^2 \rangle\rangle = \langle\langle |b_-|^2 \rangle\rangle$, where $\langle\langle\ \rangle\rangle$ denotes mean value over the ensemble of initial states $|0,\alpha\rangle_A$ of A.

Equation (3) describes a mechanism of the measurement process in which von Neumann's dilemma is not present. Relativistic quantum mechanics, in the form of scattering theory of quantum field theory, is a more correct theory than the non-relativistic Schrödinger equation, as used in the 1930s, and we choose to use Equation (3) as our starting point.

In the Feynman-diagram language of quantum field theory, transitions between the two channels, $+$ and $-$, are possible via returns to the initial state. This is a way to understand how the proportions of the channels can change as described by Equation (3). A formulation based on perturbation theory to all orders, leads to an explicitly unitary description of the whole process. (This is shown in Appendix B)

In scattering theory, transition rate (transition probability per unit time) is a central concept as we have reviewed in Appendix A. The transition rate from the initial state (1) to the final state (3) is $(2\pi)^{-1}w(\alpha)$, where $w(\alpha)$ is the squared modulus of (3),

$$w(\alpha) = |\psi_+|^2|b_+(\alpha)|^2 + |\psi_-|^2|b_-(\alpha)|^2 \,. \tag{4}$$

Each term in (4) represents the partial transition rate for the corresponding channel. Because of our assumption of common mean values for $|b_\pm(\alpha)|^2$, the mean value of (4) is the same, $\langle\langle w \rangle\rangle = \langle\langle |b_\pm|^2 \rangle\rangle$.

For equation (3) to properly represent a measurement process, i.e., a bifurcation that leads to a final state with μ in either of the eigenstates of σ_3, it is necessary that the squared moduli of the amplitudes satisfy either $|b_+(\alpha)|^2 >> |b_-(\alpha)|^2$ or $|b_-(\alpha)|^2 >> |b_+(\alpha)|^2$. If this holds for (almost) all microstates α in the resulting ensemble of final states, then it can function as a mechanism for the bifurcation of the measurement process.

Part of the basis for the von Neumann dilemma was the assumption that A is in a given initial state $|0,\alpha\rangle_A$. Before the μA-interaction, A can be in any of the states of the available initial ensemble. These states are ready to influence the recording process in different ways. To reach a final state, given by Equation (3), they compete with their transition rates, $(2\pi)^{-1}w(\alpha)$, which can differ widely between different values of α. The competition can lead to a selection and to a statistical distribution over α of the final states that is very different from the distribution in the initial ensemble.

In the following section, we will construct a mathematical model of how A influences the μA-interaction, including a description of the ensemble of possible initial states α. We then make a statistical analysis to show how both the bifurcation and the proper weights for the different measurement results can be understood in this simple setting.

3. Mathematical Model of the μA-interaction

We shall now model the amplitudes describing the μA-interaction, leading to the final state (3), and how it depends on the initial state $|0,\alpha\rangle_A$.

To have a generic model, we think of our system A as consisting of N independent subsystems, each interacting with μ, resulting in amplitudes that are products of N factors [15,16]. Since only factors resulting in differences between the two amplitudes are important, we assume

$$|b_j(\alpha)|^2 = \prod_{n=1}^{N} \left(1 + j\kappa_n(\alpha)\right) , \quad \text{with } j = + \text{ or } - \,, \tag{5}$$

where $\kappa_n(\alpha)^* = \kappa_n(\alpha)$. Small deviations from unity in the factors are characterized by a zero mean, $\langle\langle \kappa_n \rangle\rangle = 0$, while the independence between the subsystems is expressed by $\langle\langle \kappa_n \kappa_{n'} \rangle\rangle = \delta_{nn'}\chi^2$, and $0 < \chi << 1$. We have followed the convention, used in stochastic dynamics (as for instance in Ref. [5]), to calculate to second order in κ_n and then replace $\kappa_n\kappa_{n'}$ by its mean $\delta_{nn'}\chi^2$. This model reflects the unbiased character of the measurement device, and it guarantees that on average the squared moduli of the amplitudes are identical and equal to unity, $\langle\langle |b_j(\alpha)|^2 \rangle\rangle = 1$.

As an illustration, in Appendix C, we describe a situation where μ is a fast charged particle emerging from some process and then interacting electrically with the system A. Here A consists of a chain of small cylinders of ionizable material along the track where μ is passing in one of its state components. We show how the amplitude factorizes in this case.

We have chosen to keep each factor in the model close to unity in order to illustrate that even very small variations in how the subsystems interact with the system μ may result in one of the channels (one of the amplitudes), dominating over the other one, depending on the microstate α of the device. This makes it necessary to have a very large number N of subsystems. The critical assumptions are (i) the unbiased character of the device, i.e., not favoring any of the channels; and (ii) the independence of the subsystems of the device. The statistics of the interaction is treated in the following section.

4. Statistical Theory of the Transition to the Final State

We are now ready to investigate the statistical consequences of the μA-interaction modelled in the previous section. We introduce the total variance of the parameters in Equation (5), $\Xi = N\chi^2$, and define an aggregate variable $Y = Y(\alpha)$ of A, suitably normalized,

$$Y(\alpha) = \frac{1}{\Xi} \sum_{n=1}^{N} \kappa_n(\alpha) \tag{6}$$

to represent the overall degree of enhancement/suppression (so that $Y > 0$ for net enhancement of $+$ and $Y < 0$ for net enhancement of $-$). It follows that Y is characterized by mean and variance $\langle\langle Y \rangle\rangle = 0$ and $\langle\langle Y^2 \rangle\rangle = \Xi^{-1}$. Then, for sufficiently small κ_n, we can rewrite (5) as

$$|b_j(\alpha)|^2 = e^{\sum_n \log(1+j\kappa_n)} = e^{\Xi j Y(\alpha) - \frac{1}{2}\sum_n \kappa_n^2} = e^{\Xi(j Y(\alpha) - \frac{1}{2})} , \tag{7}$$

with $j = +$ or $-$. Here, in the exponent, we have done the calculation to second order in κ_n and we have replaced $\sum_n \kappa_n^2$ by $N\chi^2$.

Since all factors in the product (5) are independent, the distribution $q(Y)$ over the aggregate variable $Y = Y(\alpha)$, defined by Equation (6), in the ensemble of initial states of A, is well described by the Gaussian distribution,

$$q(Y) = \sqrt{\frac{\Xi}{2\pi}}\, e^{-\frac{1}{2}\Xi Y^2} . \tag{8}$$

centered around $Y = 0$ with variance Ξ^{-1}.

Initial states differ in their efficiency in leading to a transition to a final state, since the total transition rate may depend strongly on α. The transition to the final state (3) with $|b_j|^2$ given by (7) has the rate $(2\pi)^{-1}w(Y)$ where

$$w(Y) = |\psi_+|^2 e^{\Xi(Y-\frac{1}{2})} + |\psi_-|^2 e^{\Xi(-Y-\frac{1}{2})} , \tag{9}$$

with $\langle\langle w(Y) \rangle\rangle = 1$. The terms in (9) are the partial transition rates for the $+$ and $-$ channels.

The total transition rate (9) depends strongly on Y. We shall now go into the statistics of the final states which is strongly influenced by $w(Y)$. To get the distribution $Q(Y)$ over Y for the *final states*, corresponding to $q(Y)$ for the initial states, we must multiply $q(Y)$ by the transition rate (9) which is normalized in the sense that its mean value is 1. This is the standard approach in scattering theory, see, e.g., Ref. [17]. Here, it can be interpreted as a selection process, as previously discussed, that favors initial states which are efficient in leading to a transition, with a selective fitness being proportional to the transition rate (9). Thus, the distribution over final states can be written (see Figure 2)

$$\begin{aligned} Q(Y) &= q(Y)w(Y) = |\psi_+|^2 Q_+(Y) + |\psi_-|^2 Q_-(Y) , \\ Q_\pm(Y) &= \sqrt{\frac{\Xi}{2\pi}}\, e^{-\frac{1}{2}\Xi(Y\mp 1)^2} . \end{aligned} \tag{10}$$

The normalized partial distributions, $Q_+(Y)$ and $Q_-(Y)$, also with variance Ξ^{-1}, are centered around $Y = 1$ and $Y = -1$ and refer to μ ending up in the state $|+\rangle_\mu$ and $|-\rangle_\mu$, respectively. The coefficients of $Q_+(Y)$ and $Q_-(Y)$ in $Q(Y)$ are $|\psi_+|^2$ and $|\psi_-|^2$, expressing Born's rule explicitly.

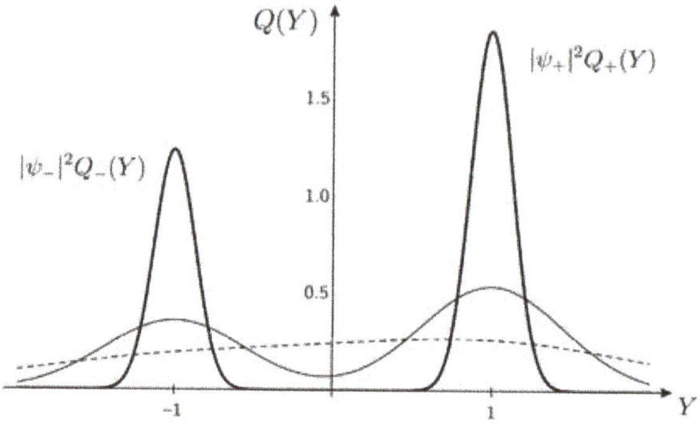

Figure 2. The distribution $Q(Y)$ over Y of transitions taking place in μA-interaction for increasing size of A corresponding to $\Xi = 1$ (broken line), $\Xi = 5$ (thin line), and $\Xi = 60$ (thick line). $Q(Y)$ is composed of two distributions $Q_+(Y)$ and $Q_-(Y)$ with weights $|\psi_+|^2$ and $|\psi_-|^2$, respectively. These distributions become separated as Ξ increases. Each initial state of A, $|0,\alpha\rangle_A$, is represented by a certain $Y = Y(\alpha)$. As the size of A increases and Ξ becomes larger, states that are efficient in leading to a transition are found around $Y = -1$ and $Y = +1$, respectively. These initial states then lead to μ ending up in either $|-\rangle_\mu$ or $|+\rangle_\mu$, respectively, with probabilities confirming the Born rule.

It is instructive to follow the distribution $Q(Y)$ with growing Ξ. For small Ξ $(= N\chi^2)$ it is broad and unimodal; it then turns broad and bimodal with narrowing peaks. For large Ξ, it is split into two well separated distributions with sharp peaks, weighted by the squared moduli of the state components of μ, $|\psi_+|^2 Q_+(Y)$ and $|\psi_-|^2 Q_-(Y)$, at $Y = 1$ and $Y = -1$, respectively. They represent two different sub-ensembles of final states (see Equation (2)). Other values of Y correspond to non-competitive processes. The aggregate variable Y is "hidden" in the fine unknown details of A that can influence the μA-interaction.

From Equation (7) we see that the dominance of either channel is characterized by $|b_+(\alpha)|^2/|b_-(\alpha)|^2 = e^{2\Xi Y}$ being either very large or very small. For a small system, i.e., small N and hence small Ξ, this ratio does not deviate much from unity which means that we have an entangled superposition of the two final states. As Ξ increases, the ratio deviates more strongly from unity and one of the channels starts to dominate. When Ξ is of the order of 10, the sub-distributions, $Q_+(Y)$ and $Q_-(Y)$, are essentially non-overlapping, $Q(Y)$ is concentrated around ± 1, and the ratio of dominance between the channels is of the order of $e^{20} \approx 10^{10}$.

The initial state for μ in (1) is a superposition, a '*both-and* state', and it ends up in (2) which is again a product state, with μ in *either* $|+\rangle_\mu$ *or* $|-\rangle_\mu$. The initial states of A vary widely in their efficiency to lead to a final state. When one transition-rate term in (9) is large, the other one is small. The selection of a large transition rate therefore also leads to a bifurcation with one of the terms in (3) totally dominating the final state.

5. Concluding Remarks

The main contribution in our work is that we have demonstrated that the initial stage of quantum measurement can be described within reversible quantum mechanics. The key components are (i) a scattering theory formulation with inverse processes that both guarantee unitarity and allow for a non-linear mechanism leading to the bifurcation; and (ii) a statistical analysis that reveals how initial states that are efficient in leading to a transition to a final state have a selective advantage and how this results in the correct probabilities of the measurement results as stated by Born's rule.

In our description, we want the system A to be big enough for a bifurcation to take place, i.e., for $\Xi = N\chi^2$ to be sufficiently large. Our idea has been to follow the qualitative recipe given by Bell who formulated a principle concerning the position of the Heisenberg cut [10], i.e., the boundary of the system A, interacting with μ according to quantum dynamics (Ref. [10], p.124):

> *put sufficiently much into the quantum system that the inclusion of more would not significantly alter practical predictions*

On the other hand, the system A should not be so large that $\mu \cup A$ cannot be described by deterministic quantum mechanics. In the model that we have described, the bifurcation of measurement takes place in the reversible stage of the interaction between μ and A before irreversibility sets in and fixes the result. In this respect, our analysis is very different from decoherence analysis [11,18].

Beyond A, the measurement apparatus must be considered to be an open system with its dynamics described by a Lindblad equation [19]. The starting point for the development here is one of the final states before the Heisenberg cut, i.e., $|+,\beta_+(\alpha)\rangle_A$ or $|-,\beta_-(\alpha)\rangle_A$, in one of the sub-ensembles described by $Q_+(Y)$ or $Q_-(Y)$. Thus, the open dynamics continues only in the channel that happens to have been chosen, $+$ or $-$.

For future work, a more detailed description is needed of a typical μA-interaction, including the statistics of the initial states and the selection of one state $|0,\alpha\rangle_A$ with a large transition amplitude, leading to a final state (2) with μ in one eigenstate, $|+\rangle_\mu$ or $|-\rangle_\mu$. An important task is to construct a detailed physical model of a non-biased measurement apparatus. The model of Appendix C is a beginning in this respect, but the mathematical assumptions in Equation (3) should be directly tied to physical properties of A. In particular, the non-bias property of A should be analyzed.

The system A should be neither too small nor too large. Then it is reasonable to describe it as mesoscopic, but Bell's principle that we have quoted above gives no indication of its actual size. In the development of realistic models, questions of limits and the accuracy of approximations will have to be handled in more detail.

In practical scientific research, there is a common working understanding of quantum mechanics. Physicists have a common reality concept for a quantum-mechanical system when it is not observed, a kind of pragmatic quantum ontology with the *quantum-mechanical state* of the studied system as the basic concept. Development of this state in time then constitutes the quantum dynamics. If quantum mechanics now can also be used to describe the measurement process, this pragmatic quantum ontology can have a wider validity than has been commonly expected.

Author Contributions: Conceptualization, K.-E.E. and K.L.; methodology, K.-E.E.; software, K.L.; formal analysis, K.-E.E. and K.L.; investigation, K.-E.E. and K.L.; writing–original draft preparation, K.-E.E. and K.L.; writing–review and editing, K.-E.E. and K.L.; visualization, K.-E.E. and K.L.; project administration, K.L.

Funding: This research received no external funding.

Acknowledgments: We thank Erik Sjöqvist and Martin Cederwall for fruitful collaboration in an earlier phase of this project [16]. Financial support from The Royal Society of Arts and Sciences in Gothenburg was important for this collaboration. We are also grateful to Andrew Whitaker for several constructive discussions. We thank two referees, whose critical comments have led us to make several improvements of the paper.

Conflicts of Interest: The authors declare no conflict of interest.

Appendix A. Scattering Matrix S and Transition Matrix M

The unitary (i.e., probability preserving) scattering operator S, takes an initial state $|i\rangle$ into a final state $S\,|i\rangle$. If a certain final state $|f\rangle$ is of interest to us then we calculate the scattering-matrix element $\langle f|\,S\,|i\rangle$. When dealing with particle scattering, it is convenient to do this in momentum space. Eigenstates of momentum are plane waves, i.e., states that occupy all space and cannot be normalized.

We shall be interested in final states $|f\rangle$ that are different from the initial state $|i\rangle$, so that $|f\rangle$ and $|i\rangle$ are orthogonal, i.e., $\langle f|i\rangle = 0$, and we can replace S by $S - 1$.

We use here the Quantum Electrodynamics book by Jauch and Rohrlich as our reference [17], to emphasize the development that had taken place between the physics of the 1930s and the quantum field theory of the 1950s.

To consider energy and momentum conservation, it is usual to write (Ref. [17], Equation (8)–(29))

$$\langle f|\,(S-1)\,|i\rangle = \delta(P_f - P_i)\,\langle f|\,M\,|i\rangle\ , \tag{A1}$$

where $\delta(P_f - P_i)$ is the 4-dimensional delta function over energy-momentum and M is the transition matrix.

Usually the probability for a transition into the final state $|f\rangle$, given the initial state $|i\rangle$, would be the squared modulus of (A1) but the square of a delta function does not make sense. Then one imposes a very large but finite length L in space and requires normalization for the wave-functions in the volume L^3, and, similarly, one imposes a time T for the whole process. Energy-momentum conservation is nearly exact for large L and T. One delta function in the squared modified (A1) becomes replaced by $(2\pi)^{-4}L^3T$. When normalization conventions are taken into account, the result becomes independent of L and proportional to T. After this we divide by T to get the transition probability per unit time (see Ref. [17], Equation (8)–(40)),

$$(2\pi)^{-1}\delta(P_f - P_i)|\,\langle f|\,M\,|i\rangle\,|^2\ . \tag{A2}$$

Then requesting the states $|i\rangle$ and $|f\rangle$ to have the same energy and momentum, we can interpret

$$(2\pi)^{-1}|\,\langle f|\,M\,|i\rangle\,|^2 = (2\pi)^{-1}\mathrm{Tr}[|f\rangle\,\langle f|\,M\rho^{(0)}M^{\dagger}]\ . \tag{A3}$$

as the transition probability per unit time, induced by M, from an initial state described by the density operator

$$\rho^{(0)} = |i\rangle\,\langle i| \tag{A4}$$

to a final state described by the projection operator $|f\rangle\,\langle f|$. We thus find that the transition probability-rate matrix obtained from the initial state (A4) is $(2\pi)^{-1}$ times

$$R = M\rho^{(0)}M^{\dagger}\ . \tag{A5}$$

Thus, $(2\pi)^{-1}R$ is the total transition rate times the density operator for the final state. Since the trace of a density operator is unity,

$$(2\pi)^{-1}w = (2\pi)^{-1}\,\mathrm{Tr}\,R \tag{A6}$$

is the total transition rate. The normalized final-state density matrix is then

$$\rho^{(f)} = \frac{1}{w}R = \frac{M\rho^{(0)}M^{\dagger}}{\mathrm{Tr}[M\rho^{(0)}M^{\dagger}]}\ . \tag{A7}$$

Let us consider the systems μ and A. M makes A entangled with μ without changing the state of μ. Still the transition amplitudes can differ between $+$ and $-$. This can distort the entanglement and induce changes in the relative proportions of $+$ and $-$ in the final state (Equation (2)). Thus, the proportions are no longer fixed by the von Neumann dilemma; the dilemma does not arise in the scattering theory that we are considering.

Appendix B. Calculation of Feynman Diagrams with Explicit Unitarity and Reversibility

The unitarity of the scattering matrix has not been explicitly visible in the main text. Reversibility that we have pointed out as crucial, is also not explicit. To remedy this we shall present a slightly more elaborate description of the whole process where the observed system μ is produced in its initial state

$|\psi\rangle_\mu$ by an external source B before interaction with A and absorbed by a sink D_+ or D_- in one of the possible final states after the interaction. In this version both unitarity and reversibility will be made explicit.

In this picture, the transition rate will instead be hidden and hence also the race to the final state. We therefore use the results that we have already obtained in the article, the transition rate (9) and the distribution (10) of the final states over the aggregated variable Y. The Born rule is also contained in (10).

As in the previous description, A starts in the initial state $|0,\alpha\rangle_A$ but μ is produced by B at an early time $-T$ in the state $|\psi\rangle_\mu$. After μA-interaction around the time zero, μ is absorbed in an eigenstate $|+\rangle_\mu$ or $|-\rangle_\mu$ at the time $+T$ by D_+ or D_-, leaving A in the state $|+,\beta_+(\alpha)\rangle_A$ or $|-,\beta_-(\alpha)\rangle_A$, respectively. We thus have one initial state $|0,\alpha\rangle_A$, a member of the ensemble of initial states, and three available final states, $|0,\alpha\rangle_A$ (no change), $|+,\beta_+(\alpha)\rangle_A$, and $|-,\beta_-(\alpha)\rangle_A$; The system μ takes part only in intermediate states.

Schematic Feynman-diagram elements for the action of the source B, the transition matrix M in Equation (3) and the sinks D_+ and D_- are shown in Figure A1, and the factors corresponding to them, J^*, $b_\pm\psi_\pm$ and $F_\pm$. We represent μ by a thin line and A by a thick line. As in Figure 1, the interaction between μ and A described by the transition matrix M, is represented by a shaded circle. Reversibility is included through the actions of the Hermitian or complex conjugates, J, $M^\dagger$, and F_j^*.

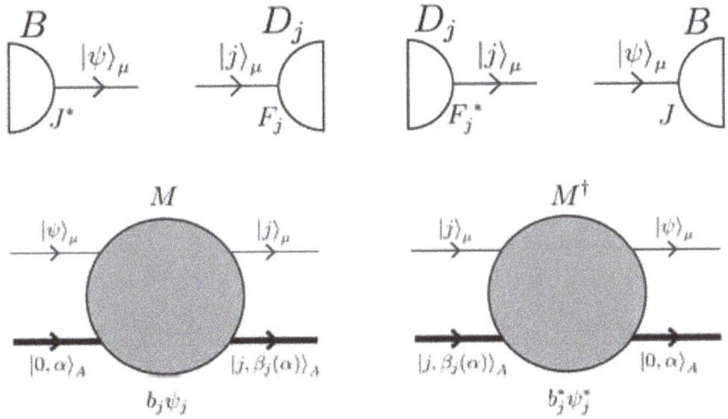

Figure A1. Schematic Feynman-diagram elements for the action of the source B, the transition matrix M and the sinks D_j $(j = \pm)$ and their conjugates.

We use perturbation theory to compute the final-state density matrix,

$$S\,|0,\alpha\rangle_{A\ A}\langle 0,\alpha|\,S^\dagger\,. \tag{A8}$$

We use the method of Nakanishi [20] to calculate this bilinear quantity directly rather than the state vector $S\,|0,\alpha\rangle_A$, simply because it makes normalization easy.

The diagrams of perturbation theory are shown in Figure A2. The zero-order no-change term is only an A-line corresponding to a contribution equal to 1 (Figure A2a). Figure A2b shows the diagram corresponding to that of Figure 1 with the source B and one sink D_j $(j = +,-)$. The inverse of this diagram is that of Figure A2c. The two taken together into one diagram represents a reduction of the no-change component due to transitions to the other states (Figure A2d). This can be repeated any number of times. All these diagrams leading back to the initial state (Figure A2e) contribute a geometrical series, representing the total no-change component of the final state,

$$1-\sum_{j=+,-} J\,\psi_j^* b_j^* F_j^* F_j b_j \psi_j J^* + \Big(\sum_{j=+,-} J\,\psi_j^* b_j^* F_j^* F_j b_j \psi_j J^*\Big)^2 \pm \ldots = \tag{A9}$$

$$\frac{1}{1+\left(|F_+|^2|\psi_+|^2|b_+|^2+|F_-|^2|\psi_-|^2|b_-|^2\right)|J|^2} = \frac{1}{1+|J|^2|F|^2\left(|\psi_+|^2 e^{\Xi(Y-\frac{1}{2})}+|\psi_-|^2 e^{\Xi(-Y-\frac{1}{2})}\right)}\,.$$

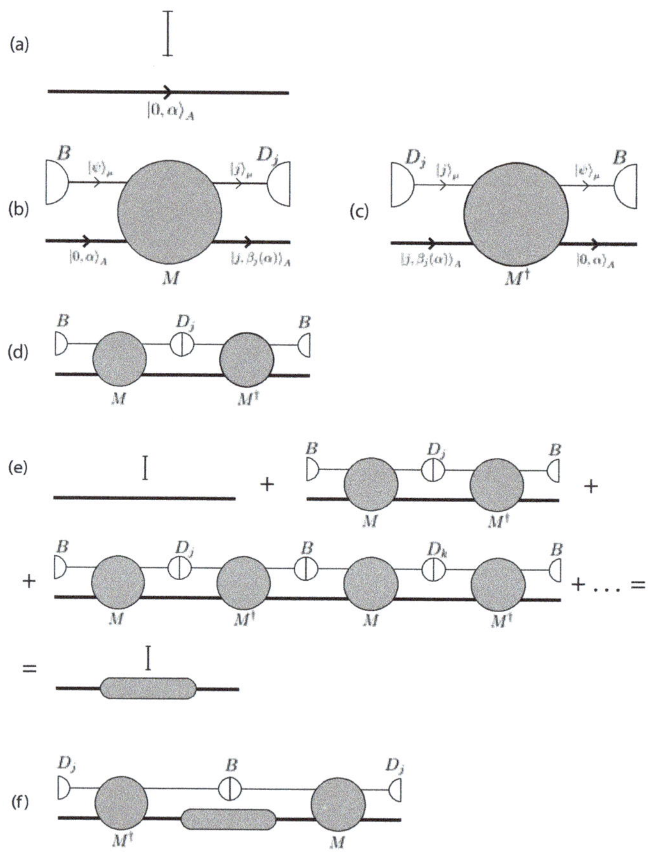

Figure A2. Schematic Feynman diagrams: (**a**) zero-order diagram for no change (the I-like sign above the A-line symbolizes "no μ-system"); (**b**) lowest order diagram for transition to a state with A marked by μ in the j state (see Figure 1); (**c**) inverse diagram of b; (**d**) diagrams b and c combined to a no-change correction; (**e**) summation over d repeated any number of times, i.e., summation of no-change diagrams to all orders; (**f**) the full perturbation expansion of the diagonal elements of the final-state density matrix with A marked by μ in the state $|j\rangle_\mu$.

Here we have used the expressions for the amplitudes in Equation (7) and given equal strength F to the two sinks D_+ and D_-. The total scattering probability, i.e., the probability of A being marked by μ is

$$
\begin{aligned}
&1 - \frac{1}{1+|J|^2|F|^2\left(|\psi_+|^2 e^{\Xi(Y-\frac{1}{2})} + |\psi_-|^2 e^{\Xi(-Y-\frac{1}{2})}\right)} = \\
&J\psi_+{}^* e^{\frac{1}{2}\Xi(Y-\frac{1}{2})} F^* \frac{1}{1+|J|^2|F|^2\left(|\psi_+|^2 e^{\Xi(Y-\frac{1}{2})} + |\psi_-|^2 e^{\Xi(-Y-\frac{1}{2})}\right)} F e^{\frac{1}{2}\Xi(Y-\frac{1}{2})} \psi_+ J^* + \\
&J\psi_-{}^* e^{\frac{1}{2}\Xi(-Y-\frac{1}{2})} F^* \frac{1}{1+|J|^2|F|^2\left(|\psi_+|^2 e^{\Xi(Y-\frac{1}{2})} + |\psi_-|^2 e^{\Xi(-Y-\frac{1}{2})}\right)} F e^{\frac{1}{2}\Xi(-Y-\frac{1}{2})} \psi_- J^* \,.
\end{aligned}
\tag{A10}
$$

The two terms on the right side of (A10) are the probabilities for the final states $|+, \beta_+(\alpha)\rangle_A$ and $|-, \beta_-(\alpha)\rangle_A$, corresponding to the diagrams of Figure A1f for the remaining diagonal elements of the density matrix. For large Ξ, the no-change contribution (A9) becomes negligible. The same is true for the non-diagonal elements of the density matrix. The diagonal terms for + and − in (A10) become

$$
p_\pm = \frac{|\psi_\pm|^2 e^{\pm\Xi Y}}{|\psi_+|^2 e^{\Xi Y} + |\psi_-|^2 e^{-\Xi Y}} \,. \tag{A11}
$$

For $Y = +1$, $p_+ = 1$ and the + channel takes everything and for $Y = -1$, $p_- = 1$ and the − channel takes everything. The norm is preserved, i.e., S is unitary. Reversibility is also clearly visible: J^*, M and $F_\pm$ are active together with their conjugates that represent inverse processes.

Appendix C. Factorization of the Transition Amplitudes

We can think of the interaction between the small system μ and the measurement apparatus as an electromagnetic interaction with small energy and momentum transfer. In Quantum Electrodynamics (QED), it is described in terms of an exchange of soft photons. Emission and exchange of soft photons is an old and well-known example of factorizable processes in QED.

To show the factorization of soft photon exchange, we consider an outgoing electron (charge $-e$, mass m) with final momentum p, described by a spinor $\overline{u}(p)$ (we follow rather closely the conventions of Ref. [17]),

$$
p^2 + m^2 = 0 \,, \quad \overline{u}(p)(ip\cdot\gamma - m) = 0 \,, \tag{A12}
$$

after emitting two soft photons with momenta k_1, k_2, and polarizations τ_1, τ_2,

$$
\begin{aligned}
&k_1^2 = k_2^2 = 0\,; \quad k_1\cdot\tau_1 = k_2\cdot\tau_2 = 0\,; \\
&|\mathbf{k_1}|\,,\ |\mathbf{k_2}| << m\,.
\end{aligned}
\tag{A13}
$$

In the evaluation of the Feynman diagram of Figure A3, the spinor $\overline{u}(p)$ for the outgoing electron of an original diagram (without soft photons) is replaced by an expression proportional to

$$
\begin{aligned}
&e^2\overline{u}(p)\Big[\tau_1\cdot\gamma\frac{i(p+k_1)\cdot\gamma+m}{(p+k_1)^2+m^2}\tau_2\cdot\gamma + (1\leftrightarrow 2)\Big]\frac{i(p+k_1+k_2)\cdot\gamma+m}{(p+k_1+k_2)^2+m^2} \approx \\
&e^2\frac{1}{2(p\cdot k_1+p\cdot k_2)}\overline{u}(p)\Big[\frac{\tau_1\cdot\gamma(ip\cdot\gamma+m)\tau_2\cdot\gamma(ip\cdot\gamma+m)}{2p\cdot k_1} + (1\leftrightarrow 2)\Big] = \\
&e^2\frac{-p\cdot\tau_1 p\cdot\tau_2}{p\cdot k_1+p\cdot k_2}\Big(\frac{1}{p\cdot k_1}+\frac{1}{p\cdot k_2}\Big)\overline{u}(p) = (s(k_1)\cdot\tau_1)(s(k_2)\cdot\tau_2)\overline{u}(p)\,,
\end{aligned}
\tag{A14}
$$

where we have used the basic relation for the Dirac gamma matrices, $\gamma_{\mu\nu} + \gamma_{\nu\mu} = 2g_{\mu\nu}$, where $g_{\mu\nu}$ is the metric tensor. In (A14), $s_\mu(k)$ is the Fourier transform of the current density of a classical point charge $-e$ moving from $\mathbf{x} = 0$ at time zero with the velocity $\mathbf{p}/p_0$,

$$s_\mu(k) = -e\frac{ip_\mu}{p \cdot k} = -e\int_0^\infty dt \int d^3\mathbf{x}\, e^{i(\mathbf{k}\cdot\mathbf{x}-|\mathbf{k}|t)}\, \delta\Big(\mathbf{x} - \frac{\mathbf{p}}{p_0}t\Big)\frac{p_\mu}{p_0}\,. \tag{A15}$$

The contribution of the diagram that μ comes from is unchanged in the limit of small k_1, k_2. Equation (A14) states that the emission of the two photons is described by one scalar emission factor for each photon. This can be extended to also include absorption.

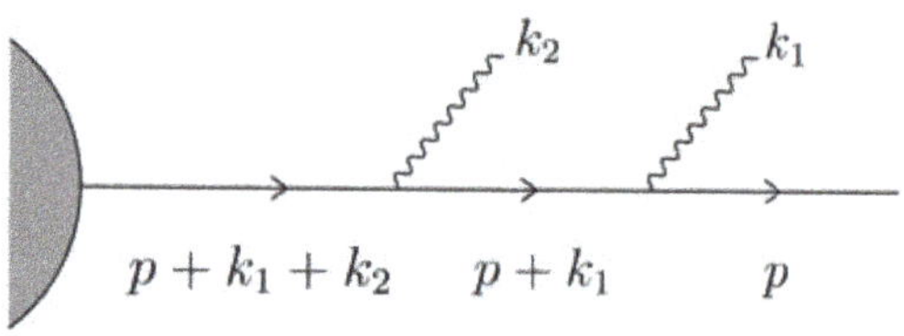

Figure A3. Feynman diagram for the emission of two soft photons.

The case of only one photon is, of course, similar and even simpler with just one emission factor. We took the example of two photons to show how the algebra gives the two factors also in this case. For the n-photon case one uses the algebraic identity

$$\sum_{(i_1 i_2 \ldots i_n)} \frac{1}{a_{i_1}(a_{i_1} + a_{i_2})\ldots(a_{i_1} + a_{i_2} + \ldots + a_{i_n})} = \frac{1}{a_1 a_2 \ldots a_n}\,. \tag{A16}$$

Thus, we can think of the classical current density

$$j_\mu(k) = -e\,\delta\Big(\mathbf{x} - \frac{\mathbf{p}}{p_0}t\Big)\frac{p_\mu}{p_0} \tag{A17}$$

as representing the electron, i.e., the system μ as felt by other systems. μ can come as a very small wave-packet travelling along the x_1-axis ($\mathbf{p} = (p_1, 0, 0)$) through a substance that can be ionized. Then we take A to be a thin cylinder of this substance around the path of the μ wave-packet.

It is convenient to consider A as consisting of a chain of N shorter cylinders $A_1, A_2, \ldots, A_N$ along the x_1-axis with A_k defined by

$$\begin{aligned} &x_1^{(0)} + \frac{k-1}{2}\Delta l \le x_1 \le x_1^{(0)} + \frac{k+1}{2}\Delta l\,, \\ &x_2^2 + x_3^2 \le \Delta r^2\,, \end{aligned} \tag{A18}$$

where Δl and Δr are small.

For our model, we can neglect the interaction between the small cylinders and we can consider μ to interact with A_k only during its passage, i.e., during the time interval

$$\frac{p_0}{p_1}\Big(x_1^{(0)} + \frac{k-1}{2}\Delta l\Big) < t \le \frac{p_0}{p_1}\Big(x_1^{(0)} + \frac{k+1}{2}\Delta l\Big)\,. \tag{A19}$$

Because of their independence, each of the cylinders acted on by μ via the current density (A17), contributes an independent factor to the total transition rate. In the mean, the factor from the μA_k-interaction should not change anything but in the single case, it can contribute an unknown factor close to one, as assumed in Equation (5). Thus, we have given here a rationale for this assumption.

References

1. Nauenberg, M. Does Quantum Mechanics Require A Conscious Observer? *J. Cosmol.* **2011**, *14*. Available online: http://journalofcosmology.com/Consciousness139.html (accessed on 26 August 2019).
2. Everett, H. "Relative State" Formulation of Quantum Mechanics. *Rev. Mod. Phys.* **1957**, *29*, 454. [CrossRef]
3. DeWitt, B.S. Quantum mechanics and reality. *Phys. Today* **1970**, *23*, 30–35. [CrossRef]
4. Gisin, N. Quantum measurements and stochastic processes. *Phys. Rev. Lett.* **1984**, *52*, 1657. [CrossRef]
5. Gisin, N.; Percival, I.C. The quantum-state diffusion model applied to open systems. *J. Phys. A Math. Gen.* **1992**, *25*, 5677–5691. [CrossRef]
6. Percival, I.C. Primary state diffusion. *Proc. R. Soc. A* **1994**, *447*, 189–209. [CrossRef]
7. Ghirardi, G.C.; Rimini, A.; Weber, T. Unified dynamics for microscopic and macroscopic systems. *Phys. Rev. D* **1986**, *34*, 470. [CrossRef] [PubMed]
8. Ghirardi, G.C.; Pearle, P.; Rimini, A. Markov processes in Hilbert space and continuous spontaneous localization of systems of identical particles. *Phys. Rev. A* **1990**, *42*, 78. [CrossRef] [PubMed]
9. Bohm, D. A suggested interpretation of the quantum theory in terms of "hidden" variables. I. *Phys. Rev.* **1952**, *85*, 166. [CrossRef]
10. Bell, J.S. Quantum Mechanics for Cosmologists. In *Speakable and Unspeakable in Quantum Mechanics*; Cambridge University Press: Cambridge, UK, 2004.
11. Zeh, H.D. On the interpretation of measurement in quantum theory. *Found. Phys.* **1970**, *1*, 69–76. [CrossRef]
12. Zurek, W.H. Quantum theory of the classical: Quantum jumps, Born's Rule and objective classical reality via quantum Darwinism. *Philos. Trans. R. Soc. A* **2018**, *376*, 20180107. [CrossRef] [PubMed]
13. Rovelli, C. Relational quantum mechanics. *Int. J. Theor. Phys.* **1996**, *35*, 1637–1678. [CrossRef]
14. Zwirn, H. The measurement problem: Decoherence and convivial solipsism. *Found. Phys.* **2016**, *46*, 635–667. [CrossRef]
15. Eriksson, K.E. Measurement as soft final-state interaction with a stochastic system. *J. Phys. B At. Mol. Opt. Phys.* **2009**, *42*, 085001. [CrossRef]
16. Eriksson, K.E.; Cederwall, M.; Lindgren, K.; Sjöqvist, E. Bifurcation in Quantum Measurement. *arXiv* **2017**, arXiv:1708.01552v2.
17. Jauch, J.M.; Rohrlich, F. *The Theory of Photons and Electrons*; Addison-Wesley: Boston, MA, USA, 1955; pp. 163–167.
18. Schlosshauer, M. Decoherence, the measurement problem, and interpretations of quantum mechanics. *Rev. Mod. Phys.* **2005**, *76*, 1267–1305. [CrossRef]
19. Lindblad, G. On the generators of quantum dynamical semigroups. *Commun. Math. Phys.* **1976**, *48*, 119–130. [CrossRef]
20. Nakanishi, N. General theory of infrared divergence. *Prog. Theor. Phys.* **1958**, *19*, 159–168. [CrossRef]

entropy

MDPI

Article

On the Rarefied Gas Experiments

Róbert Kovács [1,2,3]

1 Department of Energy Engineering, Faculty of Mechanical Engineering, Budapest University of Technology and Economics (BME), 1111 Budapest, Hungary; kovacs.robert@wigner.mta.hu

2 Department of Theoretical Physics, Wigner Research Centre for Physics, Institute for Particle and Nuclear Physics, 1121 Budapest, Hungary

3 Montavid Thermodynamic Research Group, 1112 Budapest, Hungary

Received: 6 July 2019; Accepted: 22 July 2019; Published: 23 July 2019

Abstract: There are limits of validity of classical constitutive laws such as Fourier and Navier-Stokes equations. Phenomena beyond those limits have been experimentally found many decades ago. However, it is still not clear what theory would be appropriate to model different non-classical phenomena under different conditions considering either the low-temperature or composite material structure. In this paper, a modeling problem of rarefied gases is addressed. The discussion covers the mass density dependence of material parameters, the scaling properties of different theories and aspects of how to model an experiment. In the following, two frameworks and their properties are presented. One of them is the kinetic theory based Rational Extended Thermodynamics; the other one is the non-equilibrium thermodynamics with internal variables and current multipliers. In order to compare these theories, an experiment on sound speed in rarefied gases at high frequencies, performed by Rhodes, is analyzed in detail. It is shown that the density dependence of material parameters could have a severe impact on modeling capabilities and influences the scaling properties.

Keywords: rarefied gases; non-equilibrium thermodynamics; kinetic theory

---

1. Introduction

The classical material laws such as Fourier and Navier-Stokes are acceptable for tasks concerning homogeneous materials, dense gases, and far from low-temperatures (20 K). In the engineering practice, these constitutive equations are well-known and widely used. Nevertheless, there are situations where some generalizations must be applied. Such a case could occur on small (micro or nano) length scales, short time scales, near low-temperature or far from equilibrium.

It is easier to understand the origin of the present continuum model of non-equilibrium thermodynamics with internal variables (NET-IV) for rarefied gases together with its properties if a purely heat conduction problem is presented first, since the essential attributes are inherited. Moreover, the most visible differences are analogous in both cases, for instance, the available degrees of freedom, the structure of the equations and the interpretation of the parameters. All these differences originate at the roots of these approaches.

Considering only heat conduction, various forms of heat propagation are experimentally found [1–9]. These are called second sound and ballistic propagation [9–12]. Their modeling background is diverse, and one can find many extended heat conduction equations with many different interpretations in the literature [13–20]. One of them is related to the approach of Rational Extended Thermodynamics (RET) [9,21], it considers kinetic theory rigorously and uses phonon hydrodynamics to describe these deviations from Fourier's law [22,23]. Another approach uses non-equilibrium thermodynamics with internal variables and current multipliers (NET-IV) [12]. Both are tested on the same heat conduction experiment, and the latter one seems to be more effective [23].

The main difference between these two approaches is routed to the physics that lies behind the system of constitutive equations. Using kinetic theory, one always has to assume apriori a mechanism occurring between the particles and describe the interaction among them. On the other side, non-equilibrium thermodynamics is phenomenological, the derivation of constitutive equations does not require any assumption regarding the microstructure, which makes the model more general and, in parallel, offers more degrees of freedom by not restricting the coupling coefficients. In the kinetic theory, due to the prescribed interaction model, most of the coefficients can be calculated, and only a few of them have to be fitted to the experimental data. Although its mathematical structure is advantageous, it is symmetric hyperbolic [21,24], the fixed parameters lead to its weakness: e.g., in a previously mentioned heat conduction problem, one has to use at least 30 momentum equations with increasing tensorial order to obtain the ballistic propagation speed approximately. The approach of NET-IV can resolve this problem, also preserving the structure of momentum equation; however, in order to fit, it requires more parameters [12,22,23,25]. All these approaches have advantages and disadvantages, and their detailed comparison is presented in [26].

In the case of investigating room temperature non-Fourier phenomenon, the phonon picture is not applicable [25]. One advantage of NET-IV is that it is applicable and tested on room temperature experiments that show over-diffusive type non-Fourier heat propagation [27–29]. It makes the kinetic approach of heat conduction more challenging to apply for practical problems; however, there are situations where its predictive power is useful (e.g., estimating transport coefficients). Such a situation is related to the topic of rarefied gases [30]. In some senses, the behavior of a rarefied gas (i.e., a gas under low pressure) is analogous with a rarefied phonon gas that applied in case of heat conduction. The difference among them is the type of the particle and the interpretation of some physical quantities. In order to understand the analogy, the ballistic conduction must be defined.

Using phonon hydrodynamics, the ballistic heat conduction is interpreted as non-interacting particles that scatter on the boundary only, i.e., traveling through the material without any collision [9]. It is important to emphasize that the following Equations (1) and (2) describe not merely a ballistic phenomenon but together with the diffusion and second sound propagation modes. This assumption leads to the system of equations in one spatial dimension:

$$\begin{aligned} \partial_t e + c^2 \partial_x p &= 0, \\ \partial_t p + \frac{1}{3}\partial_x e + \partial_x N &= -\frac{1}{\tau_R} p, \\ \partial_t N + \frac{4}{15} c^2 \partial_x p &= -\left(\frac{1}{\tau_R} + \frac{1}{\tau_N}\right) N, \end{aligned} \tag{1}$$

where e being the energy density, p is momentum density, c stands for the Debye speed, τ_R and τ_N are the relaxation times referring to the resistive and normal processes [9], furthermore, ∂_t denotes the partial time derivative, applied for a rigid heat conductor. Here, N is the deviatoric part of the pressure tensor. In phonon hydrodynamics, it can be identified as a current density of the heat flux. The key aspect to include ballistic contributions into the modeling is achieving coupling between the heat flux and the pressure. This is one merit of this approach: such coupling was not realized in any other theories before. That was the motivation for the approach of NET-IV, this coupling is obtained using current multipliers [31], and the same structure can be reproduced [12,25]:

$$\begin{aligned} \rho c \partial_t T + \partial_x q &= 0, \\ \tau_q \partial_t q + q + \lambda \partial_x T + \kappa \partial_x Q &= 0, \\ \tau_Q \partial_t Q + Q + \kappa \partial_x q &= 0, \end{aligned} \tag{2}$$

where Q plays the role of N, q is the heat flux, c denotes the specific heat and the coefficient κ is not fixed on contrary to (1), this property allows to adjust the exact propagation speed using only

3 equations instead of 30. The properties of the models above are discussed deeply by Jou et al. [32], Alvarez et al. [33] and Guo et al. [34].

Despite the numerous differences between phonons and real molecules, the situation is similar for rarefied gases, at least at the level of entropy; Equation (3) does not contain restrictions about the type of the fluid, i.e., there is an "entropic equivalence" between them. Here, a gas under low pressure consists few enough particles to observe the ballistic contribution. In NET-IV, the starting point is the generalization of entropy density and its current:

$$s(e,\rho,q_i,\Pi_{ij}) = s_e(e,\rho) - \frac{m_1}{2}q_iq_i - \frac{m_2}{2}\Pi_{\langle ij\rangle}\Pi_{\langle ij\rangle} - \frac{m_3}{6}\Pi_{ii}\Pi_{jj},$$
$$J_i = (b_{\langle ij\rangle} + b_{kk}\delta_{ij}/3)q_j, \tag{3}$$

then exploiting the entropy production inequality of second law [12], one obtains a continuum model compatible with the kinetic theory to model rarefied gases [25,26,35]. Einstein's summation convention is applied. Here Π_{ij} is an internal variable [36–38], it is identified as the viscous pressure, $\Pi_{ij} = P_{ij} - p\delta_{ij}$ with p being the hydrostatic pressure, in accordance with EIT [18,19]. This is the usual assumption in theories of Extended Thermodynamics, as a consequence of the compatibility with kinetic theory [21,32], it also includes Meixner's theory [39], the first extension of Navier-Stokes equation. Besides, b_{ij} is called Nyíri-multiplier (or current multiplier) [31] which permits obtaining coupling between the heat flux and the pressure. Furthermore, the form of entropy flux (3) is compatible with the one proposed by Sellitto et al. [40], where the gradient of heat flux acts as a multiplier. Since the proper description requires the separation of deviatoric and spherical parts, in Equation (3) $\langle\rangle$ denotes the traceless part of the pressure. Equation (3) presents the same generalization as used for modeling complex heat conduction processes that include diffusive and wave propagation modes together, thus, hereinafter it is called *non-local generalization* of entropy and its current density [25]. The linearized-generalized Navier-Stokes-Fourier system reads in one dimension [25]:

$$\begin{aligned}\tau_q\partial_t q + q + \lambda\partial_x T - \alpha_{21}\partial_x\Pi_s - \beta_{21}\partial_x\Pi_d &= 0,\\ \tau_d\partial_t\Pi_d + \Pi_d + \nu\partial_x v + \beta_{12}\partial_x q &= 0,\\ \tau_s\partial_t\Pi_s + \Pi_s + \eta\partial_x v + \alpha_{12}\partial_x q &= 0,\end{aligned} \tag{4}$$

where the lower indices d and s denote the deviatoric and spherical parts, respectively. The η is the bulk viscosity, ν denotes the shear viscosity, α_{ab}, β_{ab} $(a,b = 1,2)$ are the coupling parameters between the heat flux and the pressure and τ_m $(m = q,d,s)$ are the relaxation times, here the coupling parameters and the relaxation times are to be fit. This structure is equivalent to the 1D linearized version model from RET [41–43]:

$$\begin{aligned}\tau_q\partial_t q + q + \lambda\partial_x T - RT_0\tau_q\partial_x\Pi_d + RT_0\tau_q\partial_x\Pi_s &= 0,\\ \tau_d\partial_t\Pi_d + \Pi_d + 2\nu\partial_x v - \frac{2\tau_d}{1+c_v^*}\partial_x q &= 0,\\ \tau_s\partial_t\Pi_s + \Pi_s + \eta\partial_x v + \frac{\tau_s(2c_v^*-3)}{3c_v^*(1+c_v^*)}\partial_x q &= 0,\end{aligned} \tag{5}$$

with R being the gas constant and c_v^* denotes the dimensionless specific heat: $c_v^* = c_v/R$. As it is apparent, only the relaxation times are free parameters, all the other coefficients are fixed. It is interesting to note that the system (5) is derived by considering a doubled hierarchy of balance equations [24,44]. The reason behind that fact is related to the more degrees of freedom within polyatomic gases [26]. It is also important to note that it is not the only way for the kinetic theory: Lebon and Cloot derived a possible generalization using gradient terms as new variables [45] to model nonlocal phenomena. In order to obtain a complete (closed) system of equations, beside the constitutive equations above, one has to use the balance laws as well:

$$\begin{aligned} \partial_t \rho + \rho_0 \partial_x v &= 0, \\ \rho_0 \partial_t v + \partial_x \Pi_d + \partial_x \Pi_s + RT_0 \partial_x \rho + R\rho_0 \partial_x T &= 0, \\ \rho_0 c \partial_t T + \partial_x q + R\rho_0 T_0 \partial_x v &= 0, \end{aligned} \tag{6}$$

i.e., the mass, momentum and energy balances, respectively.

It is worth mentioning the earlier works of Lebon and Cloot [45] and Carrassi and Morro [46,47] where a similar comparison is performed. In these papers, other experiments are analyzed that are conducted by Meyer and Sessler [48], which slightly differ from the following one.

Before discussing the experimental observations about rarefied gases, one must define what a rarefied gas is. According to Klimontovich, a density parameter ε should be small for rarefied gases: $\varepsilon << 1$. It expresses the ratio of the occupied volume by the molecules and the overall available volume. Using the air properties at atmospheric pressure and room temperature, it turns out that $\varepsilon \approx 10^{-4}$ [49]. In other words, air at 10 atm is also rarefied or at least close to a rarefied state. Eventually this definition is not appropriate as it takes the volume corrections only into account, leaving the Knudsen number out of sight. The validity limit of the classical transport equations can be given more appropriately using the Knudsen number since it includes the mean free path as a characteristic quantity of a process. Above $Kn \approx 0.05 - 0.1$ the generalizations of the Navier-Stokes-Fourier equations must be applied [30,35].

In the following, the particular experimental observations of Rhodes are presented. That experiment highlights two essential aspects which are not independent of each other, namely, the density dependence of material parameters and the frequency/pressure (ω/p) scaling properties of the RET and NET-IV models. The discussion aims to present the necessary requirements of obtaining ω/p-dependence from continuum point of view. At the end, that measurement is evaluated using the framework of NET-IV and compared to the approach of RET.

2. Experiments

As in the case of heat conduction [23], the experimental results are considered as a benchmark problem in order to test the validity and feasibility of the corresponding generalized model. Here, one measurement performed by Rhodes [50] is discussed in detail. There are many other data in the literature [51–54], but this one is going to be sufficient to present all the necessary conclusions and difficulties arising in that field, i.e., how the scaling properties appear, the interpretation of the experiments and more importantly, the role of the material parameters.

A sonic interferometer [55] is used to measure the sound speed for various frequency-pressure ratios [50], see Figure 1 for typical data. The interferometer is placed in a dewar to maintain a constant temperature within.

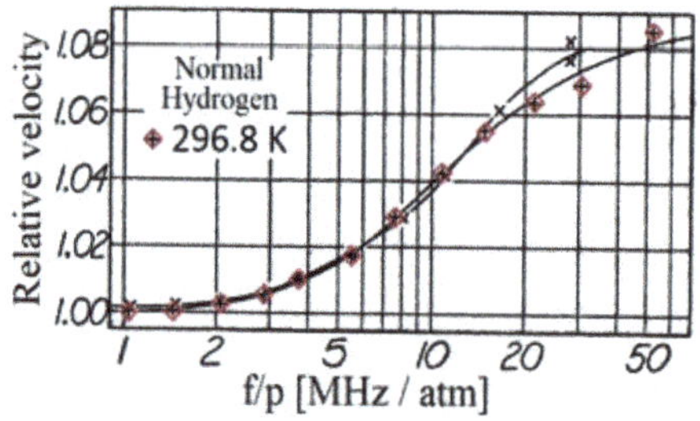

Figure 1. Speed of sound measurement performed by Rhodes [50]. The vertical axis denotes the relative speed of sound, i.e., v/v_0, where v_0 is the speed of sound related to the normal state. The original data can be found in [50]. The relevant points are emphasized by red squares.

It has to be emphasized that the frequency was constant as well in the experiments [50], i.e., the pressure is varied over the whole interval. More appropriately, it was the density that changed during the experiment when the constant temperature has maintained. In Figure 1, the results related to normal Hydrogen is presented. The measurement is also performed using pure para-Hydrogen and the 50–50 mixture of para-ortho Hydrogen [50]. Now choosing the curve from Figure 1 corresponding to 296.8 K. Before making any advancement with the extended models, two essential aspects must be discussed. The first one is to investigate the density dependence of material parameters. Then, one can calculate the dispersion relation for the relating model (4)–(6) or (5) and (6) to model the experiment and analyze the frequency-pressure dependency, too.

2.1. Density Dependence of Material Parameters

Despite the fact that the experimental data are recorded as a function of ω/p only, it is also emphasized in the related paper of Rhodes [50] that the frequency was constant all along the measurement in an isothermal environment. It means that the pressure is varied by changing the density of the gas only. That is, changing the state of the gas from normal (or dense) state to a rarefied one must reflect the role of density dependence of material parameters.

Indeed, this is an efficient way to demonstrate the validity region of the classical Navier-Stokes-Fourier equations. As the experiment shows, some effects become essential when the gas reaches its rarefied state. Density-dependent material coefficients could represent it: some of them make the related memory and nonlocal effects (couplings) negligible for dense states and worthwhile to account in rarefied states while the others change accordingly. This is a natural expectation from theoretical point of view.

Considering the RET approach of Arima et al. [43], one can notice the following:

- the viscosities are constant: $\nu = p_0\tau_d$ for shear viscosity and $\eta \sim p_0\tau_s$ for the bulk part,
- the thermal conductivity is also constant: $\lambda \sim cp_0\tau_q$ (in which c being the specific heat),
- as a consequence of the above, the relaxation times are inversely proportional with mass density: $\tau \sim \frac{1}{\rho}$.

All the other parameters are fixed and do not depend on the mass density in any way. It is important to emphasize that the essential material parameters used in their analysis are constant for very different pressures, like 10^3 or 10^5 Pa. These viscosities are derived on kinetic theory considerations (see, e.g., [56–58]) and are independent of the mass density. Since it is a theoretical value, in the following it is referred to be "physical" or theoretical quantity. It is needed to be underlined that only the "effective" or apparent properties are measurable which may differ from the theoretical ones. As Michalis et al. [59] draw the attention to the "effective" viscosity, the theoretical one must be corrected for rarefied gas flows as a function of the Knudsen number. These corrections are devoted to facilitating the phenomenological descriptions and can be compared to the above-mentioned measurements [59–63].

As the measured effective viscosity shows mass dependence, it requires corrections in both directions: from the rarefied state to the extremely dense states (up to the magnitude of 10^3 MPa). One example is the Enskog-type correction [63–65]. It is in good agreement with particular experiments that are devoted to measuring the density dependence of shear viscosity for dense states [64,66–68]. These measurements do not aim to investigate low-pressure behavior. Extrapolating the "dense data" to zero, they show the presence of non-zero viscosities at zero density (see Figure 2 for details) [56,60,66,69].

On the other hand, the measurements of Itterbeek et al. [70–72] demonstrate decreasing viscosity by decreasing the pressure. It can be only piecewise linear, its steepness changes drastically at very low pressures (1–10 Pa), and the viscosity tends to zero (Figure 3). However, it is extremely difficult to perform viscosity measurements at such a rarefied state. The outcome of the experiment depends on the size of the apparatus and could influence the results. Furthermore, evaluating such viscosity measurement that corresponds to high Kn number, the classical Navier-Stokes theory may be insufficient and a non-local theory should be used. So to say, there could be some uncertainty regarding the values of the viscosities. From practical point of view, the density dependence seems to be natural and the measurements of Itterbeek et al. also strengthen this expectation: at zero density, there is no viscosity. From a theoretical point of view, this is contradictory to the kinetic theory in the sense of the non-zero value for viscosity in the zero-density limit. Beskok and Karniadakis [73], to overcome that contradiction, suggested a correction that is inversely proportional with the Knudsen number. The correction of the "physical" viscosity is improved by Roohi and Darbandi [74], too.

From a practical point of view again, these effective quantities are essential for modeling, for instance see [59,75–79]. In these papers, generalized constitutive laws are proposed in which apparent quantities play a central role and are used as being the coefficients in the constitutive equations, this is the case also in NET-IV. These referred problems (rheology, non-Newtonian fluids, biological materials) demonstrates that the apparent transport coefficients can depend on various quantities, especially in complex materials. Since the theoretical coefficients differ from the apparent one, at least in the sense of density dependence, it could influence the scaling properties of a model. It is discussed in the following.

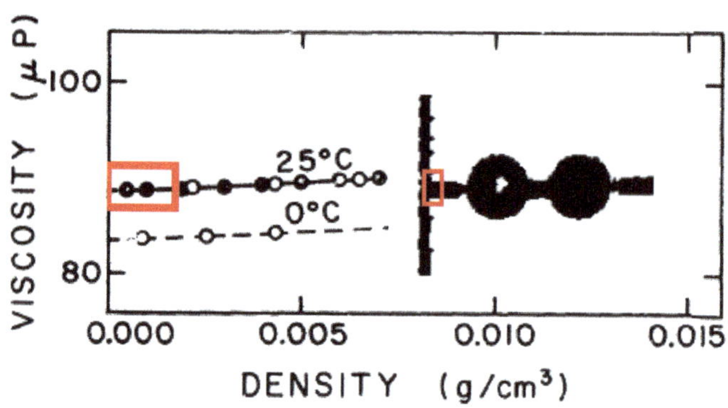

Figure 2. Density dependence of viscosity for dense gases when the non-zero viscosity at zero density appears. The original measurements can be found in [66]. Here, the red boxes show the region of interest together with the extrapolation to zero density.

p mm	$10^7 \cdot \eta$ or $10^7 \cdot \eta'$
1 Atm	889
0,0211	69,1
0,01042	39,3
0,00529	23,3
0,00267	12,0

Figure 3. Pressure dependence of viscosity for rarefied gases at room temperature. The original data can be found in [72] which is only partially depicted here.

For the sake of complete comparison with the work of Arima et al., the same assumptions are used, i.e.,

- both viscosities and the thermal conductivity are constant: $\nu = 8.82 \times 10^{-6}$ Pas, $\eta = 326 \times 10^{-6}$ Pas and $\lambda = 0.182$ W/(mK), respectively.
- all relaxation times and the coupling coefficients have $1/\rho$ dependence.

These follow from a scaling requirement which is discussed in the next section.

2.2. Frequency-Pressure Dependence

It is stated frequently in the early experimental papers [51–53] that the behavior of a gas depends on the ratio of frequency and pressure alone. From the point of view of kinetic theory, this scaling property is natural and follows from the Boltmann equation.

However, it is not that straightforward from a continuum point of view. Although this scaling is correct based on the experimental data [50], it requires constant transport coefficients, $1/\rho$ dependence in the new parameters (relaxation times and coupling coefficients) and ideal gas state equation. These assumptions work for the corresponding evaluations; it could not be valid for an extensive pressure (or density, accordingly) domain, e.g., from 10 Pa to 10^8 Pa as the apparent (It is worth to note again that the continuum models consist apparent (or measurable) coefficients in the constitutive equations.) viscosities and the thermal conductivity do depend on the pressure. Moreover, it is not clear how that scaling would appear using a more general equation of state.

Furthermore, it would worth investigating the scaling of relaxation times as the particle-wall interaction starts to dominate the process instead of the particle-particle collisions. In this kind of process, the characteristics of relaxation times are changed and thus changing the scaling properties of the equations. This could be the validity limit of the pure $1/\rho$ dependence. For example, in the experiments of Meyer and Sessler the lower pressure limit is around 0.2 Pa in which such particle-wall constribution can be especially important to consider.

This scaling property can be easily demonstrated for the classical Navier-Stokes-Fourier model by calculating the dispersion relation using the previous assumptions. Then, there no one will find terms containing the frequency ω and the pressure p separately, as follows.

Assuming the common $e^{i(\omega t-kx)}$ plane wave solution of the system (7) with the usual wave number k and frequency ω,

$$\begin{aligned}
\partial_t\rho + \rho_0\partial_x v &=0,\\
\rho_0\partial_t v + \partial_x\Pi_d + \partial_x\Pi_s + RT_0\partial_x\rho + R\rho_0\partial_x T &=0,\\
\rho_0 c_V\partial_t T + \partial_x q + R\rho_0 T_0\partial_x v &=0,\\
q + \lambda\partial_x T &-0,\\
\Pi_d + \nu\partial_x v &=0,\\
\Pi_s + \eta\partial_x v &=0,
\end{aligned} \tag{7}$$

and omitting the detailed derivation, one obtains the following expression for phase velocity $v_{ph} = \frac{\omega}{k}$:

$$\begin{aligned}
v_{ph}^2 =& \frac{cRT\rho^2 + R^2T\rho^2 + ic\eta\rho\omega + i\lambda\rho\omega + ic\nu\rho\omega}{2c\rho^2} + \\
&+ i\frac{\sqrt{\rho^2\left(-4c\lambda\omega(-iRT\rho + (\eta+\nu)\omega) + (iR^2T\rho - \lambda\omega + c(iRT\rho - (\eta+\nu)\omega))^2\right)}}{2c\rho^2}.
\end{aligned} \tag{8}$$

Expanding all the terms within Equation (8), the $v_{ph} = v_{ph}(\omega/p)$ dependence becomes visible and all the experimental data can be evaluated without calculating the pressure (or the mass density) independently from the frequency. In the case of the generalized NSF model, the situation is the same, and the previous assumptions ensure such scaling. Here, the final remark is made from an experimental point of view: the frequency and the pressure are separately controlled and should be documented in this way. Then, in a continuum model, the pressure dependence in any parameter could be implemented without any problem, and the model would be free from assumptions that may be made unconsciously. Moreover, it could extend the validity region of this modeling approach.

2.3. *Evaluations, Comparisons and Conclusions*

First, let us consider the results of Arima et al. [24,43], see Figure 4 for details. There are some important remarks on their evaluation method:

1. Dimensionless frequency $\Omega = \tau_d\omega$ is used instead of ω/p, moreover, $p\tau_d\omega/p = \nu\omega/p$ hence the shear viscosity ν is used to rescale the experimental data. Moreover, the papers [24,43] do not reflect the fact that the frequency was constant. It could be confusing hence it hides that the mass density ρ is the real independent variable in the equations in which all new coefficients (relaxation times and coupling parameters) depend on ρ.
2. Regarding the temperature, 295.15 K is used instead of 296.8 K. It is seemingly a small difference; however, when one attempts to calculate the mass density from the data ω/p, it leads to a different value, i.e., slightly inaccurate the data in [24]. As a consequence, even the speed of sound is slightly inaccurate that used for vertical scale.
3. In [24,43], only certain ratios of relaxation times are fitted. One has to know the pressure in order to determine their values.
4. One single parameter set is used to fit the data from papers [50,53,80] (Figure 4). The relevant data is the following: $\tau_q/\tau_d = 1.46$, $\tau_s/\tau_d = 144$, since the coupling coefficients are also proportional with the relaxation times. It is apparent from Figure 4 that for other measurements, even on the same material, these ratios may be different.

Figure 4 demonstrates that kinetic theory can model the behavior of the gas in the rarefied state.

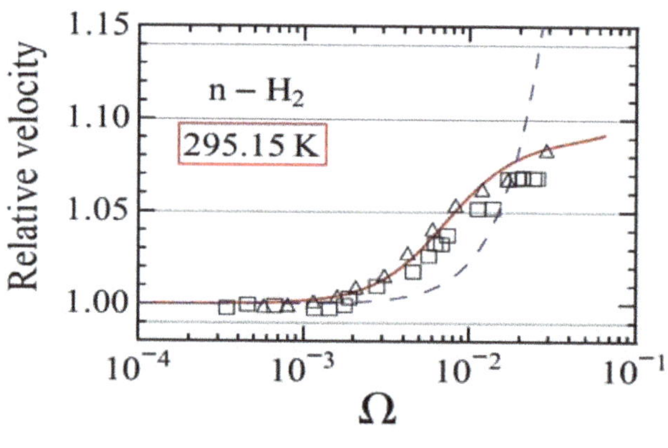

Figure 4. Calculations of Arima et al. [24]. The solid red line shows the prediction, the squares and triangles are referring to different experimental data; here, the triangles represent the data from Rhodes [50]. The dashed line shows the behavior of the Navier-Stokes-Fourier equations.

Here, using the NET-IV continuum model, only the experiment related to $T = 296.8$ K is considered for demonstrational reasons. It is not intended to evaluate the complete series of measurements. In Figure 5, two horizontal scales are used that intend to indicate the one-to-one correspondence between the ω/p and ρ. It is always possible if the frequency and the temperature are known. Although the fitting procedure is conducted by hand, it is clear that the NET-IV model is also applicable to these problems. However, it is more difficult to do due to more degrees of freedom. Tables 1 and 2 show the corresponding values of each parameter. For simplicity, in the fitting procedure the ratio of relaxation times was constrained to be the same as for RET, i.e., $\tau_q/\tau_d = 1.46$, $\tau_s/\tau_d = 144$.

Table 1. Fitted relaxation time coefficients for continuum model.

$\tau_q = \frac{t_1}{\rho}, t_1 = \left[\frac{kg\cdot s}{m^3}\right]$	$\tau_d = \frac{t_2}{\rho}, t_2 = \left[\frac{kg\cdot s}{m^3}\right]$	$\tau_s = \frac{t_3}{\rho}, t_3 = \left[\frac{kg\cdot s}{m^3}\right]$	τ_q/τ_d	τ_s/τ_d
4.526×10^{-9}	3.1×10^{-9}	4.464×10^{-7}	1.46	144

Table 2. Fitted coupling coefficients for continuum model.

$\alpha_{12} = \frac{a_{12}}{\rho}, a_{12} = \left[\frac{kg\cdot s}{m^3}\right]$	$\beta_{12} = \frac{b_{12}}{\rho}, b_{12} = \left[\frac{kg\cdot s}{m^3}\right]$	$\alpha_{21} = \frac{a_{21}}{\rho}, a_{21} = \left[\frac{kg}{m\cdot s}\right]$	$\beta_{21} = \frac{b_{21}}{\rho}, b_{21} = \left[\frac{kg}{m\cdot s}\right]$
1.7×10^{-6}	1.27×10^{-6}	1.3×10^{-4}	1.55×10^{-5}

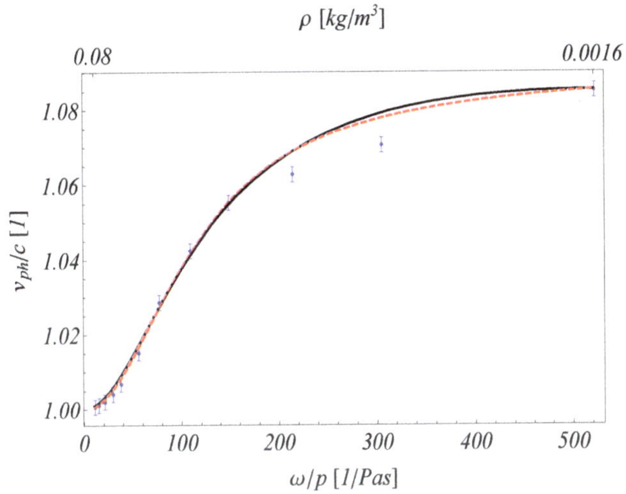

Figure 5. Evaluation using NET-IV (thick black line). The pressure starts at 1 atm and decreases to 2000 Pa, $\omega = 1$ MHz. Error bars are placed for each measurement point to indicate the uncertainty of digitalizing data, its magnitude is ± 2.5 m/s. The red dashed line shows the results of Arima et al. [24].

3. Discussion

The models originated from RET and NET-IV are briefly introduced and tested on a particular experiment performed by Rhodes. It is apparent from the experimental data that the rarefaction in a Hydrogen gas shows substantial deviation from its dense state. Here, the speed of sound data can be evaluated without any obstacles in NET IV as well, but this evaluation highlights some crucial aspects.

First, we note the difference between the theoretical and measured properties which has great importance in kinetic theory. In contrast, a continuum model does not propose this distinction, it is not possible to calculate the "physical" (theoretical) coefficient without a detailed micromechanism. Moreover, especially from practical point of view, the NET-IV model contains the "effective" (measurable) quantities which have density dependence as well, beside the temperature, according to the referred literature. Since the continuum approach does consist of the measurable transport coefficients, it keeps the continuum model on a more general level that is not restricted specifically, in contrast to the kinetic theory. In the present experimental evaluation, constant viscosities and thermal conductivity are used in order to keep the model compatible with the kinetic theory.

Second, it is advantageous if all the data are given in the experiment; the frequency-pressure ratio could be insufficient, especially when the effective transport coefficients are not constant respect to the pressure. In continuum theory, it does matter what is changed: the frequency, the pressure, or both. In that sense, it is confusing to use dimensionless frequency, especially when all the necessary data are given for the appropriate scale. Besides that fact, the application of dimensionless quantities is still valid, but their use makes it a bit more difficult to interpret the experimental data. Moreover, in the end, even the kinetic approach requires the knowledge about the pressure in order to evaluate the relaxation times and the coupling coefficients.

Moreover, it is also shown that besides the frequency/pressure scaling of experimental data, it is not necessarily obtained in the dispersion relations of a continuum model, merely by restrictive assumptions of constant coefficients. However, it is worth noting that if every experimental data are given appropriately, that is, the frequency and pressure are given separately, then the experimental data become evaluable even if the ω/p scaling is not visible in the dispersion relations. Furthermore, recalling the experimental data of Itterbeek and Gracki et al. in which the viscosity depends on the mass density, this is clear that its inclusion into the models would strongly influence the scaling properties as well. Thus, one question remains: which transport property is important from the aspect of the scaling, the theoretical one or the measurable one?

The difference between the presented approaches originates in the preassumptions. Using kinetic theory, a detailed interaction is assumed, and it restricts some degrees of freedom. On the other hand, in NET-IV, it is not necessary to make any preassumption regarding the type of the fluid, while in kinetic theory it is fixed as a first step, and the derived model such as Equation (5) will be valid only for this restricted case, in the price of the number of free coefficients. As mentioned in the introduction, one of the main difficulties is the fitting of free parameters in the model of NET-IV (4), that is, 7 coefficients are to be fitted instead of 3 that presented by Equation (5). It can be reduced if one adopts some knowledge from the kinetic approach and applies in the continuum model, such as the ratio of relaxation times. This disadvantage could be an advantage if the number of equations is still enough to describe a three-dimensional process on the contrary to the kinetic theory where the momentum expansion generates a large system of equations for a more general situation, for instance in the low temperature heat conduction problems.

As a final remark, it is essential to realize that these approaches extend each other from different directions. While NET-IV keeps the models as general as possible, RET builds a detailed one, with much more knowledge about the coefficients. Although the underlying physical picture is different, the resulting system of equations can be compatible with each other.

Funding: This research was funded by National Research, Development and Innovation Office—NKFIH K116197, K124366 and KH130378. The research reported in this paper was also supported by the Higher Education Excellence Program of the Ministry of Human Capacities in the frame of Nanotechnology research area of Budapest University of Technology and Economics (BME FIKP-NANO).

Acknowledgments: The author is thankful to Henning Struchtrup and Péter Ván for valuable discussions.

Conflicts of Interest: The author declares no conflict of interest.

References

1. Chester, M. Second sound in solids. *Phys. Rev.* **1963**, *131*, 2013–2015. [CrossRef]
2. Guyer, R.A.; Krumhansl, J.A. Thermal Conductivity, Second Sound, and Phonon Hydrodynamic Phenomena in Nonmetallic Crystals. *Phys. Rev.* **1966**, *148*, 778–788. [CrossRef]
3. Jackson, H.E.; Walker, C.T.; McNelly, T.F. Second sound in NaF. *Phys. Rev. Lett.* **1970**, *25*, 26–28. [CrossRef]
4. Rogers, S.J. Transport of heat and approach to second sound in some isotropically pure alkali-halide crystals. *Phys. Rev. B* **1971**, *3*, 1440. [CrossRef]
5. Narayanamurti, V.; Dynes, R.C. Observation of second sound in bismuth. *Phys. Rev. Lett.* **1972**, *28*, 1461–1465. [CrossRef]
6. Gyarmati, I. On the wave approach of thermodynamics and some problems of non-linear theories. *J. Non-Equilib. Thermodyn.* **1977**, *2*, 233–260. [CrossRef]
7. Joseph, D.D.; Preziosi, L. Heat waves. *Rev. Mod. Phys.* **1989**, *61*, 41. [CrossRef]
8. Joseph, D.D.; Preziosi, L. Addendum to the paper on heat waves. *Rev. Mod. Phys.* **1990**, *62*, 375–391. [CrossRef]

9. Dreyer, W.; Struchtrup, H. Heat pulse experiments revisited. *Contin. Mech. Thermodyn.* **1993**, *5*, 3–50. [CrossRef]
10. McNelly, T.F.; Rogers, S.J.; Channin, D.J.; Rollefson, R.J.; Goubau, W.M.; Schmidt, G.E.; Krumhansl, J.A.; Pohl, R.O. Heat pulses in NaF: Onset of second sound. *Phys. Rev. Lett.* **1970**, *24*, 100–102. [CrossRef]
11. McNelly, T.F. Second Sound and Anharmonic Processes in Isotopically Pure Alkali-Halides. Ph.D. Thesis, Cornell University, Ithaca, NY, USA, 1974.
12. Kovács, R.; Ván, P. Generalized heat conduction in heat pulse experiments. *Int. J. Heat Mass Transf.* **2015**, *83*, 613–620. [CrossRef]
13. Ván, P. Weakly nonlocal irreversible thermodynamics—The Guyer-Krumhansl and the Cahn-Hilliard equations. *Phys. Lett. A* **2001**, *290*, 88–92. [CrossRef]
14. Ván, P.; Fülöp, T. Universality in heat conduction theory—Weakly nonlocal thermodynamics. *Annalen der Physik (Berlin)* **2012**, *524*, 470–478. [CrossRef]
15. Chen, G. Ballistic-diffusive heat-conduction equations. *Phys. Rev. Lett.* **2001**, *86*, 2297–2300. [CrossRef]
16. Cimmelli, V.A. Different thermodynamic theories and different heat conduction laws. *J. Non-Equilib. Thermodyn.* **2009**, *34*, 299–333. [CrossRef]
17. Ván, P. Theories and heat pulse experiments of non-Fourier heat conduction. *Commun. Appl. Ind. Math.* **2016**, *7*, 150–166. [CrossRef]
18. Jou, D.; Casas-Vázquez, J.; Lebon, G. *Extended Irreversible Thermodynamics*, 4th ed.; Springer: Berlin, Germany, 2010.
19. Sellitto, A.; Cimmelli, V.A.; Jou, D. *Mesoscopic Theories of Heat Transport in Nanosystems*; Springer: Berlin, Germany, 2016.
20. Szücs, M.; Fülöp, T. Kluitenberg-Verhás rheology of solids in the GENERIC framework. *arXiv* **2019**, arXiv:1812.07052.
21. Müller, I.; Ruggeri, T. *Rational Extended Thermodynamics*; Springer: Berlin, Germany, 1998.
22. Kovács, R.; Ván, P. Models of Ballistic Propagation of Heat at Low Temperatures. *Int. J. Thermophys.* **2016**, *37*, 95. [CrossRef]
23. Kovács, R.; Ván, P. Second sound and ballistic heat conduction: NaF experiments revisited. *Int. J. Heat Mass Transf.* **2018**, *117*, 682–690. [CrossRef]
24. Ruggeri, T.; Sugiyama, M. *Rational Extended Thermodynamics Beyond the Monatomic Gas*; Springer: Berlin, Germany, 2015.
25. Kovács, R. Heat Conduction beyond Fourier's Law: Theoretical Predictions and Experimental Validation. Ph.D. Thesis, Budapest University of Technology and Economics (BME), Budapest, Hungary, 2017.
26. Kovács, R.; Madjarević, D.; Simić, S.; Ván, P. Theories of rarefied gases. *arXiv* **2018**, arXiv:1812.10355.
27. Both, S.; Czél, B.; Fülöp, T.; Gróf, G.; Gyenis, Á.; Kovács, R.; Ván, P.; Verhás, J. Deviation from the Fourier law in room-temperature heat pulse experiments. *J. Non-Equilib. Thermodyn.* **2016**, *41*, 41–48. [CrossRef]
28. Ván, P.; Berezovski, A.; Fülöp, T.; Gróf, G.; Kovács, R.; Lovas, Á.; Verhás, J. Guyer-Krumhansl-type heat conduction at room temperature. *EPL* **2017**, *118*, 50005. [CrossRef]
29. Fülöp, T.; Kovács, R.; Lovas, Á.; Rieth, Á.; Fodor, T.; Szücs, M.; Ván, P.; Gróf, G. Emergence of non-Fourier hierarchies. *Entropy* **2018**, *20*, 832. [CrossRef]
30. Struchtrup, H. *Macroscopic Transport Equations for Rarefied Gas Flows*; Springer: Berlin, Germany, 2005.
31. Nyíri, B. On the entropy current. *J. Non-Equilib. Thermodyn.* **1991**, *16*, 179–186. [CrossRef]
32. Jou, D.; Casas-Vázquez, J.; Lebon, G. Extended Irreversible Thermodynamics. *Rep. Prog. Phys.* **1988**, *51*, 1105. [CrossRef]
33. Alvarez, F.X.; Jou, D.; Sellitto, A. Phonon hydrodynamics and phonon- boundary scattering in nanosystems. *J. Appl. Phys.* **2009**, *105*, 014317. [CrossRef]
34. Guo, Y.; Wang, M. Phonon hydrodynamics and its applications in nanoscale heat transport. *Phys. Rep.* **2015**, *595*, 1–44. [CrossRef]
35. Struchtrup, H. Resonance in rarefied gases. *Contin. Mech. Thermodyn.* **2012**, *24*, 361–376. [CrossRef]
36. Berezovski, A.; Ván, P. Microinertia and internal variables. *arXiv* **2015**, arXiv:1504.03485.
37. Berezovski, A.; Ván, P. *Internal Variables in Thermoelasticity*; Springer: Basel, Switzerland, 2017.
38. Verhás, J. *Thermodynamics and Rheology*; Springer: Dordrecht, The Netherlands, 1997.
39. Meixner, J. Absorption und Dispersion des Schalles in Gasen mit Chemisch Reagierenden und Anregbaren Komponenten. I. Teil. *Annalen der Physik* **1943**, *435*, 470–487. (In German) [CrossRef]

40. Sellitto, A.; Cimmelli, V.A.; Jou, D. Entropy flux and anomalous axial heat transport at the nanoscale. *Phys. Rev. B* **2013**, *87*, 054302. [CrossRef]
41. Arima, T.; Taniguchi, S.; Ruggeri, T.; Sugiyama, M. Extended thermodynamics of dense gases. *Contin. Mech. Thermodyn.* **2012**, *24*, 271–292. [CrossRef]
42. Arima, T.; Taniguchi, S.; Ruggeri, T.; Sugiyama, M. Extended thermodynamics of real gases with dynamic pressure: An extension of Meixner's theory. *Phys. Lett. A* **2012**, *376*, 2799–2803. [CrossRef]
43. Arima, T.; Taniguchi, S.; Ruggeri, T.; Sugiyama, M. Dispersion relation for sound in rarefied polyatomic gases based on extended thermodynamics. *Contin. Mech. Thermodyn.* **2013**, *25*, 727–737. [CrossRef]
44. Pavić, M.; Ruggeri, T.; Simić, S. Maximum entropy principle for rarefied polyatomic gases. *Phys. A Stat. Mech. Appl.* **2013**, *392*, 1302–1317. [CrossRef]
45. Lebon, G.; Cloot, A. Propagation of ultrasonic sound waves in dissipative dilute gases and extended irreversible thermodynamics. *Wave Motion* **1989**, *11*, 23–32. [CrossRef]
46. Carrasi, M.; Morro, A. A modified Navier-Stokes equation, and its consequences on sound dispersion. *Il Nuovo Cimento B* **1972**, *9*, 321–343. [CrossRef]
47. Carrasi, M.; Morro, A. Some remarks about dispersion and absorption of sound in monatomic rarefied gases. *Il Nuovo Cimento B* **1973**, *13*, 281–289. [CrossRef]
48. Meyer, E.; Sessler, G. Schallausbreitung in gasen bei hohen frequenzen und sehr niedrigen drucken. *Zeitschrift für Physik* **1957**, *149*, 15–39. (In German) [CrossRef]
49. Klimontovich, Y.L. *Statistical Theory of Open Systems: A Unified Approach to Kinetic Description of Processes in Active Systems*; Springer: Dordrecht, The Netherlands, 1995.
50. Rhodes, J.E., Jr. The velocity of sound in hydrogen when rotational degrees of freedom fail to be excited. *Phys. Rev.* **1946**, *70*, 932. [CrossRef]
51. Sette, D.; Busala, A.; Hubbard, J.C. Energy transfer by collisions in vapors of chlorinated methanes. *J. Chem. Phys.* **1955**, *23*, 787–793. [CrossRef]
52. Greenspan, M. Propagation of sound in five monatomic gases. *J. Acoust. Soc. Am.* **1956**, *28*, 644–648. [CrossRef]
53. Sluijter, C.G.; Knaap, H.F.P.; Beenakker, J.J.M. Determination of rotational relaxation times of hydrogen isotopes by sound absorption measurements at low temperatures I. *Physica* **1964**, *30*, 745–762. [CrossRef]
54. Sluijter, C.G.; Knaap, H.F.P.; Beenakker, J.J.M. Determination of rotational relaxation times of hydrogen isotopes by sound absorption measurements at low temperatures II. *Physica* **1965**, *31*, 915–940. [CrossRef]
55. Stewart, J.L. A variable path ultrasonic interferometer for the four megacycle region with some measurements on air, co2, and h2. *Rev. Sci. Instrum.* **1946**, *17*, 59–65. [CrossRef] [PubMed]
56. Truesdell, C.; Muncaster, R.G. *Fundamentals of Maxwel's Kinetic Theory of a Simple Monatomic Gas: Treated as a Branch of Rational Mechanics*; Academic Press: Cambridge, MA, USA, 1980; Volume 83.
57. Pollard, W.G.; Present, R.D. On gaseous self-diffusion in long capillary tubes. *Phys. Rev.* **1948**, *73*, 762. [CrossRef]
58. Chapman, S.; Cowling, T. *The Mathematical Theory of Non-uniform Gases*, 3rd ed.; Cambridge University Press: New York, NY, USA, 1970.
59. Michalis, V.K.; Kalarakis, A.N.; Skouras, E.D.; Burganos, V.N. Rarefaction effects on gas viscosity in the Knudsen transition regime. *Microfluid. Nanofluidics* **2010**, *9*, 847–853. [CrossRef]
60. Cohen, Y.; Sandler, S.I. The viscosity and thermal conductivity of simple dense gases. *Ind. Eng. Chem. Fundam.* **1980**, *19*, 186–188. [CrossRef]
61. van der Gulik, P.S.; Trappeniers, N.J. The viscosity of argon at high densities. *Phys. A Stat. Mech. Appl.* **1986**, *135*, 1–20. [CrossRef]
62. van der Gulik, P.S.; Trappeniers, N.J. Application of Enskog theory on the viscosity of argon. *Physica B + C* **1986**, *139*, 137–139. [CrossRef]
63. van der Gulik, P.S.; ten Seldam, C.A. Density dependence of the viscosity of some noble gases. *Int. J. Thermophys.* **2002**, *23*, 15–26. [CrossRef]
64. Dymond, J.H. Corrections to the Enskog theory for viscosity and thermal conductivity. *Physica B* **1987**, *144*, 267–276. [CrossRef]
65. Umla, R.; Vesovic, V. Viscosity of liquids—Enskog-2σ model. *Fluid Phase Equilib.* **2014**, *372*, 34–42. [CrossRef]
66. Gracki, J.A.; Flynn, G.P.; Ross, J. *Viscosity of Nitrogen, Helium, Hydrogen, and Argon from −100 to 25 c up to 150–250 Atmospheres*; Project SQUID Technical Report; Purdue University: Lafayette, IN, USA, 1969; 33p.

67. Gracki, J.A.; Flynn, G.P.; Ross, J. Viscosity of Nitrogen, Helium, Hydrogen, and Argon from −100 to 25 c up to 150–250 atm. *J. Chem. Phys.* **1969**, *9*, 3856–3863. [CrossRef]
68. Haynes, W.M. Viscosity of gaseous and liquid argon. *Physica* **1973**, *67*, 440–470. [CrossRef]
69. Liboff, R.L. *Kinetic Theory: Classical, Quantum, and Relativistic Descriptions*; Springer Science & Business Media: Basel, Switzerland, 2003.
70. van Itterbeek, A.; Keesom, W.H. Measurements on the viscosity of helium gas between 293 and 1.6 k. *Physica* **1938**, *5*, 257–269. [CrossRef]
71. van Itterbeek, A.; Claes, A. Measurements on the viscosity of hydrogen-and deuterium gas between 293 K and 14 K. *Physica* **1938**, *5*, 938–944. [CrossRef]
72. van Itterbeek, A.; van Paemel, O. Measurements on the viscosity of gases for low pressures at room temperature and at low temperatures. *Physica* **1940**, *7*, 273–283. [CrossRef]
73. Beskok, A.; Karniadakis, G.E. Report: A model for flows in channels, pipes, and ducts at micro and nano scales. *Microscale Thermophys. Eng.* **1999**, *3*, 43–77.
74. Roohi, E.; Darbandi, M. Extending the Navier–Stokes solutions to transition regime in two-dimensional micro-and nanochannel flows using information preservation scheme. *Phys. Fluids* **2009**, *21*, 082001. [CrossRef]
75. Galindo-Rosales, F.J.; Rubio-Hernández, F.J.; Sevilla, A. An apparent viscosity function for shear thickening fluids. *J. Non-Newton. Fluid Mech.* **2011**, *166*, 321–325. [CrossRef]
76. Møller, P.C.F.; Fall, A.; Bonn, D. Origin of apparent viscosity in yield stress fluids below yielding. *Europhys. Lett.* **2009**, *87*, 38004. [CrossRef]
77. Falls, A.H.; Musters, J.J.; Ratulowski, J. The apparent viscosity of foams in homogeneous bead packs. *SPE Reserv. Eng.* **1989**, *4*, 155–164. [CrossRef]
78. Lipowsky, H.H.; Usami, S.; Chien, S. In vivo measurements of "apparent viscosity" and microvessel hematocrit in the mesentery of the cat. *Microvasc. Res.* **1980**, *19*, 297–319. [CrossRef]
79. Metzner, A.B.; Otto, R.E. Agitation of non-Newtonian fluids. *AIChE J.* **1957**, *3*, 3–10. [CrossRef]
80. Winter, T.G.; Hill, G.L. High-temperature ultrasonic measurements of rotational relaxation in hydrogen, deuterium, nitrogen, and oxygen. *J. Acoust. Soc. Am.* **1967**, *42*, 848–858. [CrossRef]

entropy

MDPI

Communication

A Note on the Entropy Force in Kinetic Theory and Black Holes

Rudolf A. Treumann [1,†] and Wolfgang Baumjohann [2,*,†]

1 International Space Science Institute, 3012 Bern, Switzerland
2 Space Research Institute, Austrian Academy of Sciences, Schmiedlstr. 6, 8042 Graz, Austria
* Correspondence: Wolfgang.Baumjohann@oeaw.ac.at
† These authors contributed equally to this work.

Received: 2 June 2019; Accepted: 19 July 2019; Published: 23 July 2019

Abstract: The entropy force is the collective effect of inhomogeneity in disorder in a statistical many particle system. We demonstrate its presumable effect on one particular astrophysical object, the black hole. We then derive the kinetic equations of a large system of particles including the entropy force. It adds a collective therefore integral term to the Klimontovich equation for the evolution of the one-particle distribution function. Its integral character transforms the basic one particle kinetic equation into an integro-differential equation already on the elementary level, showing that not only the microscopic forces but the hole system reacts to its evolution of its probability distribution in a holistic way. It also causes a collisionless dissipative term which however is small in the inverse particle number and thus negligible. However it contributes an entropic collisional dissipation term. The latter is defined via the particle correlations but lacks any singularities and thus is large scale. It allows also for the derivation of a kinetic equation for the entropy density in phase space. This turns out to be of same structure as the equation for the phase space density. The entropy density determines itself holistically via the integral entropy force thus providing a self-controlled evolution of entropy in phase space.

Keywords: entropy force; non-equilibrium phenomena; kinetic theory; entropic phase space density; black hole entropy

1. Introduction: Entropy Force

About thirty years ago, Prigogine [1] attempted a microscopic theory of entropy assuming that, by some quantum process, seeds of entropy could be generated. Such a hypothetical process would, in the early universe, possibly lay down the direction of time. Unfortunately, so far, such microscopic sources of entropy have not been confirmed. It seems that they can hardly be expected because quantum uncertainty itself is a stochastic process, which by its own nature does not contain any direction. It is hard to believe that it could lead to entropy production if not aided by some kind of dissipative interaction. Entropy is a thermodynamic concept, which by itself requires an underlying dynamics, which allows for the presence of many states that a system consisting of many subsystems, components, particles would be able to occupy.

More recently, it has been speculated [2] that that kind of a mesoscopic entropy in quantum string theory could cause gravity to emerge from the action of a quantum entropic force as a gradient of entropy generated in string interactions, intended to provide a physical basis for the so-called modified Newtonian gravity, which proposes that Newton's law should be corrected on the large scales to eliminate the problem of dark matter in astronomy.

From a completely different point of view, the idea of an entropy force has been picked up in the discussion of maximum entropy methods in prediction theory [3,4] in open systems where the probabilistic version of entropy depends on space and time, propagates into the future and, thus, has a finite gradient in space and time, which is interpreted as force. It apparently is capable of allowing, based on maximization of entropy, predicting the time evolution of the system, an interesting and possibly far-reaching predictive concept. In a sufficiently small closed system, it necessarily must describe the evolution of entropy towards a finite thermal state of maximum entropy. Recently, entropy forces have also been applied to molecular dynamics in proteins ([5] and the references therein). Spatial smallness is required by causality to enable synchronization. Therefore, the concept applies to the universe on the cosmological timescale only in order to allow for homogenization of entropy. On any local scale, the entropy produced in the classical system represents a localized excess in entropy. If not artificially confined, this excess tends to expand and affect its environment. This necessarily generates a local entropy force, a classical force that should not be mixed up with the above-mentioned entropic force in string systems. This force follows from the first law in thermodynamics:

$$dE = TdS - PdV \tag{1}$$

which relates the three different forms of energy E, pressure PV, and entropy TS. Gradients in energy, pressure, and temperature are known to be forces, and the gradient of volume causes dispersion, flows, and forces, for instance in charged systems.

In a similar vein, a gradient in entropy corresponds to a collective macroscopic effect as the entropy tends to expand and maximize. This is a purely macroscopic effect indeed because, similar to density/volume and pressure, the entropy S is defined only for macroscopic systems, consisting of a large number of subsystems, to which finite temperature and density can be assigned and which occupy a finite volume. In the first law, it is only the energy E that maintains its meaning also in the microscopic world down to only one particle, to which assigning temperature makes no sense. The entropy potential $U = TS$ indeed is not just a thermodynamic potential; it is also a real potential always being positive and thus repulsive. The entropy force is then given as its gradient:

$$\mathbf{F} = -\nabla U \tag{2}$$

as usually taken negative. It consist of two parts, a thermal force $-S\nabla T$, which is of no interest here, and the genuine entropy force:

$$\mathbf{F}_S = -T\nabla S \tag{3}$$

This might look trivial; however, it is not, as we will demonstrate below with a particular example: the black hole.

However, before proceeding, we recall that, since both T and S are positive definite, the entropy force is repulsive in the direction negative to the gradient of entropy. This means that an accumulation of entropy at some location, if not artificially confined to a box, will act outward. Adopting an interpretation of entropy as disorder, which by no means is generally justified, thus implies that disorder tends to infect its external region. It has the tendency to expand.

With temperature T in energy units, the entropy S has no dimension. Moreover, the product of temperature and entropy is a scalar function with the dimension of a potential. For scalar temperature, i.e., at temperature isotropy, S is also a scalar. Under conditions of anisotropic temperature, the inverse temperature becomes a vector [6], and thus, S becomes a vector as well (more generally, both become tensors). In the interest of simplicity, we do not consider this case in the following.

This entropy force does not depend on particle mass or charge, at least not explicitly. Mass is contained in temperature and energy, but there is no explicit reference to it in the definition of the entropy force. Thus, for a given temperature, all particles independent of their properties will be subject to the same entropy force. In this sense, the entropy force is a general mechanical force seeking to restore smoothness in disorder on a higher level of disorder, completely independent of which kind of particles have contributed to the inhomogeneity in disorder.

By its nature, the above entropy force is a long-range force. It does not compete with the Coulomb force on the short scales. From the first law, one realizes that the main force it competes with is the pressure gradient. Both are proportional to the temperature, which thus drops out when comparing the forces. Both are proportional to the density gradient. Thus, in the presence of changing volume, the entropy force adds to or diminishes the effect of the pressure force.

2. Entropy Force of Schwarzschild Black Holes

Let us turn to our example, the Schwarzschild black hole, which we chose for demonstration because of its simplicity and cleanness compared to Kerr or charged Nordstrom black holes. Black holes are known to carry entropy [7–12]. More correctly, since the interior of the black hole is not accessible, it is the black hole horizon that carries an entropy. This came as a surprise, as it implies that the horizon possesses a temperature and therefore must be considered as a macrosystem, which occupies a large number of states. Microscopically, this puzzle has not been resolved until today, even though a large number of attempts have been put forward to elucidate the internal structure of the horizon (see [13–17] and several others). Such considerations were based on the Bekenstein–Hawking entropy and the Hawking radiation of a black hole [11], which is attributed to its finite entropy and thus finite temperature. It implies the existence of a thermodynamic for the black hole horizon with the implication that the horizon physics involves a very large number of states that can be occupied. Jacobson [15] extended this concept to horizons in general in order to develop a thermodynamics of gravitational horizons from which he found that Einstein's gravitational field equations formally play the role of equations of state. This concept was reviewed and extended subsequently by Padmanabhan [16] to speculate about the general importance of horizon physics in general relativity and cosmology, suggesting that all the physics is holographically contained in the physics of horizons.

Schwarzschild black holes are in the first place classical objects. However, their entropy includes the quantum nature of matter at the horizon (cf., e.g., [13]), which is induced by the sharpness of the horizon and indicates that black holes are not purely classical. Let us ask what the entropy force related to the presence of the horizon would be.

2.1. Schwarzschild Constant

A Schwarzschild black hole of mass M has energy Mc^2, radius $R_S = 2GM/c^2$, and spherical surface $A_{BH} = 4\pi R_S^2$. Forming the ratio of the total black hole energy and the Schwarzschild radius yields:

$$\mathcal{F}_S = Mc^2/R_S = c^4/2G = 6.053 \times 10^{43} \quad \mathrm{N} \tag{4}$$

a constant that has the dimension of a force and that we call the Schwarzschild constant. This is a universal constant, whose value is independent of any property of the black hole, a force. This force is the Planck force, which so far has not been given any physical meaning. We prefer to call it the Schwarzschild constant as the black hole is the only place where it naturally arises.

2.2. Horizon Entropy Force

The entropy of the black hole horizon is the (dimensionless) Bekenstein–Hawking entropy:

$$S_{BH} = \frac{A_{BH}}{4\lambda_P^2} = \frac{\pi R_S^2 c^3}{G\hbar} \tag{5}$$

with λ_P the Planck length, and its corresponding black-body radiation temperature is the Hawking temperature:

$$T^{BH} = k_B T_H = \hbar c^3/8\pi GM \tag{6}$$

here given in energy units. This yields trivially the Bekenstein–Hawking energy $E_{BH} = T^{BH} S_{BH} = \frac{1}{2}Mc^2$ of the horizon, just half the black hole energy. For a classical black hole, the horizon has no width, suggesting an infinite gradient when crossing it. In order to obtain the force, the relevant distance taken for the gradient is the diameter $2R_S$ of the black hole, yielding for the modulus of the outward directed entropy force:

$$F_S^{BH} \sim \frac{T^{BH} S_{BH}}{2R_S} = \frac{c^4}{8G} = \frac{\mathcal{F}_S}{4} \approx 1.5 \times 10^{43}\,\mathrm{N} \tag{7}$$

a quarter of the Schwarzschild constant. A more precise calculation would correct for the numerical factor, which, however, is of order $O(1)$. Formally, the Schwarzschild constant, and thus also the entropy force at the horizon, is in fact a very strong force. Its presence, if real, at the horizon is rather surprising. It suggests that the physics of what happens inside the black hole is not really well enough understood.

Forming the ratio of the gravitational force $F_G^{BH} = -GmM/R_S^2$ any particle of mass m experiences when approaching and touching the black hole horizon to this horizon entropy force, one obtains:

$$\left| F_G^{BH} / F_S^{BH} \right| \sim m/M \tag{8}$$

For any massive black hole and any normal mass particle, this is a small number. A light particle $m \ll M$ will barely overcome this repulsion when hitting the horizon. To overcome it, it requires the collision of two black holes of nearly equal mass $M_1 \sim M_2$, which would make the ratio $m/M \to M_1/M_2 \approx 1$. Collisions of such nearly-equal mass black holes have only recently been detected by the spectacular observation of gravitational waves.

At its horizon, the entropy force of a massive black hole $M \gg m$ compensates by far for the black hole's gravitational attraction on m. This is a consequence of the enormous sharpness of the entropy gradient at the horizon where the entropy is restricted to the surface of the horizon only, whose width is not precisely given, but as generally assumed, is of the order of a few Planck lengths λ_P only. This force is remarkable only at the horizon itself when the mass m gets into contact with the horizon. It will not be susceptible at some larger finite distance.

This follows from the fact that there is no known classical entropy field that would allow the entropy force to extend a distance ahead of the black hole into the surrounding space and is conjectured from the complete absence of any radial dependence of the force outside the horizon. In this picture, the entropy gradient is felt only locally across the horizon of the black hole when the particle touches it, an instant that is never seen or experienced by an external observer for whom the time the particle approaches the horizon stretches out to infinity. The particle, however, does in fact experience the presence of the black hole and, assuming that it remains intact having survived the enormous attraction during its inward spiraling motion, in its proper frame at proper time, really touches the horizon and wants to cross it. Shortly before this instant, however, the horizon entropy comes into play and stops the particle.

The gravitational force on the particle of mass m (assuming it retains its mass till reaching the horizon, which is certainly not the case) would overcome the entropic force still only at a small fraction of the radius given by:

$$\frac{\Delta r}{R_S} \approx \left(\frac{M_\odot}{M}\right)^{\frac{1}{2}} \left(\frac{m}{M_\odot}\right)^{\frac{1}{2}} \approx 3 \times 10^{-28} \left(\frac{M_\odot}{M}\right)^{\frac{1}{2}} \tag{9}$$

where on the right, we assumed a proton. For instance, this distance for a proton and a $M = 10^8 M_\odot$ massive black hole is of the order of only $\Delta r \sim 10^{-23}$ m, deep inside the submicroscopic domain, though ten orders of magnitude larger than the Planck length. If it applies, then it would cause accumulation of matter in a film of roughly this width only.

The classical picture does not inform about the microscopic physics going on when this happens. Elucidating the real physics requires a quantum electrodynamic calculation for instance along the paths drawn by Hawking when calculating the black-body black hole radiation. Referring to Hawking's results implies that the horizon will be surrounded by a dilute and thin radial dust film of newly- and continuously-created virtual particles, which sustain and support the weak Hawking radiation when tunneling into reality. The radial extension of this dust film implies a softening of the radial entropy gradient corresponding to a finite radial extension of the action region of the entropy force. It would be this radial domain where the light particle in its inward spiraling motion becomes trapped and retarded and is ultimately stopped and prevented from entering the interior of the black hole.

2.3. Body Entropy

What happens to the entropy inside the black hole would be important to know (cf. [18] for a discussion of Hawking radiation inside black hole geometry) in order to resolve the puzzle. It is rather improbable that the entropy would be constant inside the black hole, as this would require that the interior is in thermal equilibrium, which it is certainly not when being under the conditions of collapsing matter under gravitational attraction. One might speculate that towards deeper inside, the entropy decreases with decreasing radius, because the surface decreases as $\sim(r/R_S)^2$. Assigning a Hawking temperature to each shell of such a radius, the corresponding Hawking temperature would increase only as $\sim R_S/r$. Thus any entropy-force potential should decrease towards the interior like $\sim r/R_S$. The outer black hole horizon becomes the black hole shell of maximum entropy, the radius where the black hole entropy maximizes. The interior entropy force, the gradient of the potential, remains constant throughout the entire interior volume of the black hole with the exclusion of the singularity.

Notably, this entropy force points towards the interior of the hole, i.e., towards the singularity. It thus adds to the already existing gravitational acceleration being felt throughout the entire interior. By pointing inside towards decreasing radius r, it would push any existing massive particle that made it across the horizon into the singularity up in energy. This probably means that classically, no massive particle can make it across the horizon. It can only be non-massive radiation that crosses inward: photons and gluons, the massless bosons of electrodynamics and chromodynamics. Whether massive particles like electrons and quarks can indeed tunnel across the horizon remains a question that cannot be answered in the realm of classical physics.

Admittedly, these considerations are rather speculative as long as the evolution of entropy with increasing radial distance from the horizon towards inside and also outside the black hole has not been microscopically inferred. In any case, the question of the horizon representing a sharp surface remains a question that probably only quantum gravity can give an ultimate answer to, as it must proceed on scales close to the Planck scale λ_P. This is not our concern here.

2.4. Visibility and Matter Digestion

Naked isolated black holes are invisible except for their weak and so far inaccessible Hawking radiation. The question why black holes, which are embedded into surrounding matter, when accreting become visible at all is comparably easy to answer. Any mass flow approaching the horizon before encounter feels the gravitational field of the black hole, spirals in, accelerates, heats up, becomes partially transformed into radiation, and starts radiating violently. General relativity indicates that this process stretches time to infinity. Hence, even though the matter starts as material particles that cannot be digested by the black hole, because matter cannot pass the horizon due to the barrier the classical entropic force provides for massive particles, the emitted radiation is visible for long. The latter is a well-known fact, and though radiation from accreting black hole suspects has been observed for decades already, the observational proof has only very recently been given when a particular black hole signature could be resolved in radio emission.

During inward spiraling, the matter irradiates, which happens for all the matter that consists of much smaller mass particles (gaseous clouds, dust, stars) than the black hole. The total mass of the matter that hits the horizon at each instant is much less than M. The radiation produced in this process may be considered isotropic because there is no remarkable beaming until the matter becomes charged during gravitational compression, heating, and ionization. It then via a dynamo process generates its proper magnetic field, which tangentially surrounds the black hole horizon and funnels the irreducible to radiation charged particles into two approximately symmetric jets. This self-generated magnetic field provides the outflow channel for the escape of light not irradiated charged matter, which the entropy force rejects from crossing the horizon. Matter accreted by a massive black hole does not arrive at the very horizon as matter, but as charge and massless radiation: mostly photons, possibly gluons, depending on the strength of the gravitational force (i.e., on the mass M of the black hole whether or not it would be large enough to overcome gluon confinement, which is rather unbelievable).

The fraction of radiative energy that hits the black hole and gets trapped consists of photons. These are massless and do not feel the entropy force when encountering the horizon, because the entropy force acts on finite mass particles only. The photons feel, however, the gravitational black hole potential, which is acting on their energy and thus gravitationally deflects their orbits. The photon paths become spirally warped until they ultimately hit the horizon. When this happens, the photons make it across the horizon and enter the interior of the black hole. Looked at from the outside, this takes infinitely long again. It is an open question as to what happens to them inside the horizon, whether or not they collapse, and whether a singularity forms at all if only photons are available. We do not ponder about those interesting questions here.

The implication is that the mass influx into the hole proceeds via irradiation of matter as radiative inflow, not as matter inflow. The black hole is fed by photons. Feeding a black hole with small portions of matter in this view proceeds via transformation into radiation. Those parts of matter that do not transform into radiation, protons and the required neutralizing electrons, become expelled along the newly-formed magnetic funnels into space in the form of jets before touching the horizon. The jets either disperse in interaction with distant matter or become part of cosmic radiation. The process of how radiation may tunnel across the horizon is answered by the quantum electrodynamics of this process including the positive entropy potential drop at the horizon the radiation passes when hitting the black hole, which however barely affects the uncharged and massless photons.

Another question concerns the merging of two equal mass massive black holes. This case is of substantial interest because it has been observed in the first detections of gravitational radiation. If there is just a small mass difference, then probably the two almost equally-strong forces would produce a deformation of the horizons at contact, causing a bubble to evolve, like in the encounter of two soap bubbles. Merging of the horizons takes place at the circumference where the gradients of the entropy become tangential. The holes would start here to merge until the horizon encompasses both holes, with a trapped bubble forming in its common interior and thus becoming invisible to the external observer.

Finally, what happens when asking for the mysterious planckions, Planck particles of mass $M \sim 10^{-8}$ kg ($\sim 10^{19}$ GeV), which may have been created in the Big Bang and are believe to be Planck scale black holes? According to Hawking radiation theory, they should have evaporated in a Planck time of $\sim 10^{-43}$ s already after production, though it is not clear whether at the Planck scale, one can speak at all of black holes, as inside the planckion, quantum gravity necessarily comes into play, and Hawking's quantum electrodynamical calculations should become invalid. Looked at from the outside, a planckion is its own horizon and thus is fuzzy because its radius and diameter equal spatial uncertainty. Assuming that one still could speak about their surface, entropy, and entropy force, their entropy would be of the order of $S \sim O(1)$, while the entropy force would remain huge, equal to the Schwarzschild constant, outrunning the gravitational attraction force. Does this mean that planckions would neither radiate, nor be able to merge, keeping one another at a distance and in larger numbers causing some crystal-like texture? In this case, they could have survived (cf., e.g., [19] for contras) since the Big Bang and accumulated in agglomerations like clusters of galaxies where they could well serve (see [20] for pros) as a dark matter candidate.

3. Microscopic Phase-Space Density and the Entropy Force

So far, we just discussed the effect of the entropy force on a particular object: Schwarzschild black holes in astrophysics. We now turn to the general kinetic problem of the microscopic evolution of the particle distribution in many-particle physics. We restrict solely to classical systems, i.e., to systems that are described on the microscopic level by the classical Liouville equation, respectively its Klimontovich [21] equivalent in Equation (12) given below, and its hydrodynamic generalization [22].

Liouville's equation describes the evolution of the microscopic phase space density in N-dimensional phase space. On the classical elementary level of indistinguishable point charges, which have some properties like mass m_a, possibly some charge e of different sign, and are distributed over a spatial volume V with volume element d^3q and the momentum volume of element d^3p can be described alternatively [21,22] by an exact known phase space density:

$$\begin{aligned}\mathcal{N}_a^m(\mathbf{p},\mathbf{q},t) &= \sum_{i=1}^{N_a}\delta(\mathbf{p}-\mathbf{p}_{ai}(t))\delta(\mathbf{q}-\mathbf{q}_{ai}(t)) \\ &\equiv \sum_{i=1}^{N_a}\delta(\mathbf{x}-\mathbf{x}_{ai}(t))\end{aligned} \tag{10}$$

which simply counts the number of particles of sort a in the entire $6D$-phase space volume, such that it is normalized as:

$$N_a = \int d^3p\, d^3q\, \mathcal{N}_a^m(\mathbf{p},\mathbf{q},t) \tag{11}$$

For a constant particle number, the time dependence is implicit in the particle trajectories $\mathbf{p}_{ai}(t), \mathbf{q}_{ai}(t)$ such that integration has to be performed along all of them. One may note that the microscopic phase space density $\mathcal{N}_a^m$ is otherwise dimensionless. This is seen from the definition of the delta-functions, which in the integration over phase space simply count numbers, which of course means that the normalization to space and momentum is implicit to them. Later, we will make the normalization more explicit, as this will be required by reference to the entropy.

Since the assumption is that the particles are classical, then in the absence of any particle sources or losses, the particle number in phase space is conserved along all the dynamical trajectories of the particles under their mutual, as well as external forces. In this case, the continuity equation of the particles, i.e., the microscopic Liouville equation in the N_a-particle $6D$-phase space [21], reads simply:

$$\dot{\mathcal{N}}_a^m \equiv \frac{\partial\mathcal{N}_a^m}{\partial t} + \frac{\mathbf{p}}{m_a}\cdot\nabla_{\mathbf{q}}\mathcal{N}_a^m + \frac{d\mathbf{p}}{dt}\cdot\frac{\partial\mathcal{N}_a^m}{\partial\mathbf{p}} = 0 \tag{12}$$

Of course, here, $\dot{\mathbf{p}} = \mathbf{F}$ is the total force that acts on the particles at their location $\mathbf{q} = \mathbf{q}_{ai}(t)$ and thus on the phase space density, and the two last terms together constitute the Poisson bracket $[\ldots]$ in the Liouville equation, which in N_a-phase space, the $6D$-phase space that within, the N_a particles perform their trajectories, is a tautology.

The entropy force can be compared with other more conventional forces. Let, for simplicity, the total force $\mathbf{F} = \mathbf{F}_Q + \mathbf{F}_S$ be the sum of the entropy force and of another potential force $\mathbf{F}_Q = -\nabla_q U$, where $U(\mathbf{q},t)$ is the force potential. The entropy force just adds the potential $TS(\mathbf{q},t)$ to the force potential U. Note that the entropy-force potential is always positive, as already made use of above, because there are neither negative temperatures [23] (The absence of negative temperatures is immediately clear from the definition of the temperature T as proportional to the mean ensemble averaged square of the momentum fluctuations $T \sim \langle(\delta\mathbf{p})^2\rangle$ of all particles in the volume, which clearly, is a positive definite quantity. Negative temperatures would require imaginary momenta or particle mass. There are no candidates for such particles, though experiments of neutrino oscillations provide negative mean square masses, which, however, are interpreted differently.), nor are there negative entropies. Clearly, for strong forces acting on the particles and weak entropy gradients, the entropy force is negligible. This might be the usual case. On the other hand, if on the large scale the inter-particle forces compensate, the entropy force will remain because there is no obvious counterpart that could compensate it. For instance, when dealing with electrostatic interactions only in the absence of any external fields and forces, the microscopic force $\mathbf{F}^m_Q(\mathbf{q},t) = \sum_a e_a \mathcal{E}^m(\mathbf{q},t)$ is the Coulomb force acting on the charges $e_a = ae$ with $a = +,-$ in the microscopic electrostatic field $\mathcal{E}^m(\mathbf{q},t)$ obeying Maxwell–Poisson's equations:

$$\nabla_q \cdot \mathcal{E}^m = \frac{1}{\epsilon_0} \sum_a \rho^m_{ae}(\mathbf{q},t), \quad \mathcal{E}^m = -\nabla_{\mathbf{q}} \Phi^m_e(\mathbf{q},t) \tag{13}$$

with electrostatic potential Φ^m_e, and thus, $U = \sum_a e_a \Phi^m_e$. On the microscopic level in phase space, the microscopic electric space charge (not the charge density) of species a is:

$$\rho^m_{ae}(\mathbf{q},t) = e_a \int d^3p\, \mathcal{N}^m_a(\mathbf{p},\mathbf{q},t), \quad \int d^3q \rho^m_{ae} = e_a N_a \tag{14}$$

It simply counts all charges in the total volume not relating them to the spatial volume V_a yet. Summing over all species a, the total space charge is obtained. On average, it will be zero. The charges are moving, and there is a microscopic current:

$$\mathbf{j}^m_{ae}(\mathbf{q},t) = \frac{e_a}{m_a} \int d^3p\, \mathbf{p}\, \mathcal{N}^m_a(\mathbf{p},\mathbf{q},t) = e_a \mathbf{v}_a(\mathbf{q},t) N_a \tag{15}$$

with $\mathbf{v}_a(\mathbf{q},t)$ the average velocity of particles in group a. It gives rise to an internal magnetic field, which, in the electrostatic approximation, is relativistically small and is thus neglected (e.g., [21]), though this is not completely correct, because in a linear theory of fluctuations, it should be taken into account.

Electrostatic interactions have been the subject of exhaustive investigations in the literature. Here, they serve only as another force field against which the entropy force can be compared. The striking difference is that for the entropy force, no field is generated because there is no entropy charge comparable to e_a and, hence, no singularity that would act as the source of the entropy field. In other words, the entropy field is, in contrast to the electric field, not related to field equations and thus lacks a field theory. Disorder lacks any elementary source not being a field, at least in classical physics.

The entropy of a system entering the first law of total energy conservation is an integral quantity. In order to refer to it on the elementary level of the microscopic kinetic equation in $6D$-phase space, one has to return to its microscopic definition as the phase space average of the probability distribution.

It is convenient to define an entropy phase space density by referring to Gibbs–Boltzmann's definition of entropy through the probability density. Entropy density will then be obtained by integrating out the momentum space coordinates in the usual way. In the definition of the phase space density of entropy, we will at this point not yet make the assumption that the phase space volume is constant, but include the spatial dependence as well. This is advantageous because it allows making use of phase space densities. Integrating out the volume can be done at a later stage. With this in mind, the "microscopic Boltzmann entropy phase-space density" of species a becomes (A number of other definitions or generalizations of entropy different from Boltzmann–Gibbs have been put forward in the near past [24–30], the physical, not the statistical meaning of which is not entirely clear. Though the theory could be extended to include those, we will neither refer to, nor use them in this note.):

$$\mathcal{S}^m_{aB}(\mathbf{p},\mathbf{q},t) = -\log \mathcal{N}'^m_a(\mathbf{p},\mathbf{q},t), \quad \mathcal{N}'^m_a = \mathcal{N}^m_a / N_a \tag{16}$$

where the phase space density has been normalized to the total number N_a of particles of species a. This makes the argument of the logarithm smaller than one, of which the negative sign takes care. A definition like this leans on Boltzmann's proposal. It is incomplete on the microscopic level because the entropy is a collective quantity, which is obtained by integrating over momentum space with the microscopic phase space density $\mathcal{N}_a$ as the weight. One thus has as microscopic N-particle entropy phase-space density in $(\mathbf{p}, \mathbf{q})$-space:

$$\mathcal{S}_a^m(\mathbf{p}, \mathbf{q}, t) = -\mathcal{N}_a^m(\mathbf{p}, \mathbf{q}, t) \log \mathcal{N}_a'^m(\mathbf{p}, \mathbf{q}, t) \tag{17}$$

This microscopic phase-space density of the entropy is not the entropy itself, which is a function solely of the space coordinates. The N_a-particle entropy of sort a is explicitly obtained by the integration of (17) over the entire momentum phase space:

$$\begin{aligned} S_a^m(\mathbf{q}, t) &= \int d^3p\, \mathcal{S}_a^m(\mathbf{q}, \mathbf{p}, t) \\ &\equiv \int d^3p' d^3q' \delta(\mathbf{q} - \mathbf{q}')\, \mathcal{S}_a^m(\mathbf{q}', \mathbf{p}', t) \end{aligned} \tag{18}$$

and is always positive, as is easily seen from the definition of the microscopic phase space density, a positive quantity, and the above choice of entropy. Summing over all particle species a then gives the total entropy. Moreover, because information is transported via some field, for instance the electromagnetic field, the time under the integral in Equation (17) is the retarded time $t^R = t - |\mathbf{q} - \mathbf{q}'|/c$ where c is the velocity of signal/information transport between the particles at locations $\mathbf{q}$ and $\mathbf{q}'$ in the real-space subspace of the $6D$-phase space [31,32]. In conventional kinetic theory, retardation is neglected because c is the velocity of light, and the distances between particles are usually less than ct. This is also assumed in the following.

There is a direct correspondence between this real space microscopic entropy density and the real space charge density $\rho^m(\mathbf{q}, t)$. Both enter the force term via taking the spatial gradient. The difference is that for the electric charge density, this step passes through the electric field $\mathcal{E}^m$, which is generated by the space charges. Repeated again, for the entropy, there is no such field, nor field equation in classical physics. Entropy is not a charge of some entity and thus does not generate a field. Taking its spatial gradient directly provides the force that acts on the particle at location $\mathbf{q}$.

4. Kinetic Equation with Entropy Force

The entropy force acting on species a is the negative gradient of Equation (18). This leads to a repulsive force, independent of any charge. It adds to the potential U in Klimontovich's equation Thus, taking it into account in Equation (12), it becomes clear that it does not affect the particle number and thus does not imply any important change in the microscopic N_a-particle phase space density $\mathcal{N}_a^m$. The main interest is in its effect on the one-particle kinetic phase space distribution function $f_a(\mathbf{x}, t)$. This is defined through the ensemble-averaged N_a-particle phase space density:

$$\frac{N_a}{V_a} f_a(\mathbf{x}, t) = \langle \mathcal{N}_a^m(\mathbf{x}, t) \rangle \tag{19}$$

where $\langle \dots \rangle$ indicates the ensemble average, and explicitly for the one-particle distribution:

$$f_a(\mathbf{x}_{a1}, t) = V_a \int f_N d^6\mathbf{x}_{a2} \dots d^6\mathbf{x}_{aN_a} \prod_{b \neq a} d^6\mathbf{x}_{b1} \dots d^6\mathbf{x}_{bN_b} \tag{20}$$

$$\langle \mathcal{N}_a^m(\mathbf{x}, t) \rangle = N_a \int \delta(\mathbf{x} - \mathbf{x}_{a1}) f_N \prod_a d^6\mathbf{x}_{a1} \dots d^6\mathbf{x}_{aN_a} \tag{21}$$

with $V_a \equiv V$ the spatial volume occupied by the indistinguishable particle sort a. f_N is the N-particle distribution function, and the integration is with respect to all indistinguishable particles $N - 1$, but one, the particle with coordinates $\mathbf{x}_{a1}$, as has been defined by Klimontovich [21]. In fact, the distribution function f_N is not explicitly given. It can be resolved on the way of sequentially stepping up the ladder from the one-particle distribution function to higher order distribution functions, which depend on one, two, three, or more indistinguishable particles.

Before proceeding to rewriting the Klimontovich Equation (12), it is necessary to investigate what happens to the entropy when performing the ensemble average implied in the former equations. We do actually not need the entropy itself, rather its spatial gradient, i.e., we need the spatial gradient of the entropy-phase space density (17). For this, we have:

$$-\nabla_{\mathbf{q}} S_a^m = \left(1 + \log \mathcal{N}_a'^m\right) \nabla_{\mathbf{q}} \mathcal{N}_a^m \tag{22}$$

The entropy force is the integral of the gradient of Equation (18) over the primed phase space:

$$\begin{aligned} \mathbf{F}_S^a(\mathbf{q}, t) &= T\nabla_{\mathbf{q}} \int d^3p' d^3q' \delta(\mathbf{q} - \mathbf{q}') \times \\ &\times \mathcal{N}_a^m(\mathbf{p}', \mathbf{q}', t) \log \mathcal{N}_a'^m(\mathbf{p}', \mathbf{q}', t) \end{aligned} \tag{23}$$

Reduction of the entropy-force term in Klimontovich's equation requires performing the ensemble average of the term:

$$\mathbf{F}_S^a(\mathbf{q}, t) \cdot \frac{\partial}{\partial \mathbf{p}} \mathcal{N}_a^m(\mathbf{q}, \mathbf{p}, t) \tag{24}$$

In order to do so, we need to consider different groups of particles such that:

$$\begin{aligned} \mathbf{F}_S(\mathbf{q}, t) &= T\sum_b \nabla_{\mathbf{q}} \int d^3p' d^3q' \delta(\mathbf{q} - \mathbf{q}') \times \\ &\times \mathcal{N}_b^m(\mathbf{p}', \mathbf{q}', t) \log \mathcal{N}_b'^m(\mathbf{p}', \mathbf{q}', t) \end{aligned} \tag{25}$$

This produces formally the entropy force contribution to the Klimontovich equation:

$$\begin{aligned} \mathbf{F}_S &\cdot \frac{\partial}{\partial \mathbf{p}} \mathcal{N}_a^m = T\nabla_{\mathbf{q}} \sum_b \int d^3p' d^3q' \delta(\mathbf{q} - \mathbf{q}') \cdot \\ &\cdot \frac{\partial}{\partial \mathbf{p}} \left\langle \mathcal{N}_a^m(\mathbf{p}, \mathbf{q}, t) \mathcal{N}_b^m(\mathbf{p}', \mathbf{q}', t) \log \mathcal{N}_b'^m(\mathbf{p}', \mathbf{q}', t) \right\rangle \end{aligned} \tag{26}$$

where $\langle \dots \rangle$ indicates the ensemble average, and we have used Equation (22). The momentum differentiation affects only terms containing the phase space density. This leads to the appearance of the logarithmic term on the right and introduces a third-order correlation term. The $(N-1)$-particle ensemble-averaged term provides problems because it contains the logarithm of the phase space density. In a somewhat severe approximation, we may assume that the logarithm is a slowly-varying function. Its argument is smaller than one such that it can be expanded, which yields:

$$\begin{aligned} &\left\langle \mathcal{N}_a^m(\mathbf{p}, \mathbf{q}, t) \mathcal{N}_b^m(\mathbf{p}', \mathbf{q}', t) \log \mathcal{N}_b'^m(\mathbf{p}', \mathbf{q}', t) \right\rangle \\ \approx &\left\langle \mathcal{N}_a^m(\mathbf{p}, \mathbf{q}, t) \mathcal{N}_b^m(\mathbf{p}', \mathbf{q}', t) \left(\mathcal{N}_b'^m(\mathbf{p}', \mathbf{q}', t) - 1 \right) \right\rangle \end{aligned} \tag{27}$$

This generates the ensemble-averaged Klimontovich equation:

$$\begin{aligned} \frac{\partial \langle \mathcal{N}_a^m \rangle}{\partial t} &+ \frac{\mathbf{p}}{m_a} \cdot \nabla_q \langle \mathcal{N}_a^m \rangle - T\nabla_q \sum_{b \neq a} \int d^6x' \, \delta(\mathbf{q} - \mathbf{q}') \\ &\cdot \frac{\partial}{\partial \mathbf{p}} \left\langle \mathcal{N}_a^m(\mathbf{x}, t) \, \mathcal{N}_b^m(\mathbf{x}', t) \right\rangle = -\left\langle \mathcal{C}_a^S(\mathbf{x}, t) \right\rangle \end{aligned} \tag{28}$$

The average purely entropic collision term on the right collects the third-order correlations:

$$\begin{aligned}\left\langle \mathcal{C}_a^S(\mathbf{x},t)\right\rangle &= T\nabla_q \sum_{b\neq a}\int d^6x'\,\delta(\mathbf{q}-\mathbf{q}') \\ &\cdot \frac{\partial}{\partial \mathbf{p}}\left\langle \mathcal{N}_a^m(\mathbf{x},t)\,\mathcal{N}_b^m(\mathbf{x}',t)\,\mathcal{N}_b^{\prime m}(\mathbf{x}',t)\right\rangle\end{aligned}$$

In these expressions, we have, for simplicity of writing, only included the entropy force term. One trivially adds the microscopic Coulomb or any other force term to this if required (Note, however, that adding the microscopic gravitational force causes problems because it remains uncompensated (As in any kinetic theory, this is an important difference between gravitation and any other force. It implies that in kinetic theory gravitation can only be included consistently in a general relativistic quantum gravitation where gravitation is balanced by quantum fluctuations.).). The entropy force term resembles the latter, but lacks a charge singularity. This is replaced by the spatial derivative of the delta-function, which appears under the integral.

The main difference is that already on this very basic level, the presence of the entropy force contributes a purely entropic dissipative term $\langle \mathcal{C}_a^S(\mathbf{x},t)\rangle$, which has been transferred to the right in the above expression. This term arises due to the generation of entropy in the system. It is a three-particle correlation term, as will become clear below. It is caused by the logarithm in the entropy, the continuous growth of entropy in a many-particle system. Whether it can be neglected as being of higher order is a subtle question. It causes collisionless dissipation in the presence of entropy. Since this effect is non-collisional, when neglecting particle collisions, one must take care whether its neglect is allowed. Below, we show that, however, dissipation is proportional to the inverse particle number N_a^{-1} and can in most cases for very large numbers of particles be neglected.

The next step in this theory is to relate the last equation to the one-particle distribution function defined in Equation (19). Following Klimontovich [21], this is achieved via considering the fluctuations:

$$\delta\mathcal{N}_a^m(\mathbf{x},t) = \mathcal{N}_a^m(\mathbf{x},t) - \left\langle \mathcal{N}_a^m(\mathbf{x},t)\right\rangle \tag{29}$$

When ensemble-averaged, these deviations from the mean phase-space density vanish, and we have:

$$\begin{aligned}\left\langle \mathcal{N}_a^m(\mathbf{x},t)\mathcal{N}_b^m(\mathbf{x}',t)\right\rangle &= \left\langle \mathcal{N}_a^m(\mathbf{x},t)\right\rangle\left\langle \mathcal{N}_b^m(\mathbf{x}',t)\right\rangle \\ &+ \left\langle \delta\mathcal{N}_a^m(\mathbf{x},t)\,\delta\mathcal{N}_b^m(\mathbf{x}',t)\right\rangle\end{aligned} \tag{30}$$

We can now make use of the definition of the one-particle distribution function $f_a(\mathbf{x},t)$ by Klimontovich [21]. Define the particle density $n_a = N_a/V_a$ to obtain:

$$\begin{aligned}\left\langle \mathcal{N}_a^m(\mathbf{x},t)\mathcal{N}_b^m(\mathbf{x}',t)\right\rangle &= n_a n_b\Big[f_a(\mathbf{x},t)f_b(\mathbf{x}',t) \\ +g_{ab}(\mathbf{x},\mathbf{x}',t)\Big] &+ \delta_{ab}\delta(\mathbf{x}-\mathbf{x}')n_a f_a(\mathbf{x},t)\end{aligned} \tag{31}$$

Here, $g_{ab}(\mathbf{x},\mathbf{x}',t)$ is the two-particle correlation function, which results from the ensemble-averaged product of the fluctuations $\delta\mathcal{N}^m$ of the phase space density in the last term on the right in Equation (30). The three terms in the expression (31) are of the same structure as in the ordinary one-particle kinetic theory [21]. One may note that the last term, which is linear in the distribution function, simply becomes absorbed in the convective term in the kinetic equation. In non-relativistic, theory it just causes a translation. We can immediately write down the one-particle kinetic equation including the entropy force. One must, however, take care of to which terms the gradient and momentum operations apply. This yields the result:

$$\begin{aligned} &\frac{\partial f_a}{\partial t} + \frac{\mathbf{p}}{m_a} \cdot \nabla_{\mathbf{q}} f_a - T\, \nabla^b_{\mathbf{q}} \sum_b n_b \int d^6x' \\ &\times \delta(\mathbf{q}-\mathbf{q}') \cdot \frac{\partial}{\partial \mathbf{p}} \Big[f_a(\mathbf{x},t) f_b(\mathbf{x}',t) \Big] = \Big(\mathcal{G}^{S(\mathrm{x},t)}_{ab} - \Big\langle \mathcal{C}^{S(\mathrm{x},t)}_a \Big\rangle \Big)(\mathbf{x},t) \end{aligned} \tag{32}$$

which, when integrating over the primed spatial coordinate, simplifies to:

$$\begin{aligned} &\frac{\partial f_a}{\partial t} + \frac{\mathbf{p}}{m_a} \cdot \nabla_{\mathbf{q}} f_a - T \frac{\partial}{\partial \mathbf{p}} f_a(\mathbf{q},\mathbf{p},t) \\ &\cdot \nabla_{\mathbf{q}} \sum_b n_b \int d^3p'\, f_b(\mathbf{q},\mathbf{p}',t) = \Big(\mathcal{G}^{S(\mathrm{x},t)}_{ab} - \Big\langle \mathcal{C}^{S(\mathrm{x},t)}_a \Big\rangle \Big)(\mathbf{x},t) \end{aligned} \tag{33}$$

In this expression on the right, the term $\mathcal{G}_{ab}$ results from the two-particle correlation term $g_{ab}(\mathbf{x},\mathbf{x}',t)$. It corresponds to what in kinetic theory is understood as direct particle collisions. The last expression contains the integral over the primed momentum space. Only the distribution f_b depends on this integration. It is therefore convenient to define the number density ρ_a of species a as:

$$\rho_a(\mathbf{q},t) = n_a \int d^3p\, f_a(\mathbf{q},\mathbf{p},t) \tag{34}$$

and the last expression just includes the global entropy force term:

$$\begin{aligned} \frac{\partial f_a}{\partial t} &+ \frac{\mathbf{p}}{m_a} \cdot \nabla_{\mathbf{q}} f_a - T \Big(\nabla_{\mathbf{q}} \sum_b \rho_b(\mathbf{q},t) \Big) \cdot \frac{\partial f_a}{\partial \mathbf{p}} \\ &= \Big(\mathcal{G}^{S(\mathrm{x},t)}_{ab} - \Big\langle \mathcal{C}^{S(\mathrm{x},t)}_a \Big\rangle \Big)(\mathbf{x},t) \end{aligned} \tag{35}$$

The sum is over all particle components, implying the total number density. Thus, the entropy force term simply adds to any other potential force term in the kinetic equation. This is true already to first order in the expansion of the logarithmic term in the definition of the entropy. In the case of charged particles, such a force is the Coulomb force or the Lorentz force, when including magnetic fields. The difference is, however, that this force term does not depend on charge while acting on the microscopic particle phase space distribution. It resembles the gravitational force, but does not contain its inverse square dependence on the inter-particle distance. This is advantageous as it releases from the necessity of compensation. On the other hand, the new force term introduces another non-linearity contained in the density, which itself is the integral of the distribution function.

The entropy force resembles a pressure force on the kinetic level. With zero right-hand side in the kinetic equation, it conserves particle number. This is a rather simple result, which, of course, could have been anticipated, without reference to any complicated derivation from first principles as done here, by adding a macroscopic entropy force to the force terms.

The ensemble-averaged term $\langle \mathcal{C}^S_a \rangle$ is a purely entropic lowest order (in the smallness of $\mathcal{N}'^{m}_a$) dissipation term for which, in conventional kinetic theory, no equivalence arises. This term is, however, small and thus negligible, as will be shown in the next section.

In the collisionless kinetic theory of forces between particles, any non-collisional dissipation term caused by particle interactions via their fields yields correlations, which can be neglected, respectively discussed away by comparing dissipation and collisionless scales. The entropic dissipation term instead remains because it is not caused by particle collisions, nor wave–particle interactions. There is no entropy source field that leads to the correlations between particles. Rather, it is the inhomogeneity in the macroscopic disorder that is responsible for the fluctuations and the appearance of the dissipative entropic correlations between the fluctuations leading to the dissipation term. Hence, this term remains even under completely collisionless conditions. Once disorder exhibits spatial structure, it will always be present. In the next section, we provide the explicit versions of these two terms.

5. Dissipative Terms

In order to complete the theory, one needs to express the two dissipative terms in the final kinetic Equation (32). The collision term $\mathcal{G}_{ab}$ is of the same structure as the Coulomb collision term [21,33]. It adds to the latter:

$$\mathcal{G}^S_{ab} = T\sum_b n_b \nabla_{\mathbf{q}} \cdot \int d^6x' \delta(\mathbf{q}-\mathbf{q}') \frac{\partial}{\partial \mathbf{p}} g_{ab}(\mathbf{x},\mathbf{x}',t) \tag{36}$$

In the particular case that the correlation g_{ab} does not contain any singularity, this expression has no singularity at $\mathbf{q}=\mathbf{q}'$ other than that in the derivative of the delta-function, which replaces $\mathbf{q}' \to \mathbf{q}$ in the correlation function g_{ab} when the integration is carried out. The remaining expression becomes:

$$\mathcal{G}^S_{ab}(\mathbf{q},\mathbf{p},t) = T\frac{\partial}{\partial \mathbf{p}} \cdot \sum_b n_b \int d^3p' \, \nabla_{\mathbf{q}} g_{ab}(\mathbf{q},\mathbf{p},\mathbf{p}',t) \tag{37}$$

The presence of the entropy force thus contributes to the collision term via the particle correlation function. Clearly, due to the strong Coulomb force at short distances, the particle interaction on the short scales is dominated by the Coulomb force. However, at distances larger than the Coulomb collision length, the entropic collisional interaction remains. In a charge collisionless plasma, for instance, the Coulomb term causes charge screening felt inside the Debye sphere and eliminates the microscopic electric field between the charges on scales larger than the Debye length λ_D. On such scales, entropic dissipation might enter the scene. Since it is proportional to temperature T and also number density ρ, it has the character of a collisional contribution of the pressure in the inhomogeneities of the entropy.

One may take notice that the spatial gradient operator can be taken out of the integral in the last expression. This allows writing:

$$\mathcal{G}^S_{ab}(\mathbf{q},\mathbf{p},t) = T\,\nabla_{\mathbf{q}} \cdot \frac{\partial}{\partial \mathbf{p}} G^S_a(\mathbf{q},\mathbf{p},t) \tag{38}$$

where we introduced the entropic correlation integral:

$$G^S_a(\mathbf{q},\mathbf{p},t) = \sum_b n_b \int d^3p' \, g_{ab}(\mathbf{q},\mathbf{p},\mathbf{p}',t) \tag{39}$$

We will return to the discussion of this correlation integral below, because it contains the most interesting effect introduced by the entropy force.

In general, the correlation will contain contributions from the forces that depend on local charges. This leads from the field equations to singularities in the correlation function, as the example of the Coulomb force suggests. The simplified form of the correlation term in the dissipation function retains the form in Equation (36) and must be explicitly spelled out. Exchanging the derivatives, this can be written as:

$$\mathcal{G}^S_{ab} = T\frac{\partial}{\partial \mathbf{p}} \cdot \sum_b n_b \nabla_{\mathbf{q}} \int d^6x' \delta(\mathbf{q}-\mathbf{q}') g_{ab}(\mathbf{x},\mathbf{x}',t) \tag{40}$$

Let us now turn to the remaining term $\langle \mathcal{C}^S_a \rangle$. From Equations (27) and (28), one realizes that it contains the product of three microscopic phase space densities before taking the ensemble average. This complicates its calculation. In analogy to Equations (30) and (31), it requires the introduction of higher order correlations. Formally, this is quite simple as it has been pioneered by Klimontovich [21] how one would have to deal with it in this case. We need the third-order ensemble average, which becomes in the same way as (31):

$$\begin{aligned}\left\langle \mathcal{N}_a^m \mathcal{N}_b^m \mathcal{N}_c^m \right\rangle &= n_a n_b n_c f_{abc}(\mathbf{x},\mathbf{x}',\mathbf{x}'') \\ &+\delta_{ab} n_a n_c \delta(\mathbf{x}-\mathbf{x}') f_{ac}(\mathbf{x},\mathbf{x}'') \\ &+\delta_{ac} n_a n_b \delta(\mathbf{x}-\mathbf{x}'') f_{ab}(\mathbf{x},\mathbf{x}') \\ &+\delta_{bc} n_a n_c \delta(\mathbf{x}'-\mathbf{x}'') f_{ac}(\mathbf{x},\mathbf{x}'') \\ &+\delta_{ab}\delta_{bc}\delta(\mathbf{x}-\mathbf{x}')\delta(\mathbf{x}-\mathbf{x}'') f_a(\mathbf{x})\end{aligned} \tag{41}$$

For convenience, we dropped the common variable t. The two- and three-particle distribution functions f_{ab}, f_{abc} read:

$$\begin{aligned} f_{ab}(\mathbf{x},\mathbf{x}') &= f_a(\mathbf{x}) f_b(\mathbf{x}') + g_{ab}(\mathbf{x},\mathbf{x}') \\ f_{abc}(\mathbf{x},\mathbf{x}',\mathbf{x}'') &= f_a(\mathbf{x}) f_b(\mathbf{x}') f_c(\mathbf{x}'') \\ &+ f_a(\mathbf{x}) g_{bc}(\mathbf{x}',\mathbf{x}'') + f_b(\mathbf{x}') g_{ac}(\mathbf{x},\mathbf{x}'') \\ &+ f_c(\mathbf{x}'') g_{ab}(\mathbf{x},\mathbf{x}') + g_{abc}(\mathbf{x},\mathbf{x}',\mathbf{x}'') \end{aligned} \tag{42}$$

With their help, the dissipation function can be constructed. However, its structure simplifies substantially because in our case, on the left in the first line in Equation (41), the microscopic phase space densities of index b and c are identical, and only the f_{ab} contributes. Hence, the ensemble average becomes:

$$\left\langle \mathcal{N}_a^m \mathcal{N}_b^m \mathcal{N}_c^{\prime m} \delta_{bc}\delta(\mathbf{x}'-\mathbf{x}'') \right\rangle = n_a n_b f_{ab}(\mathbf{x},\mathbf{x}') \frac{1}{N_b} \tag{43}$$

Therefore, only the two-particle distribution function f_{ab} would be relevant in the determination of the dissipative term, i.e., in the first line in Equation (42). This is, however, the same as what we already used in Equation (31). To this result, one has to apply the operation of space and momentum differentiation. Hence, the collisionless dissipative term contributed by the entropy force is of the same kind as the collision term $\mathcal{G}_{ab}^S$ it contributes, though being of a different sign. In other words, the two terms would cancel to first order if there were not the normalization to particle number N_b. Since $N_b \approx N_a \gg 1$, we find that the collisionless dissipation due to the entropy force $\langle \mathcal{C}_a^S \rangle \ll \mathcal{G}_{ab}^S$ is small and can be neglected in comparison with the entropic collision term.

Thus, it is the collisional correlation term $\mathcal{G}_{ab}^S(\mathbf{x},t)$ (37) that is retained as a long-range collisional dissipation introduced by the presence of the entropy force. It adds to the Coulomb collisions and might become important on the large scales much larger than the Debye scale or any other inter-particle interaction scale. this important result suggests that the entropic dissipation is a mesoscale, respectively macro effect. We should, however, point out here that we are still dealing with a non-relativistic theory. At large scales, transport and propagation of information, respectively entropy, cannot be neglected anymore, and the theory has to given a covariant relativistic formulation.

6. Kinetic Equation for Fluctuations

The remaining problem is the behavior of fluctuations. These are defined as deviations in the one-particle phase space distribution f_a from its mean "equilibrium" value $\bar{f}_a$ as:

$$\delta f_a = f_a - \bar{f}_a, \qquad \overline{\delta f}_a = 0 \tag{44}$$

The evolution equation of the fluctuations is obtained from Equation (33) via subtracting the averaged kinetic equation:

$$\frac{\partial \bar{f}_a}{\partial t} + \frac{\mathbf{p}}{m_a} \cdot \nabla_{\mathbf{q}} \bar{f}_a - T \sum_b n_b \int d^3p' \times \\ \times \nabla^b_{\mathbf{q}} \cdot \frac{\partial}{\partial \mathbf{p}} \left[\bar{f}_a(\mathbf{q}, \mathbf{p}, t) \bar{f}_b(\mathbf{q}, \mathbf{p}', t) + \overline{\delta f_a \delta f_b} \right] = \overline{\mathcal{G}^S_{ab}} \tag{45}$$

The mean collision term on the right contains all the contributions of the correlations of the mean and fluctuating quantities. Being interested only in linear fluctuations and assuming that the collisions are weak enough to not contribute to the evolution of fluctuations, we drop this term in the following. Subtracting from the complete kinetic equation, the fluctuations obey the non-collisional equation:

$$\frac{\partial \delta f_a}{\partial t} + \frac{\mathbf{p}}{m_a} \cdot \nabla_{\mathbf{q}} \delta f_a - T \sum_b n_b \int d^3p' \\ \times \nabla^b_{\mathbf{q}} \cdot \frac{\partial}{\partial \mathbf{p}} \left[\delta f_a(\mathbf{q}, \mathbf{p}, t) \bar{f}_b(\mathbf{q}, \mathbf{p}', t) \right] = \\ T \sum_b n_b \int d^3p' \nabla^b_{\mathbf{q}} \cdot \frac{\partial}{\partial \mathbf{p}} \left[\bar{f}_a(\mathbf{q}, \mathbf{p}, t) \delta f_b(\mathbf{q}, \mathbf{p}', t) - \overline{\delta f_a \delta f_b} \right] \tag{46}$$

This expression still contains the average $\overline{\delta f_a \delta f_b}$ of the squared fluctuations. If this is a constant on the fluctuation time scale, then the equation can be rescaled. In linear theory, it would be neglected to first order and taken into account to second order in a quasi-linear approach.

Again, carrying out the integration with respect to $\mathbf{p}'$, the last expression simplifies to:

$$\frac{\partial \delta f_a}{\partial t} + \frac{\mathbf{p}}{m_a} \cdot \nabla_{\mathbf{q}} \delta f_a - T \frac{\partial \delta f_a}{\partial \mathbf{p}} \cdot \nabla_{\mathbf{q}} \Big(\sum_b \bar{\rho}_b(\mathbf{q}, t) \Big) \\ = T \sum_{b \neq a} n_b \int d^3p' \nabla^b_{\mathbf{q}} \cdot \frac{\partial}{\partial \mathbf{p}} \left[\bar{f}_a(\mathbf{x}, t) \delta f_b(\mathbf{q}, \mathbf{p}', t) - \overline{\delta f_a \delta f_b} \right] \tag{47}$$

where in the term on the right-hand side, we retained the fluctuation in the distribution function, not replacing it with the density fluctuation $\delta\rho_b(\mathbf{q}, t)$ for the obvious reason that this is an equation for the fluctuations in the distribution function itself. The term on the right couples all fluctuations in the different particle components $b \neq a$ to $\bar{f}_a$.

The linear theory is still complicated by the fact that it contains the sum over the particle correlations. Here, one must include all particles contained in the medium. Moreover, we have written here only those terms that result from the inclusion of the entropy force. To these terms, one must add the electromagnetic force terms. Since the electromagnetic and entropy forces superimpose, this does not produce any additional mixing, but simply adds those common and well-known terms that take care of the electromagnetic interactions. In this sense, the formal theory is complete. The ranges of the two different forces acting on the particle populations are vastly different because the entropy force is a collective force, which does not originate from any elementary charge. There is no singularity of the entropy that could give rise to an entropy field. The search for such singularities is outside classical physics.

7. Evolution of Entropic Phase Space Density

Having defined the entropic phase space density in Equation (17,) the question arises how it possibly evolves in phase space. Since the entropy is given as the phase space integral with respect to the entropic phase space density, an always positive quantity, this question is not senseless. Once knowing its evolution, the entropy can be calculated by integration. Moreover, if an equation for the phase space density can be obtained, its entropic momentum should yield an evolution equation for the entropy, which, essentially, in the long-term limit should be the fundamental thermodynamic laws, while in the short term, it should give the evolution equation of entropy with time. In order to construct the entropic phase space equation, we multiply Equation (12) by $-\log \mathcal{N}_a^{\prime m}$ to obtain:

$$\partial_t \mathcal{S}_a^m + \left[\mathcal{H}_{N_a}, \mathcal{S}_a^m\right] - \left\{\partial_t \mathcal{N}_a^m + \left[\mathcal{H}_{N_a}, \mathcal{N}_a^m\right]\right\} = 0 \tag{48}$$

The term in the braces vanishes identically, yielding ultimately:

$$\partial_t \mathcal{S}_a^m + \left[\mathcal{H}_{N_a}, \mathcal{S}_a^m\right] = 0 \tag{49}$$

We thus find the almost trivial result that the microscopic entropic phase-space density $\mathcal{S}_a^m$ itself satisfies the Liouville equation, i.e., the continuity equation for the entropic phase space density in the phase space. It thus evolves in the microscopic particle phase space like a dissipationless fluid. This is just another expression for the fact that (classically), there are no microscopic sources of entropy, nor is there any entropic field. Entropy is just disorder in the particles.

However, the microscopic entropic density in phase space is not entirely independent of any disorder. It acts back on itself via the integral entropy force term contained in the above Hamiltonian $\mathcal{H}_{N_a}$. It provides an entropy potential contribution $U_S = TS$ to the Hamiltonian with S, the momentum space integral of the entropy phase space density $\mathcal{S}_a^m\{\mathcal{N}_a^m\}$, which itself is a function of the phase space density $\mathcal{N}_a^m$. Though the structure of the kinetic equation for the entropy density $\mathcal{S}_a^m$ remains the same as that of the phase space density $\mathcal{N}_a^m$, both containing the entropy force term and becoming integro-differential equations, the phase space density is determined by the integral entropy density through the entropy force. This force is obtained by adding up all contributions over all phase space. This shows that both the kinetic equation for the particle density and the kinetic equation for the entropy density in phase space must be solved together as both are intimately related.

One can interpret this result in the way that the holographic reaction of the integral entropy on the evolution of the phase space density of the entropy appears like an elementary entropy source. This is not unsatisfactory, because it can hardly be expected that a microscopic source of entropy would exist as there are no entropy charges and no entropy fields in the world, at least not classically. Instead, the elementary source arises from the non-linear self-interaction of the entropy. This is a rather important conclusion in that, presumably, little will be changed when including quantum effects in a quantum mechanical treatment, making the transition to quantum statistical mechanics.

8. Discussion and Conclusions

In this note, we included the force that an inhomogeneous entropy might exert on the dynamics of particles in phase space. This is not an obvious step. It is a purely collective effect. So far, any such force has not yet been included in the dynamics of large numbers of particles and kinetic theory.

Collective effects of this kind are known from ponderomotive forces and pressure forces. However, the inclusion of a separate ponderomotive force or a pressure force on the microscopic level is not necessary. Ponderomotive forces are taken care of by the interaction of the electromagnetic field with the particles. They arise from correlations. Similarly, the pressure force, which is directly proportional to the gradient of the particle density on any level, is already included in the evolution of the phase space density.

The entropy force is different in the sense that it is not obvious that it is given by the gradient of density. The entropy force takes care of the chaotic disorder that is produced by the dynamics itself. Neither the pressure, nor the temperature account for it. Entropy is a function of the phase space density, not its moment like pressure and temperature. It is the cause of chaotic expansion of the phase space in the course of the dynamics. It therefore gives rise to a collective effect felt on the level of the microscopic phase space density. In many processes, this effect may be very small and negligible. This will depend on scales. Elucidating those effects requires investigation of particular cases. The present work presents the theory on which such attempts must be based.

We derived the basic kinetic equation for the one particle phase space density including the global entropy force. Since this force is a global integral one, it has no microscopic source, while it affects the dynamics of the one-particle phase space density through the interaction Hamiltonian. This gives rise to the construction of a kinetic equation for the entropic phase space density, which turns out to be of similar structure, like the Liouville (Klimontovich) equation for the phase space density. There is, however, a fundamental difference in that the entropic kinetic equation is self-referential. It determines the dynamics of the entropy density in phase space by reference to the integrated entropy of the entire system itself. This is a very important finding because it shows that the entropy density in phase space evolves holographically. It is determined by itself. It takes care of its own evolution, which in addition depends on the evolution of the matter phase space density. This can be interpreted as a self-regulation of the evolution of entropy on the microscopic level, which takes care of the total produced entropy. According to this finding, any many-particle system that in the course of its dynamics generates entropy in an inhomogeneous and time-dependent way is subject to the entropy that controls its own evolution. This we feel is the most important insight we arrived at in our analysis. Entropy generates and controls itself in this highly nonlinear way already on the microscopic level of phase space density. We conjecture that these properties remain when including quantum effects in kinetic theory on the microscopic quantum level without the need to introduce a seed source of entropy.

In order to demonstrate an effect, we in the introductory part of this note treated the astrophysical example of a Schwarzschild black hole. This led us to the definition of the Schwarzschild constant, a universal constant, which is essentially the Planck force, which so far had been formally postulated without finding a physical interpretation. Its meaning lies in the Schwarzschild constant as the entropy force at the black hole horizon. Some of its implications we have discussed briefly. The entropy force at the horizon, being independent of charge, is of only one sign. It causes a repulsive force. This is similar to the gravitational force, though counteracting it. It thus in large space may compete with the gravitational attraction, where it may become kind of an anti-gravity. Investigation of its effect on the universal expansion might also be of interest, as also the role it may play in primordial black holes and planckions, which may have been generated in the early universe, the Big Bang, and if surviving, possibly due to the anti-gravity action of the entropy force, could provide all or part of the mysterious dark matter on the scales of clusters of galaxies.

Author Contributions: Conceptualization, W.B. and R.T., formal analysis, R.T., writing—review and editing, W.B. and R.T.

Funding: This research received no external funding.

Acknowledgments: This work was part of a Visiting Scientist Programme at the International Space Science Institute (ISSI) Bern. The interest of the ISSI Directorate is acknowledged, as is in particular the friendly hospitality of the ISSI staff. Thanks are directed to the ISSI system administrator Saliba F. Saliba for technical support and to the librarians Andrea Fischer and Irmela Schweizer for access to the library and literature.

Conflicts of Interest: The authors declare no conflict of interest.

References

1. Prigogine, I. *From Being to Becoming. Time and Complexity in the Physical Sciences*; Freeman: New York, NJ, USA, 1980.
2. Verlinde, E. On the origin of gravity and the laws of Newton. *J. High Energy Phys. JHEP* **2011**, *2011*, 29. [CrossRef]
3. Kappen, H.J. Comment: Causal entropic forces. *arXiv* **2013**, arXiv:1312.4185.
4. Wissner-Gross, A.D.; Freer, C.E. Causal entropy forces. *Phys. Rev. Lett.* **2013**, *110*, 168702. OhysRevLett.110.168702. [CrossRef] [PubMed]
5. Keul, N.D.; Oruganty, K.; Bergman, E.T.S.; Beattie, N.R.; McDonald, W.E.; Kadirvelraj, R.; Gross, M.L.; Phillips, R.S.; Harvey, S.C.; Wood, Z.A. The entropic force generated by intrinsically disordered segments tunes protein function. *Nature* **2018**, *563*, 584–588. [CrossRef] [PubMed]
6. Nakamura, T.K. Relativistic equilibrium distribution by relative entropy maximization. *Europhys. Lett. EPL* **2009**, *88*, 40009. [CrossRef]

7. Bardeen, J.M.; Carter, B.; Hawking, S.W. The four laws of black hole mechanics. *Commun. Math. Phys.* **1973**, *31*, 161–170. [CrossRef]
8. Bekenstein, J.D. Black holes and entropy. *Phys. Rev. D* **1973**, *7*, 2333–2346. [CrossRef]
9. Bekenstein, J.D. Black holes and the second law. *Nuovo Cim. Lett.* **1972**, *4*, 737–740. [CrossRef]
10. Hawking, S.W. Gravitational radiation from colliding black holes. *Phys. Rev. Lett.* **1971**, *21*, 1344–1346. [CrossRef]
11. Hawking, S.W. Particle creation by black holes. *Comm. Math. Phys.* **1975**, *43*, 199–220. [CrossRef]
12. Hawking, S. Black holes and thermodynamics. *Phys. Rev. D* **1976**, *13*, 191–197. [CrossRef]
13. Brout, R.; Massar, S.; Parentani, R.; Spindel, P. A primer for black hole quantum physics. *Phys. Rep.* **1995**, *260*, 329–446. [CrossRef]
14. Doran, R.; Lobo, F.S.N.; Crawford, P. Interior of a Schwarzschild black hole revisited. *Found. Phys.* **2008**, *38*, 160–187. [CrossRef]
15. Jacobson, T. Thermodynamics of spacetime: The Einstein equation of state. *Phys. Rev. Lett.* **1995**, *75*, 1260–1263. [CrossRef] [PubMed]
16. Padmanabhan, T. Thermodynamical aspects of gravity: New insights. *Rep. Progr. Phys.* **2009**, *73*, 6901. [CrossRef]
17. Taylor, P.L.; Tabachnik, J. Entropic forces—Making the connection between mechanics and thermodynamics in an exactly soluble model. *Eur. J. Phys.* **2013**, *34*, 729. [CrossRef]
18. Hamilton, A.J.S. Hawking radiation inside a Schwarzschild black hole. *Gen. Relat. Gravit.* **2018**, *50*, 50. [CrossRef]
19. Carr, B.; Kühnel, F.; Sandstad, M. Primordial black holes and dark matter. *Phys. Rev. D* **2016**, *94*, 083504. [CrossRef]
20. Garny, M.; McCullen, S.; Sloth, M.S. Planckian interacting massive particles as dark matter. *Phys. Rev. Lett.* **2016**, *116*, 10302. [CrossRef]
21. Klimontovich, Y.L. *The Statistical Theory of Non-Equilibrium Processes in a Plasma*; The MIT Press: Cambridge, MA, USA, 1967.
22. Gerasimenko, V.I.; Shtyuk, V.O.; Zagorodny, A.G. Hydrodynamic equations for microscopic phase densities. *Centr. Eur. J. Phys.* **2011**, *9*, 71–77. [CrossRef]
23. Dunkel, J.; Hilbert, S. Consistent thermostatistics forbids negative absolute temperatures. *Nat. Phys.* **2014**, *10*, 67–69. [CrossRef]
24. Rényi, A. *Probability Theory*; North-Holland Publ. Comp.: Amsterdam, The Netherlands, 1970.
25. Tsallis, C. Possible generalization of Boltzmann-Gibbs statistics. *J. Stat. Phys.* **1988**, *52*, 479–487. [CrossRef]
26. Treumann, R.A. Kinetic theoretical foundation of Lorentzian statistical mechanics. *Phys. Scr.* **1999**, *59*, 19–26. [CrossRef]
27. Treumann, R.A.; Jaroschek, C.H.; Scholer, M. Stationary plasma states far from equilibrium. *Phys. Plasmas* **2004**, *11*, 1317–1325. [CrossRef]
28. Treumann, R.A.; Jaroschek, C.H. Gibbsian theory of power-law distributions. *Phys. Rev. Lett.* **2008**, *100*, 155005. [CrossRef] [PubMed]
29. Treumann, R.A.; Baumjohann, W. Beyond Gibbs-Boltzmann-Shannon: General entropies—The Gibbs-Lorentzian example. *Front. Phys.* **2014**, *2*, 49. [CrossRef]
30. Wehrl, A. General properties of entropy. *Rev. Mod. Phys.* **1978**, *50*, 221–260. [CrossRef]
31. Wheeler, J.A.; Feynman, R.P. Interaction with the absorber as the mechanism of radiation. *Rev. Mod. Phys.* **1945**, *17*, 157–161. [CrossRef]
32. Wheeler, J.A.; Feynman, R.P. Classical electrodynamics in terms of direct interparticle action. *Rev. Mod. Phys.* **1949**, *21*, 425–433. [CrossRef]
33. Treumann, R.A.; Baumjohann, W. Causal kinetic equation of non-equilibrium plasmas. *Ann. Geophys.* **2017**, *35*, 683–690. [CrossRef]

entropy

MDPI

Article

Dynamic Maximum Entropy Reduction

Václav Klika [1,*], Michal Pavelka [2], Petr Vágner [2,3] and Miroslav Grmela [4]

1 Department of Mathematics—FNSPE, Czech Technical University, Trojanova 13, 12000 Prague, Czech Republic
2 Mathematical Institute, Faculty of Mathematics and Physics, Charles University, Sokolovská 83, 18675 Prague, Czech Republic
3 Weierstrass Institute, Mohrenstrasse 39, 10117 Berlin, Germany
4 École Polytechnique de Montréal, C.P.6079 suc. Centre-ville, Montréal, QC H3C3A7, Canada
* Correspondence: vaclav.klika@fjfi.cvut.cz

Received: 28 June 2019; Accepted: 19 July 2019; Published: 22 July 2019

check for updates

Abstract: Any physical system can be regarded on different levels of description varying by how detailed the description is. We propose a method called Dynamic MaxEnt (DynMaxEnt) that provides a passage from the more detailed evolution equations to equations for the less detailed state variables. The method is based on explicit recognition of the state and conjugate variables, which can relax towards the respective quasi-equilibria in different ways. Detailed state variables are reduced using the usual principle of maximum entropy (MaxEnt), whereas relaxation of conjugate variables guarantees that the reduced equations are closed. Moreover, an infinite chain of consecutive DynMaxEnt approximations can be constructed. The method is demonstrated on a particle with friction, complex fluids (equipped with conformation and Reynolds stress tensors), hyperbolic heat conduction and magnetohydrodynamics.

Keywords: model reduction; non-equilibrium thermodynamics; MaxEnt; dynamic MaxEnt; complex fluids; heat conduction; Ohm's law

1. Introduction

The problem of model reduction is ubiquitous in physics and mathematics. Consider a system (physical or mathematical) that can be regarded on two levels of description, upper (more detailed level) and lower (less detailed). The state variables on the lower level contain less information than state variables on the upper level. A projection from the upper level to the lower level is necessary to state the problem of model reduction correctly. Assume, moreover, that dynamics of the state variables on the upper level is granted, but one wishes to see evolution of the lower variables. The reason can be for instance the complexity of the detailed evolution, availability of experimental observations or simplicity of the lower description. A reduction of dynamics from the upper level to the lower (less detailed) level is called model reduction.

There is no general model reduction technique applicable to all systems. However, many physically based (we do not focus on formal mathematical expansion methods although we make a certain comparison below) methods have been developed, such as the Chapman–Enskog expansion [1] or other series expansions [2], projector operator techniques [3,4], or the method of natural projector, invariant slow manifolds, entropic scalar product and Ehrenfest reduction [5–8]. A common feature of the reduction techniques is the recognition of entropy, since entropy (measuring unavailable information) grows during the passage from the more detailed level to the less detailed. In particular, states on the higher level corresponding to maximum entropy are referred to as the quasi-equilibrium manifold. This manifold is constructed by maximization of entropy on the upper level while knowing the result of the projection of the state variables to the lower level. This is the principle of Maximum Entropy (MaxEnt), see e.g., [9,10].

Apart from the relations between state variables on the two levels of description, it is necessary to find relations between vector fields generating evolution on the two levels. Indeed, evolution equations on the higher level can be seen as a motion along a given vector field (following arrows of the field) while the corresponding vector field on the lower level is to be found. For instance, in the Ehrenfest reduction, the vector field on the higher level is first prolonged by Taylor series and subsequently projected to the lower level, using MaxEnt, and closed. See [7] for various geometric techniques on how to obtain the vector field on the lower level of description.

Our approach is different. First, we recognize not only the state variables, but also conjugate variables as independent quantities, being motivated by the formulation of thermodynamics in contact geometry [11–13]. Eventually, conjugate variables become related to the state variables through derivatives of a thermodynamic potential (e.g., energy or entropy), but they are considered independent from direct variables in contact formulation and exhibit evolution towards that relation while approaching a given level. State variables between the levels can be related by MaxEnt as in [7,9,14], but conjugate variables can be exploited to find the approximation of the vector field on the higher level of description such that evolution on the lower level becomes closed while extracting key features ("measured" by entropy potential) of the upper level dynamics. In other words, the vector field on the lower level becomes tangent to the quasi-equilibrium manifold, see [15] or [14]. We refer to this method as Dynamic MaxEnt (DynMaxEnt).

Novelty of this paper lies in the following points: (i) The DynMaxEnt is introduced in the energetic representation, which simplifies the calculations, (ii) a chain or higher order DynMaxEnt approximations is identified, (iii) DynMaxEnt is compared to asymptotic expansions and (iv) it is applied to a reduction of various complex continuum dynamics to classical irreversible thermodynamics (conformation tensor, Reynolds stress, hyperbolic heat conduction and magnetohydrodynamics).

In Section 2, we first recall the usual (static) Maximum Entropy principle (MaxEnt). In Section 3, we introduce the method of Dynamic MaxEnt, which serves as a reduction from the more detailed evolution equations to less detailed, and then we demonstrate it on damped particle dynamics. In Section 4, we use the DynMaxEnt method for reduction of dynamics of complex fluids, hyperbolic heat conduction and electromagnetohydrodynamics to the Navier–Stokes–Fourier system and magnetohydrodynamics. Finally, in Section 5, we present a geometric motivation for the DynMaxEnt method in the framework of contact geometry.

2. Static MaxEnt

As a thorough understanding of (static) maximum entropy (MaxEnt) method is required, we shall recapitulate its key steps, what it means and what it provides.

Let us denote the state variables on the more microscopic level as $\mathbf{x} \in \mathcal{M}$, $\mathcal{M}$ being the manifold (often vector space) of the state variables, with conjugate variables $\mathbf{x}^*$ via entropy ${}^{\uparrow}S$. Furthermore, let us assume that there is a projection that relates two sets of variables $\mathbf{x} \in \mathcal{M}$, $\mathbf{y} \in \mathcal{N}$ via $\pi(\mathbf{x}) = \mathbf{y}$ where the latter corresponds to the more macroscopic level of description. The static MaxEnt provides an inverse mapping $\tilde{\mathbf{x}}(\mathbf{y})$ such that $\tilde{\mathbf{x}}(\mathbf{y})$ is the point of preimage $\pi^{-1}(\mathbf{y})$ with the highest entropy. This determines a manifold in $\mathcal{M}$, the MaxEnt manifold $\tilde{\mathcal{M}}$.

The inverse mapping can be achieved by maximization of entropy while keeping the constraint that $\pi(\mathbf{x}) = \mathbf{y}$, i.e., by the method of Lagrange multipliers. More geometrically, it can be also done via two consecutive Legendre transformations which together correspond to maximisation with a constraint $\mathbf{y} = \pi(\mathbf{x})$ [14,16]. In particular, as a first step, one obtains a relation $\tilde{\mathbf{x}}(\mathbf{y}^*)$ from solving

$$\mathbf{0} = \partial_{\mathbf{x}} \underbrace{\left(-{}^{\uparrow}S(\mathbf{x}) + \langle \mathbf{y}^*, \pi(\mathbf{x}) \rangle\right)}_{{}^{\uparrow}\phi} \tag{1}$$

while the lower conjugate entropy is ${}^{\downarrow}S^*(\mathbf{y}^*) = {}^{\uparrow}\phi(\tilde{\mathbf{x}}(\mathbf{y}^*), \mathbf{y}^*)$. Note that this (actually generalized) Legendre transformation can not be inverted.

Next, Legendre transformation of the lower conjugate entropy provides lower entropy and a relation $\tilde{\mathbf{y}^*}(\mathbf{y})$:

$$\mathbf{0} = \partial_{\mathbf{y}^*} \underbrace{\left(-{}^{\downarrow}S^*(\mathbf{y}^*) + \langle \mathbf{y}, \mathbf{y}^* \rangle \right)}_{{}^{\downarrow}\phi^*}, \tag{2}$$

which solution yields $\tilde{\mathbf{y}^*}(\mathbf{y})$ and ${}^{\downarrow}S(\mathbf{y}) = {}^{\downarrow}\phi^*(\mathbf{y}, \tilde{\mathbf{y}^*}(\mathbf{y}))$. Finally, the "inverse" mapping to the projection $\mathbf{y} = \pi(\mathbf{x})$ is $\mathbf{x} = \tilde{\mathbf{x}}(\tilde{\mathbf{y}^*}(\mathbf{y})) := \pi^{-1}(\mathbf{y})$. Note that it is now evident that π^{-1} is not a one-to-one mapping but rather a mapping identifying the most probable (with respect to the lower entropy) set of values of the microscale variable $\mathbf{x}$ that correspond to a given macroscale state $\mathbf{y}$. We shall refer to this method as MaxEnt and see Figure 1 for a summary of the method.

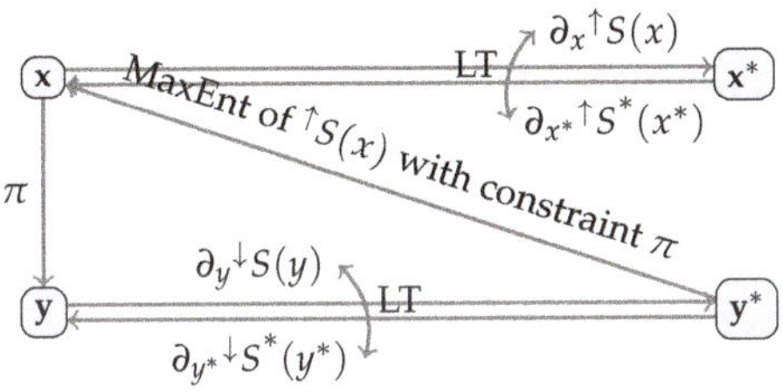

Figure 1. A summary of static MaxEnt highlighting relations between state variables on the higher level and the lower level of description and their conjugates. MaxEnt provides lower entropy ${}^{\downarrow}S(\mathbf{y})$ and a relation $\mathbf{x} = \pi^{-1}(\mathbf{y})$ from composition of $\tilde{\mathbf{x}}(\mathbf{y}^*)$ and $\tilde{\mathbf{y}^*}(\mathbf{y})$. LT denotes a relation via Legendre transformation, π stands for a projection from the microscale to the macroscale variables and by an arrow we depict a mapping (written above or below the arrow) that relates the variables in the connected nodes.

3. Dynamic MaxEnt

A form of the Dynamic MaxEnt reduction first appeared in [15] in the context of contact geometry. Here, we further develop DynMaxEnt using the energetic representation, which simplifies the procedure so that reductions, for example, from complex fluid dynamics to Navier–Stokes equation and from hyperbolic heat conduction to the Fourier law are carried out easily. Moreover, we generalize the method to an infinite chain of consecutive approximations.

The key idea behind dynamic MaxEnt is to treat conjugate variables $\mathbf{x}^{\dagger}$ as independent quantities ensuring invariance of the quasi-equilibrium manifold. This step is motivated by contact geometry, where conjugate variables are indeed granted independence and evolve towards the corresponding Gibbs–Legendre manifold, see Section 6.1.

3.1. First Order DynMaxEnt Reduction

Here, we propose an extension to the static version of MaxEnt (This extension is based on our previous work in [14]; however, we clarify, extend and elaborate on this method in this article.), which provides in addition to the lower entropy ${}^{\downarrow}S(\mathbf{y})$ and the inverse projection $\pi^{-1}(\mathbf{y})$ the dynamics on the lower level, i.e., reduced evolution equations.

Assuming the evolution on the more microscopic (higher) level can be expressed as

$$\dot{x}^i = V^i(\mathbf{x}, \mathbf{x}^{\dagger}), \tag{3}$$

where $\mathbf{x}^{\dagger}$ are conjugate variables which can be eventually identified with derivatives of energy (being the choice in this paper or e.g., [17–19]), entropy or another thermodynamic potential. Let us denote the yet unspecified functional by ${}^{\uparrow}\Phi$, i.e., $x^{\dagger}_i = {}^{\uparrow}\Phi_{x^i}$. Components of the right-hand side of the evolution equations V^i can be interpreted as elements of a vector field on the manifold of state variables $\mathcal{M}$, $\mathbf{x} \in \mathcal{M}$. With the inverse relation (we shall use simply $\tilde{\mathbf{x}}(\mathbf{y})$ instead of $\pi^{-1}(\mathbf{y})$ hereafter) at hand, which enslaves the microscale state variables $\mathbf{x}$ in terms of the macroscale (or reduced) variables $\mathbf{y}$, we may evaluate the more detailed evolution equations on the MaxEnt manifold as

$$\dot{\tilde{x}}^i = \frac{\partial \tilde{x}^i}{\partial y^a}\dot{y}^a = V^i\left(\tilde{\mathbf{x}}(\mathbf{y}), \mathbf{x}^{\dagger} = \mathbf{y}^{\dagger} \cdot \frac{\partial \pi}{\partial \mathbf{x}}\Big|_{\tilde{\mathbf{x}}(\mathbf{y})}\right), \tag{4}$$

noting that

$$\frac{\partial^{\uparrow}\Phi(\tilde{\mathbf{x}}(\pi(\mathbf{x})))}{\partial x^i}\Big|_{\tilde{\mathbf{x}}(\mathbf{y})} = \frac{\partial^{\downarrow}\Phi}{\partial \mathbf{y}} \cdot \frac{\partial \pi}{\partial \mathbf{x}}\Big|_{\tilde{\mathbf{x}}(\mathbf{y})} \tag{5}$$

for ${}^{\downarrow}\Phi(\mathbf{y}) = {}^{\uparrow}\Phi(\tilde{\mathbf{x}}(\mathbf{y}))$. By projection π, we obtain the reduced equations

$$\dot{y}^a = \frac{\partial \pi^a}{\partial x^i}\Big|_{\tilde{\mathbf{x}}(\mathbf{y})}\dot{\tilde{x}}^i = \frac{\partial \pi^a}{\partial x^i}\Big|_{\tilde{\mathbf{x}}(\mathbf{y})} V^i\left(\tilde{\mathbf{x}}(\mathbf{y}), \mathbf{x}^{\dagger} = \mathbf{y}^{\dagger} \cdot \frac{\partial \pi}{\partial \mathbf{x}}\Big|_{\tilde{\mathbf{x}}(\mathbf{y})}\right), \tag{6}$$

where it should be noted that the reduced equations have to live on the lower level. To this end, a relation $\tilde{\mathbf{x}}^{\dagger}(\mathbf{y}, \mathbf{y}^{\dagger})$ has to be identified. By comparing these last two evolution equations, it follows that

$$\frac{\partial \tilde{x}^i}{\partial y^a}\frac{\partial \pi^a}{\partial x^j}\Big|_{\tilde{\mathbf{x}}(\mathbf{y})} V^j\left(\tilde{\mathbf{x}}(\mathbf{y}), \mathbf{x}^{\dagger} = \mathbf{y}^{\dagger} \cdot \frac{\partial \pi}{\partial \mathbf{x}}\Big|_{\tilde{\mathbf{x}}(\mathbf{y})}\right) = V^i(\tilde{\mathbf{x}}(\mathbf{y}), \mathbf{x}^{\dagger}(\mathbf{y}, \mathbf{y}^{\dagger})), \tag{7}$$

which is a consistency condition entailing relations among conjugate variables $\tilde{\mathbf{x}}^{\dagger}(\mathbf{y}, \mathbf{y}^{\dagger})$. Without this condition, the evolution (4) would leave the manifold of MaxEnt states $\tilde{\mathbf{x}}(\mathbf{y})$, the vector field would be sticking out of the MaxEnt manifold $\tilde{\mathcal{M}}$. Condition (7) is actually an equation for $\mathbf{x}^{\dagger}$, the solution of which will be denoted by $\tilde{\mathbf{x}}^{\dagger}(\mathbf{y}, \mathbf{y}^{\dagger})$. After substitution into Equation (6), we obtain the reduced evolution equations for $\mathbf{y}$, which is the result of the first order DynMaxEnt reduction.

The first order DynMaxEnt reduction can be summarized as the sequence

$$\mathbf{y} \overset{\text{MaxEnt}}{\rightarrow} \tilde{\mathbf{x}}(\mathbf{y}) \overset{\text{Equation (7)}}{\rightarrow} \tilde{\mathbf{x}}^{\dagger}(\mathbf{y}, \mathbf{y}^{\dagger}), \tag{8}$$

which ends up in a closed system of equations for the reduced state variables $\mathbf{y}$. The lower level potential follows from the projection as ${}^{\downarrow}\Phi(\mathbf{y}) = {}^{\uparrow}\Phi(\tilde{\mathbf{x}}(\mathbf{y}))$.

Note, however, that the link tying $\mathbf{x}$ and $\mathbf{x}^{\dagger}$ was broken because $\tilde{\mathbf{x}}^{\dagger}$ was determined by solving Equation (7) instead of differentiating the potential ${}^{\uparrow}\Phi$ with respect to $\mathbf{x}$ at $\tilde{\mathbf{x}}(\mathbf{y})$. This leads to the higher order DynMaxEnt reduction.

3.2. Higher Order DynMaxEnt

From the first order DynMaxEnt, we have acquired independent relations among direct and conjugate variables, $\tilde{\mathbf{x}}(\mathbf{y})$ and $\tilde{\mathbf{x}}^{\dagger}(\mathbf{y}, \mathbf{y}^{\dagger})$, but at the same time direct and conjugate variables are linked via the potential ${}^{\uparrow}\Phi$. This entails that these two relations cannot be independent and some of the relations have to be violated.

There are two possible remedies of this situation both being iterative: (i) to correct the upper entropy so that the MaxEnt value is indeed a conjugate to the identified relation $\tilde{\mathbf{x}}^{\dagger}(\mathbf{y}, \mathbf{y}^{\dagger})$ on the lower level; however, this change in entropy means that MaxEnt has to be recalculated including everything that follows as well and the situation repeats itself; (ii) to correct the MaxEnt value of the direct variable so that the direct and conjugate values are now in line with the upper entropy evaluated on the lower level; however, this again modifies the dependent evolution equations on the lower level, in turn the value of upper conjugate variables and the situation repeats.

Although the former correction, the correction of the upper entropy, might seem natural, it turns out that it cannot be a general approach as the corrected entropy would fail to meet the requirement of being an even function with respect to time reversal when the reduced state variables change parity during the transition to a lower level, see Appendix A.1. We shall now develop the latter approach in detail (forming a possibly infinite chain of corrections) and compare it with asymptotic methods for upscaling evolution equations.

To repair the link between $\mathbf{x}$ and $\mathbf{x}^{\dagger}$, which remained broken after the first order DynMaxEnt reduction, an additional correction of the state variables $\mathbf{x}$ is required,

$$\left.\frac{\partial^{\uparrow}\Phi}{\partial\mathbf{x}}\right|_{\tilde{\mathbf{x}}^{(2)}} = \tilde{\mathbf{x}}^{\dagger}(\mathbf{y},\mathbf{y}^{\dagger}). \tag{9}$$

The solution to this equation gives the second iteration of the value of the state variable, $\tilde{\mathbf{x}}^{(2)}(\mathbf{y},\mathbf{y}^{\dagger})$.

However, is the consistency condition (7) satisfied at $\tilde{\mathbf{x}}^{(2)}$? Not in general. Therefore, the condition can be regarded as an equation for the second-order iteration of $\mathbf{x}^{\dagger}$, $\tilde{\mathbf{x}}^{\dagger(2)}$. This iterative chain can be summarized as

$$\mathbf{y} \overset{\text{MaxEnt}}{\rightarrow} \tilde{\mathbf{x}}(\mathbf{y}) \overset{\text{Equation (7)}}{\rightarrow} \tilde{\mathbf{x}}^{\dagger}(\mathbf{y},\mathbf{y}^{\dagger}) \overset{\text{Equation(9)}}{\rightarrow} \tilde{\mathbf{x}}^{(2)}(\mathbf{y},\mathbf{y}^{\dagger}) \overset{\text{Equation(7)}}{\rightarrow} \tilde{\mathbf{x}}^{\dagger(2)}(\mathbf{y},\mathbf{y}^{\dagger}) \rightarrow \ldots, \tag{10}$$

which can continue indefinitely. We have thus found an infinite chain of DynMaxEnt reduction, which leads to evolution equations for the reduced state variables $\mathbf{y}$ in a closed form. Note that the lower potential corresponds to the chosen step k in the infinite chain of DynMaxEnt as ${}^{\downarrow}\Phi^{(k)}(\mathbf{y}) = {}^{\uparrow}\Phi(\tilde{\mathbf{x}}^{(k)}(\mathbf{y}))$.

It is now apparent that any correction in this infinite chain of DynMaxEnt reduction leads to another correction as any of the adaptations, be it in direct or conjugate variables or even entropy, yield new disparity. Where should one end the iteration and what is the best choice of a method generating evolution equations on the lower level of description while retaining the thermodynamic structure and knowledge of the equations?

First, it should be mentioned that the aim of dynamic MaxEnt is to arrive at reasonable evolution equations for a specified level of description. We conjecture that the static MaxEnt value of direct variables $\tilde{\mathbf{x}}(\mathbf{y})$ is the best choice as it corresponds to the most probable, least biased relation [20] between direct lower and upper state variables. The conjugate variables then follow from the requirement of the dynamics being such that it does not drive the system away from the MaxEnt values of the direct variables, i.e., $\tilde{\mathbf{x}}^{\dagger}(\mathbf{y},\mathbf{y}^{\dagger})$. Finally, the lower potential is chosen as the first correction ${}^{\downarrow}\Phi^{(2)}(\mathbf{y}) = {}^{\uparrow}\Phi\left(\tilde{\mathbf{x}}^{(2)}(\mathbf{y})\right)$. The reason is twofold: (i) a correction of the lower entropy neither affects the static MaxEnt value nor does it explicitly change the evolution equations that are given in terms of direct and conjugate variables (it affects them indirectly via a resulting change of the relation of conjugate to direct variables); (ii) the corrected entropy is more tightly linked to the evolution equations rather than to the static MaxEnt which we aim to extend. Additionally, as we shall see below, in the special case of projection corresponding to relaxation of fast variables, the ${}^{\downarrow}S$ entropy is simply the upper entropy but where all the effects of fast variables are neglected while the correction ${}^{\downarrow}S^{(2)}$ includes additional (typically non-local) effects resulting from this transition between levels.

In short, direct state variables are set-up in such a way that their most probable value (with given information about the system comprised in entropy) is always kept on the lower level (although it might evolve with the evolution of the lower state variables). The choice of conjugate variables entails persistence of the direct variables exactly on their most probable values. Lower entropy corresponds to the set-up of conjugate rather than direct variables, which contain some non-trivial effects due to the transition of scales.

3.3. Prototype Example—Damped Particle

Let us now demonstrate the DynMaxEnt reduction on a prototype example—damped particle in a potential field. The state variables represent position, momentum and entropy of the particle, $\mathbf{x} = (\mathbf{r}, \mathbf{p}, s)$, and momentum is considered as the fast variable, which is to be reduced, i.e., $y = (\mathbf{r}, s)$. The projection to the lower (less detailed) level is thus $\pi : (\mathbf{r}, \mathbf{p}, s) \to (\mathbf{r}, s)$.

The more detailed evolution equations are ([14], Ch 5.3.1)

$$\dot{\mathbf{r}} = \mathbf{p}^\dagger, \tag{11a}$$

$$\dot{\mathbf{p}} = -\mathbf{r}^\dagger - \frac{1}{\tau}\frac{\mathbf{p}^\dagger}{s^\dagger}, \tag{11b}$$

$$\dot{s} = \frac{1}{\tau}\left(\frac{\mathbf{p}^\dagger}{s^\dagger}\right)^2, \tag{11c}$$

where $x^\dagger$ can be interpreted as conjugates with respect to energy

$${}^{\uparrow}e = \frac{\mathbf{p}^2}{2m} + V(\mathbf{r}) + \varepsilon(s), \tag{12}$$

consisting of kinetic energy, potential energy and internal energy. The evolution equations represent Hamilton canonical equations (for $\mathbf{r}$ and $\mathbf{p}$) equipped with friction in $\mathbf{p}$ and entropy production, c.f. [21]. Total energy is conserved by the evolution equations, $\dot{e} = \mathbf{r}^\dagger\dot{\mathbf{r}} + \mathbf{p}^\dagger\dot{\mathbf{p}} + s^\dagger\dot{s} = 0$.

3.3.1. First Order DynMaxEnt

From relation (12), it follows that entropy on the higher level reads

$${}^{\uparrow}s = s\left(e - \frac{\mathbf{p}^2}{2m} - V(\mathbf{r})\right), \tag{13}$$

$s(\bullet)$ being the inverse function to $\varepsilon(\bullet)$. Entropy attains maximum (for a given energy and position) at $\tilde{\mathbf{p}} = 0$, which is the MaxEnt value of momentum.

The consistency condition (7) becomes in this particular case

$$\begin{pmatrix} 1 & 0 \\ 0 & 0 \\ 0 & 1 \end{pmatrix} \cdot \begin{pmatrix} 1 & 0 & 0 \\ 0 & 0 & 1 \end{pmatrix} \cdot \begin{pmatrix} \mathbf{p}^\dagger \\ -\mathbf{r}^\dagger - \frac{1}{\tau}\frac{\mathbf{p}^\dagger}{\mathbf{r}^\dagger} \\ \frac{1}{\tau}\left(\frac{\mathbf{p}^\dagger}{\mathbf{r}^\dagger}\right)^2 \end{pmatrix} = \begin{pmatrix} \mathbf{p}^\dagger \\ -\mathbf{r}^\dagger - \frac{1}{\tau}\frac{\mathbf{p}^\dagger}{s^\dagger} \\ \frac{1}{\tau}\left(\frac{\mathbf{p}^\dagger}{\mathbf{r}^\dagger}\right)^2 \end{pmatrix}, \tag{14}$$

which can be simplified to

$$0 = -\mathbf{r}^\dagger - \frac{1}{\tau}\frac{\mathbf{p}^\dagger}{s^\dagger}. \tag{15}$$

The solution to this equation is the first iteration of the conjugate momentum, $\tilde{\mathbf{p}}^\dagger = -\tau s^\dagger \mathbf{r}^\dagger$. Plugging this back into the evolution equations leads to

$$\dot{\mathbf{r}} = -\tau s^\dagger \mathbf{r}^\dagger, \tag{16a}$$

$$\dot{s} = \tau(\mathbf{r}^\dagger)^2. \tag{16b}$$

These are the reduced equations obtained by the first order DynMaxEnt procedure. The † symbols denote derivative of a yet unspecified energy on the lower level of description ${}^{\downarrow}e(\mathbf{r}, s)$. Note that the energy is again conserved and that entropy is produced. To make the reduced evolution equations closed, we should identify the lower energy ${}^{\downarrow}e$ as the MaxEnt value of the higher-level energy,

$${}^{\downarrow}e = {}^{\uparrow}e(\mathbf{r}, \tilde{p}, s) = V(\mathbf{r}) + \varepsilon(s). \tag{17}$$

Equations (16) then gain an explicit form manifesting that the particle tends to the minimum of the potential V while producing entropy.

3.3.2. Second Order DynMaxEnt

By solving equation (14), we have actually broken the link between $\mathbf{p}$ and $\mathbf{p}^\dagger$, namely $\mathbf{p}^\dagger \neq \partial^\uparrow e/\partial \mathbf{p}$. To recover that link, we have to find a new value of $\mathbf{p}$ that corresponds to the obtained $\tilde{p}^\dagger$,

$$\frac{\tilde{\mathbf{p}}^{(2)}}{m} = \frac{\partial^\uparrow e}{\partial \mathbf{p}}\Big|_{\tilde{\mathbf{p}}^{(2)}} = -\tau \frac{\partial^\uparrow e}{\partial s}\frac{\partial^\uparrow e}{\partial \mathbf{r}} = -\tau \frac{\partial \varepsilon}{\partial s}\frac{\partial V}{\partial \mathbf{r}}. \tag{18}$$

Plugging this new value of $\mathbf{p}$ into energy $^\uparrow e$ gives a new energy on the lower level,

$$^\downarrow e^{(2)} = \frac{m}{2}\left(\tau \frac{\partial \varepsilon}{\partial s}\frac{\partial V}{\partial \mathbf{r}}\right)^2 + V(\mathbf{r}) + \varepsilon(s), \tag{19}$$

which can be seen as a weakly nonlocal correction of the MaxEnt lower energy $^\downarrow e$.

Once the link between $\mathbf{p}$ and $\mathbf{p}^\dagger$ through derivative of energy (Legendre transformation) has been recovered by updating $\tilde{\mathbf{p}}$ to $\tilde{\mathbf{p}}^{(2)}$, condition (14) no longer holds. To satisfy the condition, we have to find a new value of the conjugate momentum by solving (assuming that $\tau\partial\varepsilon/\partial s = \zeta = \text{const}$ for simplicity)

$$\begin{aligned} \dot{\tilde{\mathbf{p}}}^{(2)} &= -m\zeta \frac{\partial^2 V}{\partial \mathbf{r}^2}\dot{\mathbf{r}} = -m\zeta\frac{\partial^2 V}{\partial \mathbf{r}^2}\tilde{\mathbf{p}}^{\dagger(2)} \\ &= -\mathbf{r}^\dagger - \frac{1}{\zeta}\tilde{\mathbf{p}}^{\dagger(2)} = -\frac{\partial V}{\partial \mathbf{r}} - \frac{1}{\zeta}\tilde{\mathbf{p}}^{\dagger(2)}. \end{aligned} \tag{20}$$

The solution to this equation is

$$\tilde{\mathbf{p}}^{\dagger(2)} = \frac{-\zeta \frac{\partial V}{\partial \mathbf{r}}}{1 - m\zeta^2 \frac{\partial^2 V}{\partial \mathbf{r}^2}} \sim -\zeta \frac{\partial V}{\partial \mathbf{r}} - m\zeta^3 \frac{\partial V}{\partial \mathbf{r}^2} + O(\zeta)^5. \tag{21}$$

The latter contribution is obviously of the second order in the relaxation time τ while the former contribution is identical to the $\tilde{\mathbf{p}}^\dagger$ found above. This second-order correction of conjugate momentum can be plugged back into the equations for $\dot{\mathbf{r}}$ and $\dot{s}$ to obtain

$$\dot{\mathbf{r}} = \frac{-\zeta \frac{\partial V}{\partial \mathbf{r}}}{1 - m\zeta^2 \frac{\partial^2 V}{\partial \mathbf{r}^2}}, \tag{22a}$$

$$\dot{s} = \frac{\zeta}{s^\dagger}\frac{\left(\frac{\partial V}{\partial \mathbf{r}}\right)^2}{\left(1 - m\zeta^2 \frac{\partial^2 V}{\partial \mathbf{r}^2}\right)^2}, \tag{22b}$$

which is the second-order DynMaxEnt reduction. It is instructive to compare asymptotic expansion of the evolution equations for small τ/ζ with DynMaxEnt.

Note that the singularity suggested by this second order DynMaxEnt is not physically relevant but rather an invitation to a higher order as Equation (20) reveals—independence of $\mathbf{p}^{\dagger(2)}$ and $\partial_{\mathbf{r}} V = 0$. In addition, if $\tau \ll 1$, i.e., $\zeta \ll 1$ is small, DynMaxEnt generates a converging sequence of evolution laws where there is no blow-up. Hence, when the parameter ζ or τ is not small, the "corrections" stemming from higher order DynMaxEnt might be large and significant. Hence, as we shall further explore below, the higher order corrections seem to be mainly relevant when a small parameter is present.

3.3.3. Damped Particle by Asymptotic Expansions

A hallmark example of the usage of asymptotic expansions in statistical physics is the Chapman–Enskog expansion in kinetic theory [2,22].

In general, the two approaches, asymptotic expansion vs. Dynamic MaxEnt, are very different concepts of obtaining description of a system on a coarser level. The asymptotic analysis (such as the method of multiple scales, homogenisation, regular and singular perturbation methods or boundary layer analysis) does not explicitly assess the lower level of description or what exactly does the asymptotic approximation represents, but, from intuition and the dimensionless form of the evolution equations, one can use the presence of a small parameter to relate two levels of description (more precisely, two different spatial or temporal scales). The number of state variables and evolution equations are typically not changed (although in Chapman–Enskog analysis, evolution equations for several moments of the distribution function somewhat naturally appear) and a suitable choice of the form of expansion series allows a nested problem formulation on the coarser level by sequentially solving each asymptotic order. Note, however, that there is not a unique way to include the small parameter in spatial scaling, etc.

Dynamic MaxEnt, on the other hand, uses projections to the lower level of description (e.g., by relaxation of fast variables). In particular, the number of evolution equations (state variables) can be very different on the two levels in contrast to asymptotic analysis.

Let us compare the asymptotic method of solution with the Dynamic MaxEnt method on the simple problem of a damped particle where the dimensionless parameter $1/\tau$ measures the ratio of the reversible and irreversible evolution. Typically, the timescale of relaxation of dissipative processes is much shorter than the remaining evolution, hence $\tau \ll 1$. The solution to the problem can be searched in the form of asymptotic expansions

$$\mathbf{p} = \mathbf{p}_0 + \tau\mathbf{p}_1 + \tau^2\mathbf{p}_2 + O(\tau^3), \; \mathbf{r} = \mathbf{r}_0 + \tau\mathbf{r}_1 + O(\tau^2), \; s = s_0 + \tau s_1 + O(\tau^2) \tag{23}$$

and the conjugate $\mathbf{r}^\dagger$ variable has the following expansion

$$\mathbf{r}^\dagger = V_\mathbf{r}(\mathbf{r}_0 + \tau\mathbf{r}_1 + \tau^2\mathbf{r}_2) = V_\mathbf{r}(\mathbf{r}_0) + \tau\mathbf{r}_1 V_\mathbf{r}(\mathbf{r}_o) + O(\tau^2).$$

Noting that $\mathbf{p}^\dagger = \mathbf{p}/m$, the leading order solution is

$$\tau^{-1}: \quad \mathbf{p}_0 = 0,$$

while the first subleading order gives

$$\tau^0 : \mathbf{p}_1 = -ms^\dagger V_\mathbf{r}(\mathbf{r}_0), \quad \dot{\mathbf{r}}_0 = \frac{\mathbf{p}_0}{m} = 0.$$

Therefore, $\mathbf{p}_1$ is independent of time and the second subleading order reads

$$\mathbf{p}_2 = -ms^\dagger V_{\mathbf{rr}}(\mathbf{r}_0)\mathbf{r}_1 - ms^\dagger\dot{\mathbf{p}}_1 = -ms^\dagger V_{\mathbf{rr}}(\mathbf{r}_0)\mathbf{r}_1, \quad \dot{\mathbf{r}}_1 = \frac{\mathbf{p}_1}{m} = -s^\dagger V_\mathbf{r}(\mathbf{r}_0), \tag{24}$$

while, finally, $\dot{\mathbf{r}}_2 = \mathbf{p}_2/m$. In summary, the reduced evolution up to the second order can be characterised by the following set of equations:

$$\dot{\mathbf{r}}_0 = 0, \quad \dot{\mathbf{r}}_1 = -s^\dagger V_\mathbf{r}(\mathbf{r}_0), \quad \dot{\mathbf{r}}_2 = -s^\dagger V_{\mathbf{rr}}(\mathbf{r}_0)\mathbf{r}_1. \tag{25}$$

From the first subleading order, one could estimate that perhaps $\mathbf{p}_0 = 0$, $\mathbf{p}_1 = -ms^\dagger\mathbf{r}^\dagger$ and thus $\dot{\mathbf{r}} = -\tau ms^\dagger\mathbf{r}^\dagger$. We can now straightforwardly verify this by using the asymptotic expansions (23).

Hence, indeed, we have $\mathbf{p} = -\tau m s^\dagger \mathbf{r}^\dagger$ while the remaining equations can be written in the following way:

$$\dot{\mathbf{r}} = -\tau s^\dagger \mathbf{r}^\dagger, \tag{26a}$$

$$\dot{s} = \tau \left(\mathbf{r}^\dagger\right)^2, \tag{26b}$$

which means that the particle tends to the minimum of the potential $V(\mathbf{r})$. These equations are in line with Equations (16), obtained by DynMaxEnt. Additionally, the leading order solution in the asymptotic method corresponds to MaxEnt $\tilde{\mathbf{x}}(\mathbf{y})$ value (as in the Chapman–Enskog solution to the Boltzmann equation where the leading order solution corresponding to vanishing collision term is the local Maxwell distribution).

Note that we proposed the DynMaxEnt method to be the first order in state variables (both direct and conjugate) accompanied by the second order lower energy ${}^{\downarrow}e^{(2)}$. In particular, if we now compare the lower evolution equations from the asymptotic (26) and dynamic MaxEnt (16), we observe that they are identical with the exception stemming from the correction of the lower energy (conjugates in the lower evolution equations are always with respect to the lower energy). Furthermore, the comparison of the asymptotic solution $\mathbf{p}$, Equation (24), and of the dynamic MaxEnt result reveals that: (i) the structure of dynamic MaxEnt iteration resembles asymptotic expansion for a small parameter τ; (ii) the leading order solutions are the same, however, the subleading terms differ.

3.3.4. Relation to GENERIC

Evolution equations for the damped particle (11) can be seen as a particular realization of the General Equation for Non-Equilibrium Reversible-Irreversible Coupling (GENERIC) [4,14,23,24], with the following building blocks

$$\mathbf{L} = \begin{pmatrix} 0 & 1 & 0 \\ -1 & 0 & 0 \\ 0 & 0 & 0 \end{pmatrix} \quad \text{and} \quad \Xi^{(\mathbf{p})} = \frac{1}{2}\frac{1}{\tau}(\mathbf{p}^*)^2, \tag{27}$$

where the former expression defines a Poisson bivector while the latter dissipation potential (Irreversible evolution generated by a dissipation potential is also called gradient dynamics. It is in tight relation to the Steepest Entropy Ascent [25,26], which is essentially equivalent to the formulation of GENERIC with dissipative brackets [4].). The dissipation potential is naturally formulated in terms of $\mathbf{p}^*$, which can be interpreted as derivative of entropy. The evolution equation consists of reversible part $\mathbf{L} \cdot \mathrm{d}E$ and irreversible $\Xi_{\mathbf{p}^*}|_{\mathbf{p}^*=S_{\mathbf{p}}}$. In order to use only derivative w.r.t. energy, we recall the relation among the two representations $\mathbf{p}^* = -\mathbf{p}^\dagger/s^\dagger$, see [14,27] for more details (Indeed, on the Gibbs–Legendre manifold, where conjugate variables are identified with derivatives of thermodynamic potentials, one has $\left(\frac{\partial s}{\partial p_i}\right)_e = -\left(\frac{\partial e}{\partial p_i}\right)_s \left(\frac{\partial e}{\partial s}\right)_{\mathbf{p}}^{-1}$ and $\left(\frac{\partial e}{\partial s}\right)_{\mathbf{p}} = \left(\frac{\partial s}{\partial e}\right)_{\mathbf{p}}^{-1}$.) The equations are then explicitly

$$\frac{\mathrm{d}}{\mathrm{d}t}\begin{pmatrix} \mathbf{r} \\ \mathbf{p} \\ s \end{pmatrix} = \begin{pmatrix} 0 & 1 & 0 \\ -1 & 0 & 0 \\ 0 & 0 & 0 \end{pmatrix} \cdot \begin{pmatrix} \mathbf{r}^\dagger \\ \mathbf{p}^\dagger \\ s^\dagger \end{pmatrix} + \begin{pmatrix} 0 \\ -\frac{1}{\tau}\frac{\mathbf{p}^\dagger}{s^\dagger} \\ \frac{1}{\tau}\left(\frac{\mathbf{p}^\dagger}{s^\dagger}\right)^2 \end{pmatrix}, \tag{28}$$

which is the same as Equations (11). The equations thus possess the GENERIC structure.

After the relaxation of the momentum $\mathbf{p}$, expressed by Equation (15), evolution of positions becomes irreversible, given by Equation (16). Is this equation compatible with GENERIC? In other words, is there a dissipation potential generating that evolution? The answer is affirmative and actually easy to find at least in the case of the damped particle. Indeed, by evaluating dissipation potential $\Xi^{(\mathbf{p})}$ at the constitutive relation (15), we obtain dissipation potential for the lower level

$$\Xi^{(\mathbf{r})}(\mathbf{r}^*) = \Xi^{(\mathbf{p})}|_{\mathbf{p}^*=-\tau\mathbf{r}^\dagger=\tau\frac{\mathbf{r}^*}{e^*}} = \frac{\tau}{2}\left(\frac{\mathbf{r}^*}{e^*}\right)^2, \tag{29}$$

where $e^* = S_e = 1/s^\dagger$, e being total energy of the particle. Derivative of this dissipation potential w.r.t. $\mathbf{p}^*$ reads

$$\dot{\mathbf{r}} = \Xi^{(\mathbf{r})}_{\mathbf{r}^*} = \tau\frac{\mathbf{r}^*}{(e^*)^2} = -\tau s^\dagger \mathbf{r}^\dagger, \tag{30}$$

which is the reduced evolution equation (16). In other words, at least in this particular case the reduced evolution equation for $\mathbf{r}$ is generated by a dissipation potential constructed from the original dissipation potential for $\mathbf{p}$ by a projection, see also [21]. At least in the case of damped particle, the reduced evolution is a particular realization of GENERIC, and the reduced dissipation potential is obtained from the original dissipation potential.

3.4. Summary of the Dynamic MaxEnt Method

A few remarks should be pointed out:

1. MaxEnt with constraints corresponding to a chosen projection linking the two levels of description is equivalent to MinEne with the same constraints. This follows from the same argument as used in ([27], Ch 5.1) only with the addition of constraints which, crucially, describe the same manifold in the phase space of $(S, E, \mathbf{x})$.
2. It is important to consider direct and conjugate variables to be independent until reaching the Legendre manifold where they are related via appropriate entropy. This stands out during the MaxEnt procedure as noted above and in the contact-geometric formulation in Section 5.
3. Static MaxEnt should be seen as not providing a relation among conjugate variables but rather only among the direct ones. This can be appreciated in a special case of projection that corresponds to a relaxation of fast variables in the system, hence removing some of the state variables $\mathbf{x}$ when a transition to a less microscopic description is carried out. For this point of view, it is essential to consider direct and conjugate variables as independent.
4. If direct and conjugate variables are not considered independent during MaxEnt and hence MaxEnt would provide MaxEnt values for both reduced and conjugate variables, the dynamics on MaxEnt manifold would be (typically) such that its vector field would be "sticking out", i.e., driving the dynamics out of the MaxEnt manifold. The correction in finding $\tilde{\mathbf{x}}^*(\mathbf{y}, \mathbf{y}^*)$ is exactly such that the MaxEnt manifold $\tilde{\mathcal{M}}$ in direct variables is never left by the dynamics.
5. The distinction of direct and conjugate variables has several crucial benefits. First, it guarantees the thermodynamic structure of the evolution equations (potentials, reversible and irreversible parts of equations, CR-GENERIC or possibly GENERIC structure). Secondly, this distinction of state variables enables to always sustain the MaxEnt, i.e., the most probable, value of the direct variables on the lower description (as discussed above). This cannot be achieved in an asymptotic framework/approach, where such knowledge is not at hand and the solution is searched in the form of asymptotic corrections to a leading order solution.
6. Parity of the state variables with respect to time reversal typically changes during the DynMaxEnt reduction. For instance, the momentum, which was initially an odd variable, becomes proportional to the gradient of potential, which is even, or the conformation tensor (which is initially even) becomes proportional to the shear rate, which is odd. Similarly, behavior with respect to space-time transformations (e.g., Galilean boost) also changes. For instance, momentum of a particle, the value of which of course depends on the choice of inertial laboratory frame, becomes independent of Galilean boosts after the reduction (being proportional to gradient of the potential). This is compatible with the multiscale point of view of the studied systems. For instance, if one is able to measure the conjugate entropy flux $\mathbf{w}$ (see Section 4.3) directly, one can also see that Galilean boost affects it, and one should stay on the level of description

where $\mathbf{w}$ is among the state variables. On the other hand, if one only measures $\mathbf{w}$ in the relaxed state, where it is proportional to the gradient of temperature, one does not see the effect of Galilean boosts anymore, and one can safely work on the Fourier level, where $\mathbf{w}$ is no longer among the state variables. In summary, the behavior of physical quantities with respect to time reversal and space-time transformations crucially depends on the chosen level of description, and this level-dependent behavior is compatible with the multiscale point of view of physical systems.

The comparison to the asymptotic expansion methods provided further insight into the Dynamic MaxEnt method. For example, the asymptotic analysis provides corrections to the solution at each order, whereas Dynamic MaxEnt provides relations for closures/fluxes. In the particular examples above, it may seem that both methods yield the same set of leading order evolution equations but note that this is only when one can explicitly solve the asymptotic problems in each order. As noted above, typically asymptotic methods do not change the number of equations as opposed to Dynamic MaxEnt, where the number is given by the projection. Asymptotic methods also typically do not change parity with respect to time reversal, whereas DynMaxEnt does [28]. Finally, note that Dynamic MaxEnt does not rely per se on the presence of a small parameter but rather on the existence of a projection which is similar but not the same.

In summary, Dynamic MaxEnt does not have (and perhaps should not have) an aim to find other than the leading order evolution equations on a specified level. From all the observations and discussion above, we propose that the most appropriate choice for this aim is to find and keep the static MaxEnt values of direct variables exactly while identifying the conjugate state variables in such a way that evolution (dynamics) stays exactly on this MaxEnt value of direct variables; entropy is modified in such a way as to correspond to conjugate variables and the first correction of the direct variables. It seems that, if the zero-th order asymptotic solution coincides with the static MaxEnt value of the direct state variable $\tilde{\mathbf{x}}(\mathbf{y})$, the asymptotic expansion method yields the same leading order behaviour as the Dynamic MaxEnt (although without the thermodynamic structure and new phenomena linked to the change of entropy accompanying the transition of scales). Interestingly, we found in the studied example that even higher order asymptotic solutions seem to be related to the Dynamic MaxEnt method, although it is yet unclear how exactly and will be subjected to further research.

4. Applications in Continuum Thermodynamics

Let us now demonstrate the Dynamic MaxEnt on a few examples in continuum thermodynamics, namely on relaxation of conformation tensor, relaxation of Reynolds stress, and hyperbolic heat conduction. The former two examples were already discussed in [14].

4.1. *Suspension of Hookean Dumbbells*

4.1.1. Non-Equilibrium Thermodynamics of Conformation Tensor

First, let the state variables be density of matter ρ, momentum density $\mathbf{u}$, entropy density s and conformation tensor c^{ij}, which expresses correlations of dumbbell orientation and prolongation. Poisson bracket expressing kinematics of these state variables is

$$\begin{aligned}\{A,B\}^{(\mathbf{c})} &= \{A,B\}^{(FM)} + \int \mathrm{d}\mathbf{r} c_{ij}\left(\partial_k A_{c_{ij}} B_{u_k} - \partial_k B_{c_{ij}} A_{u_k}\right) \\ &\quad + \int \mathrm{d}\mathbf{r} c_{ij}\left(\left(A_{c_{kj}} + A_{c_{jk}}\right)\partial_i B_{u_k} - \left(B_{c_{kj}} + B_{c_{jk}}\right)\partial_i A_{u_k}\right),\end{aligned} \tag{31}$$

where c^{ij} was identified with c_{ij} for simplicity of notation. Bracket $\{\bullet,\bullet\}^{(FM)}$ is the fluid mechanics Poisson bracket (A3). Note that the conformation tensor is related to the left Cauchy–Green tensor $\mathbf{B}$

by $\mathbf{c} = \rho\mathbf{B}$. Reversible evolution equations for state variables $\mathbf{x} = (\rho, \mathbf{u}, s, \mathbf{c})$ implied by bracket (31) are

$$\frac{\partial \rho}{\partial t} = -\partial_i \left(\rho E_{u_i}\right), \tag{32a}$$

$$\frac{\partial u_i}{\partial t} = -\partial_j \left(u_i E_{u_j}\right) - \rho \partial_i E_\rho - u_j \partial_i E_{u_j} - s \partial_i E_s - -c_{jk}\partial_i E_{c_{jk}} + \partial_k \left(c_{kj}\left(E_{c_{ij}} + E_{c_{ji}}\right)\right), \tag{32b}$$

$$\frac{\partial s}{\partial t} = -\partial_i \left(s E_{u_i}\right), \tag{32c}$$

$$\frac{\partial c_{ij}}{\partial t} = -\partial_k \left(c_{ij} E_{u_k}\right) + c_{kj}\partial_k E_{u_i} + c_{ki}\partial_k E_{u_j}, \tag{32d}$$

where E is the total energy of the system.

With energy

$$E = \int d\mathbf{r} \left[\frac{\mathbf{u}^2}{2\rho} + \varepsilon(\rho, s, \mathbf{c})\right], \tag{33}$$

where internal energy ε still remains unspecified, evolution equation (32d) can be rewritten in terms of the upper-convected time-derivative as

$$\overset{\nabla}{\mathbf{c}} = -\mathbf{c}\nabla \cdot \mathbf{v}, \qquad \mathbf{v} = \frac{\mathbf{u}}{\rho}, \tag{34}$$

which is the reversible part of Maxwell rheological model [29].

Considering a suspension of Hookean dumbbells, entropy is

$$S = \int d\mathbf{r} \left[\frac{1}{2} n k_B \ln \det \mathbf{c} + s\left(n, e - \frac{\mathbf{u}^2}{2\rho} - \frac{1}{2} H \,\mathrm{Tr}\mathbf{c}\right)\right], \tag{35}$$

as derived for instance in [14]. Parameter H is the spring constant of the dumbbells, and n represents concentration of dumbbells. Derivative of this entropy with respect to $\mathbf{c}$ is

$$c^*_{ij} = \frac{\partial S}{\partial c_{ij}} = \frac{1}{2} k_B n c^{-1}_{ij} - \frac{1}{2}\frac{H}{T}\delta_{ij}, \tag{36}$$

which is equal to zero for

$$\tilde{\mathbf{c}} = \frac{k_B T n}{H}\mathbf{I}. \tag{37}$$

This is the MaxEnt value of $\mathbf{c}$. Note that inverse temperature T^{-1} is identified as derivative of entropy with respect to energy density.

Dissipation potential can be prescribed as

$$\Xi^{(\mathbf{c})} = \int d\mathbf{r} \Lambda_c c_{ij} c^*_{ik} c^*_{jk}, \tag{38}$$

the derivative of which is

$$\Xi^{(\mathbf{c})}_{c^*_{ij}} = 2\Lambda_c c_{ik} c^*_{kj}. \tag{39}$$

The evolution equation of $\mathbf{c}$ then gains an irreversible term,

$$\left.\frac{\partial \Xi^{(\mathbf{c})}}{\partial c^*_{ij}}\right|_{\mathbf{c}_* = S_\mathbf{c}} = -\frac{\Lambda_c H}{T}\left(c_{ij} - \frac{k_B T n}{H}\delta_{ij}\right). \tag{40}$$

After the transformation to the energetic representation (conjugates with respect to energy rather than entropy), the sum of the reversible and irreversible contributions to evolution equations for $(\rho, \mathbf{u}, \mathbf{c}, s)$ is prepared for the DynMaxEnt reduction.

4.1.2. DynMaxEnt to Hydrodynamics

Let us now apply the Dynamic MaxEnt reduction so that the conformation tensor $\mathbf{c}$ relaxes. The energetic representation reversible Equations (32) and irreversible Equations (40) together are

$$\frac{\partial \rho}{\partial t} = -\partial_i \left(\rho u_i^\dagger\right), \tag{41a}$$

$$\begin{aligned}\frac{\partial u_i}{\partial t} &= -\partial_j \left(u_i u_j^\dagger\right) - \rho \partial_i \rho^\dagger - u_j \partial_i u_j^\dagger - s\partial_i s^\dagger - \\ &\quad - c_{jk}\partial_i c_{jk}^\dagger + \partial_k \left(c_{kj}\left(c_{ij}^\dagger + c_{ji}^\dagger\right)\right),\end{aligned} \tag{41b}$$

$$\frac{\partial s}{\partial t} = -\partial_i \left(s u_i^\dagger\right) + 2\frac{\Lambda_c}{(s^\dagger)^2} c_{ij}^\dagger c_{ik} c_{kj}^\dagger, \tag{41c}$$

$$\frac{\partial c_{ij}}{\partial t} = -\partial_k \left(c_{ij} u_k^\dagger\right) + c_{kj}\partial_k u_i^\dagger + c_{ki}\partial_k u_j^\dagger - \frac{2\Lambda_c}{s^\dagger} c_{ik} c_{kj}^\dagger. \tag{41d}$$

Consider now the isothermal incompressible case (The compressible case and the origin of incompressibility were discussed in [19].), i.e., $S_e = T = \text{const}$, $n = \text{const}$ and $\nabla \cdot \mathbf{u}^\dagger = 0$. Equations (41b) and (41d) at the MaxEnt value of $\mathbf{c}$ (given by Equation (37)) become

$$\begin{aligned}\frac{\partial u_i}{\partial t} &= -\partial_j \left(u_i u_j^\dagger\right) - \rho \partial_i \rho^\dagger - u_j \partial_i u_j^\dagger - s\partial_i s^\dagger - \\ &\quad - \frac{k_B T n}{H}\partial_i \mathrm{Tr}\mathbf{c}^\dagger + \frac{k_B T n}{H}\partial_k \left(c_{ik}^\dagger + c_{ki}^\dagger\right),\end{aligned} \tag{42a}$$

$$0 = \partial_j u_i^\dagger + \partial_i u_j^\dagger - 2\frac{\Lambda_c}{T} c_{ij}^\dagger. \tag{42b}$$

The last equation has a solution

$$\mathbf{c}^\dagger = \frac{T}{2\Lambda_c}\left(\nabla \mathbf{u}^\dagger + (\nabla \mathbf{u}^\dagger)^T\right), \quad \mathrm{Tr}\mathbf{c}^\dagger = 0. \tag{43}$$

By plugging this solution into the equation for momentum density, we obtain the Navier–Stokes equation for momentum density

$$\begin{aligned}\frac{\partial u_i}{\partial t} &= -\partial_j \left(u_i u_j^\dagger\right) - \rho \partial_i \rho^\dagger - u_j \partial_i u_j^\dagger - s\partial_i s^\dagger \\ &\quad + \frac{k_B T^2 n}{H\Lambda_c}\partial_k \left(\partial_i u_k^\dagger + \partial_k u_i^\dagger\right),\end{aligned} \tag{44}$$

where the coefficient $k_B T^2 n / H\Lambda_c$ corresponds to the shear viscosity and $\mathbf{u}^\dagger = E_\mathbf{u} = \mathbf{v} = \mathbf{u}/\rho$ is the velocity.

The Dynamic MaxEnt reduction of the conformation tensor leads to the Newtonian shear stress tensor.

4.2. Reynolds Stress

We now turn to a complex fluid where momentum–momentum correlations between two neighboring particles matter, the correlation being expressed by the Reynolds stress tensor R_{ij}.

4.2.1. Non-Equilibrium Thermodynamics of Reynolds Stress

Let the state variables be $\mathbf{x} = (\rho, \mathbf{u}, s, \mathbf{R})$. The Poisson bracket expressing kinematics of $\mathbf{x}$ is

$$\begin{aligned} \{A,B\}^{(\mathbf{R})} &= \{A,B\}^{(FM)} + \int \mathrm{d}\mathbf{r} R_{ij}\left(\partial_k A_{R_{ij}} B_{u_k} - \partial_k B_{R_{ij}} A_{u_k}\right) - \\ &\quad - \int \mathrm{d}\mathbf{r} R_{ij}\left(\left(A_{R_{kj}} + A_{R_{jk}}\right)\partial_k B_{u_i} - \left(B_{R_{kj}} + B_{R_{jk}}\right)\partial_k A_{u_i}\right), \end{aligned} \tag{45}$$

see, e.g., [14,30]. The reversible evolution equations are then

$$\frac{\partial \rho}{\partial t} = -\partial_i\left(\rho E_{u_i}\right), \tag{46a}$$

$$\begin{aligned} \frac{\partial u_i}{\partial t} &= -\partial_j\left(u_i E_{u_j}\right) - \rho\partial_i E_\rho - u_j\partial_i E_{u_j} - s\partial_i E_s - \\ &\quad - R_{kj}\partial_i E_{R_{kj}} - \partial_k\left(R_{ij}\left(E_{R_{kj}} + E_{R_{jk}}\right)\right), \end{aligned} \tag{46b}$$

$$\frac{\partial s}{\partial t} = -\partial_i\left(s E_{u_i}\right), \tag{46c}$$

$$\frac{\partial R_{ij}}{\partial t} = -\partial_k\left(R_{ij} E_{u_k}\right) - R_{kj}\partial_i E_{u_k} - R_{ki}\partial_j E_{u_k}. \tag{46d}$$

Let entropy be given by

$$S^{(\mathbf{R})} = \int \mathrm{d}\mathbf{r}\left[s\left(\rho, e - \frac{\mathbf{u}^2}{2\rho} - \frac{1}{2m}\mathrm{Tr}\mathbf{R}\right) + \frac{1}{2}k_B\frac{\rho}{m}\ln\det\frac{\mathbf{R}}{Q_R}\right], \tag{47}$$

where Q_R is an appropriately chosen constant. The reason for this entropy is analogical to the entropy (35). A derivative of entropy (47) with respect to $\mathbf{R}$ is

$$R^*_{ij} = \frac{\partial S^{(\mathbf{R})}}{\partial R_{ij}} = -\frac{1}{2m}S_e\delta_{ij} + \frac{k_B\rho}{2m}(R^{-1})_{ij}, \tag{48}$$

which is equal to zero if and only if

$$R_{ij} = k_B T\rho\delta_{ij}. \tag{49}$$

This is the MaxEnt value of $\mathbf{R}$, at which the Reynolds stress is proportional to the unit matrix. Similarly as in the preceding section, we choose dissipation potential

$$\Xi^{(\mathbf{R})} = \int \mathrm{d}\mathbf{r}\Lambda_R R^*_{ij} R_{jk} R^*_{ki}, \tag{50}$$

the derivative of which is

$$\Xi^{(\mathbf{R})}_{R^*_{ij}} = 2\Lambda_R R_{jk} R^*_{ki}. \tag{51}$$

Note that R^{ij} was identified with R_{ij} and similarly for $\mathbf{R}^*$ for simplicity of notation. Evolution equation of $\mathbf{R}$ then gains an irreversible term

$$\left.\frac{\partial \Xi^{(\mathbf{R})}}{\partial R^*_{ij}}\right|_{\mathbf{R}^* = S_{\mathbf{R}}} = -\frac{\Lambda_R}{Tm}\left(\mathbf{R} - k_B T\rho\mathbf{I}\right). \tag{52}$$

By combining the reversible evolution (46) and irreversible (52), we obtain

$$\begin{aligned}
\frac{\partial \rho}{\partial t} &= -\partial_i \left(\rho E_{u_i}\right), && \text{(53a)}\\
\frac{\partial u_i}{\partial t} &= -\partial_j \left(u_i E_{u_j}\right) - \rho \partial_i E_\rho - u_j \partial_i E_{u_j} - s \partial_i E_s - \\
&\quad - R_{kj} \partial_i E_{R_{kj}} - \partial_k \left(R_{ij}\left(E_{R_{kj}} + E_{R_{jk}}\right)\right), && \text{(53b)}\\
\frac{\partial s}{\partial t} &= -\partial_i \left(s E_{u_i}\right) + 2\frac{\Lambda_R}{(E_s)^2} E_{R_{ij}} R_{jk} E_{R_{ki}}, && \text{(53c)}\\
\frac{\partial R_{ij}}{\partial t} &= -\partial_k \left(R_{ij} E_{u_k}\right) - R_{kj}\partial_i E_{u_k} - R_{ki} \partial_j E_{u_k} \\
&\quad -2\frac{\Lambda_R}{E_s} R_{jk} E_{R_{ki}}, && \text{(53d)}
\end{aligned}$$

which are the GENERIC evolution equations for fluid mechanics with Reynolds stress. For instance, the last equation can be rewritten as

$$\begin{aligned}
\frac{\partial R_{ij}}{\partial t} &= -\partial_k \left(R_{ij} v_k\right) - R_{kj}\partial_i v_k - R_{ki}\partial_j v_k \\
&\quad -\frac{\Lambda_R}{Tm}\left(\mathbf{R} - k_B T \rho \mathbf{I}\right), && \text{(54)}
\end{aligned}$$

from which the tendency to relaxation of the Reynolds stress tensor to the respective MaxEnt value is obvious.

4.2.2. DynMaxEnt to Hydrodynamics

As in the case of the conformation tensor in Section 4.1, let us now show how the Reynolds stress relaxes. The MaxEnt value (49) can be plugged into Equations (53). Assuming again isothermal incompressible flow, $\rho = \text{const}$, $\nabla \cdot \mathbf{u}^\dagger = 0$ and $S_e = T = \text{const}$, the equations become

$$\begin{aligned}
\frac{\partial u_i}{\partial t} &= -\partial_j \left(u_i u_j^\dagger\right) - \rho \partial_i \rho^\dagger - u_j \partial_i u_j^\dagger - s \partial_i s^\dagger - \\
&\quad - k_B T \rho \partial_i R^\dagger_{kk} - k_B T \rho \partial_k \left(R^\dagger_{ki} + R^\dagger_{ik}\right), && \text{(55a)}\\
0 &= -k_B T \rho \left(\partial_i u_j^\dagger + \partial_j u_i^\dagger\right) - 2\Lambda_R k_B \rho R^\dagger_{ji}. && \text{(55b)}
\end{aligned}$$

The last equation has a solution

$$\tilde{\mathbf{R}}^\dagger = -\frac{T}{2\Lambda_R}\left(\nabla \mathbf{u}^\dagger + (\nabla \mathbf{u}^\dagger)^T\right) \qquad \text{and} \qquad \mathrm{Tr}\tilde{\mathbf{R}} = 0. \tag{56}$$

Plugging this solution back into the equation for $\mathbf{u}$ leads to

$$\begin{aligned}
\frac{\partial u_i}{\partial t} &= -\partial_j \left(u_i u_j^\dagger\right) - \rho \partial_i \rho^\dagger - u_j \partial_i u_j^\dagger - s \partial_i s^\dagger \\
&\quad + \frac{k_B T^2 \rho}{\Lambda_R} \partial_k \left(\partial_k u_i^\dagger + \partial_i u_k^\dagger\right), && \text{(57)}
\end{aligned}$$

which is again the Navier–Stokes equation with shear viscosity. Relaxation of Reynolds stress thus leads to extra (also called turbulent) viscosity by means of the Dynamic MaxEnt reduction.

4.3. *Hyperbolic Heat Conduction*

4.3.1. Non-Equilibrium Thermodynamics of Heat

Kinematics of heat transfer can be thought of as kinematics of phonons, and kinematics of phonons has been successfully described by Boltzmann-like dynamics, where the distribution function of phonons plays the role of state variable, see e.g., book [31]. By the reduction from the kinetic theory to fluid mechanics, see e.g., [1,14], kinematics of phonons can be expressed in terms of the entropy density and momentum related to entropy transport, the kinematics of which is expressed by a hydrodynamic-like Poisson bracket (see [32]). Subsequent transformation to density of matter ρ, total momentum of matter and phonons $\mathbf{m}$, entropy density s and conjugate entropy flux $\mathbf{w}$, which is equal to the ratio of phonon momentum and entropy density, leads to bracket

$$
\begin{aligned}
\{F,G\}^{(Cat)} &= \{F,G\}^{(FM)}\Big|_{\mathbf{u}=\mathbf{m}} + \int d\mathbf{r}(G_{w_i}\partial_i F_s - F_{w_i}\partial_i G_s) \\
&+ \int d\mathbf{r} w_j \left(\partial_i F_{w_i} G_{m_j} - \partial_i G_{w_i} F_{m_j}\right) \\
&+ \int d\mathbf{r}\, (\partial_i w_j - \partial_j w_i) \left(F_{w_i} G_{m_j} - G_{w_i} F_{m_j}\right) \\
&+ \int d\mathbf{r} \frac{1}{s} (\partial_i w_j - \partial_j w_i) F_{w_i} G_{w_j},
\end{aligned} \tag{58}
$$

expressing kinematics of matter and heat—the Cattaneo Poisson bracket. The name Cattaneo is due to the implied hyperbolicity of heat transport [19]. The Poisson bracket (58) generates reversible evolution equations

$$\frac{\partial \rho}{\partial t} = -\partial_k(\rho E_{m_k}), \tag{59a}$$

$$
\begin{aligned}
\frac{\partial m_i}{\partial t} &= -\partial_j(m_i E_{m_j}) - \partial_j(w_i E_{w_j}) - \rho\partial_i E_\rho - m_j \partial_i E_{m_j} - s\partial_i E_s \\
&\quad - w_k \partial_i E_{w_k} + \partial_i (E_{w_k} w_k),
\end{aligned} \tag{59b}
$$

$$\frac{\partial s}{\partial t} = -\partial_k \left(s E_{m_k} + E_{w_k}\right), \tag{59c}$$

$$\frac{\partial w_k}{\partial t} = -\partial_k E_s - \partial_k (w_j E_{m_j}) + (\partial_k w_j - \partial_j w_k)\left(E_{m_j} + \frac{1}{s} E_{w_j}\right). \tag{59d}$$

These evolution equations express reversible dynamics of fluid mechanics and conjugate entropy flux $\mathbf{w}$. Note that, for the heat flux, i.e., flux of energy, the usual relation $\mathbf{q} = E_s E_{w_k} = T\mathbf{J}^{(s)}$ holds true, see [14] for more details.

Local dissipation is enforced by adopting an algebraic dissipation potential, the simplest of which is

$$\Xi(\mathbf{w}^*) = \int d\mathbf{r}\, \frac{1}{2}\frac{1}{\tau}(\mathbf{w}^*)^2 = \int d\mathbf{r}\, \frac{1}{2}\frac{1}{\tau}\left(\frac{1}{s^\dagger}\mathbf{w}^\dagger\right)^2, \tag{60}$$

where the last equality follows from the transformation between energetic and entropic representation. Then, the irreversible terms generated by this dissipation potential are added to the reversible evolution, Equations (59),

$$\frac{\partial \rho}{\partial t} = -\partial_k(\rho m_k^\dagger), \tag{61a}$$

$$\frac{\partial m_i}{\partial t} = -\partial_j(m_i m_j^\dagger) - \partial_j(w_i w_j^\dagger) - \rho \partial_i \rho^\dagger - m_j \partial_i m_j^\dagger - s\partial_i s^\dagger - w_k \partial_i w_k^\dagger + \partial_i(w_k^\dagger w_k), \tag{61b}$$

$$\frac{\partial s}{\partial t} = -\partial_k\left(s m_k^\dagger + w_k^\dagger\right) + \frac{1}{\tau (s^\dagger)^2}(\mathbf{w}^\dagger)^2, \tag{61c}$$

$$\frac{\partial w_k}{\partial t} = -\partial_k s^\dagger - \partial_k(w_j m_j^\dagger) + (\partial_k w_j - \partial_j w_k)\left(m_j^\dagger + \frac{1}{s}w_j^\dagger\right) - \frac{1}{\tau s^\dagger} w_k^\dagger . \tag{61d}$$

These are the GENERIC equations for fluid mechanics with hyperbolic heat conduction.

4.3.2. DynMaxEnt to Fourier Heat Conduction

The simplest possible dependence of entropy on the extra field $\mathbf{w}$ is quadratic (keeping in mind that S has to be a concave and even with respect to time reversal functional),

$$S(\rho, \mathbf{m}, e, \mathbf{w}) = \int \mathbf{dr}\, s\left(\rho, e - \frac{\mathbf{m}^2}{2\rho} - \frac{1}{2}\alpha \mathbf{w}^2\right) . \tag{62}$$

Consequently, entropy is highest (for given fields ρ, $\mathbf{u}$ and e) at $\mathbf{w} = 0$, which is the MaxEnt estimate $\tilde{\mathbf{w}}$. Plugging this value into Equations (61) leads to

$$\frac{\partial \rho}{\partial t} = -\partial_k(\rho m_k^\dagger), \tag{63a}$$

$$\frac{\partial m_i}{\partial t} = -\partial_j(m_i m_j^\dagger) - \rho \partial_i \rho^\dagger - m_j \partial_i m_j^\dagger - s\partial_i s^\dagger, \tag{63b}$$

$$\frac{\partial s}{\partial t} = -\partial_k\left(s m_k^\dagger + w_k^\dagger\right) + \frac{1}{\tau (s^\dagger)^2}(\mathbf{w}^\dagger)^2, \tag{63c}$$

$$0 = -\partial_k s^\dagger - \frac{1}{\tau s^\dagger} w_k^\dagger . \tag{63d}$$

Equation (63d) has the solution

$$\tilde{\mathbf{w}}^\dagger = -\tau s^\dagger \nabla s^\dagger . \tag{64}$$

Plugging this value into the rest of Equations (63), we obtain

$$\frac{\partial \rho}{\partial t} = -\partial_i(\rho E_{m_i}), \tag{65a}$$

$$\frac{\partial m_i}{\partial t} = -\partial_j(m_i E_{m_j}) - \rho \partial_i E_\rho - m_j \partial_i E_{m_j} - s\partial_i E_s, \tag{65b}$$

$$\frac{\partial s}{\partial t} = -\partial_k\left(s E_{m_k} - \tau E_s \partial_k E_s\right) + \tau(\nabla E_s)^2 , \tag{65c}$$

which are Euler equations with Fourier heat conduction. Indeed, denoting local temperature E_s as T, the entropy flux is

$$\mathbf{J}^{(s)} = -\tau T \nabla T = \frac{-\lambda \nabla T}{T} , \tag{66}$$

where $\lambda = T^2 \tau$ is the heat conductivity and $\mathbf{q} = -\lambda \nabla T$ is the heat flux.

One can also seek higher order corrections by means of the infinite DynMaxEnt chain. The corrected value of $\mathbf{w}$ implied by Equation (63d) is

$$\tilde{\mathbf{w}}^{(2)} = -\frac{\tau}{\alpha} T \nabla T, \tag{67}$$

which leads to energy

$$E = \int d\mathbf{r} \left(\frac{\mathbf{m}^2}{2\rho} + \varepsilon(\rho, s) + \frac{1}{2} \tau \alpha \varepsilon_s^2 (\nabla \varepsilon_s)^2 \right). \tag{68}$$

This is a weakly non-local energy implied by the second-order DynMaxEnt correction.

In summary, Fourier's law, which tells us that heat flows from a hotter body to a colder body, can be derived by the dynamic MaxEnt reduction from the coupled dynamics of phonons and fluid mechanics. The only irreversibility on the higher level of description is present in the evolution equation for $\mathbf{w}$. After the reduction, this irreversibility leads to irreversible terms in the equation for entropy (irreversible entropy flux and entropy production). Note that this reduction is again compatible with the asymptotic expansion carried out in [33].

4.4. *Magnetohydrodynamics*

Let us now turn to DynMaxEnt when the electromagnetic field is present.

4.4.1. Non-Equilibrium Thermodynamics of Charged Mixtures

Dynamics of charged mixtures is governed by the Maxwell equations interacting with fluid mechanics of the species, see ([14] Section 6.4). Let us start with a Poisson bracket for the binary mixture of oppositely charged species endowed with a single entropy, total momentum density, displacement field and magnetic field, that is,

$$\begin{aligned}
\{F,G\}^{(\text{EMHD-2})}(\rho_+,\rho_-,\mathbf{m},s,\mathbf{D},\mathbf{B}) &= \{F,G\}^{(\text{CIT-2})}(\rho_+,\rho_-,\mathbf{m},s) \\
\{F,G\}^{(\text{EM})}(\mathbf{D},\mathbf{B}) \Big\{ & + \int \mathrm{d}\mathbf{r} \left(F_{D_i} \varepsilon_{ijk} \partial_j G_{B_k} - G_{D_i} \varepsilon_{ijk} \partial_j F_{B_k} \right) \\
\{F,G\}^{(\text{SP})}(\mathbf{D},\mathbf{m}) \left\{ \begin{array}{l} \\ \\ \\ \end{array} \right. & \begin{aligned} &+ \int \mathrm{d}\mathbf{r} D_i \left(\partial_j F_{D_i} G_{m_j} - \partial_j G_{D_i} F_{m_j} \right) \\ &+ \int \mathrm{d}\mathbf{r} \partial_j D_j (F_{m_i} G_{D_i} - G_{m_i} F_{D_i}) \\ &+ \int \mathrm{d}\mathbf{r} D_j (F_{m_i} \partial_j G_{D_i} - G_{m_i} \partial_j F_{D_i}) \end{aligned} \\
\{F,G\}^{(\text{SP})}(\mathbf{B},\mathbf{m}) \left\{ \begin{array}{l} \\ \\ \\ \end{array} \right. & \begin{aligned} &+ \int \mathrm{d}\mathbf{r} B_i \left(\partial_j F_{B_i} G_{m_j} - \partial_j G_{B_i} F_{m_j} \right) \\ &+ \int \mathrm{d}\mathbf{r} \partial_j B_j (F_{m_i} G_{B_i} - G_{m_i} F_{B_i}) \\ &+ \int \mathrm{d}\mathbf{r} B_j (F_{m_i} \partial_j G_{B_i} - G_{m_i} \partial_j F_{B_i}), \end{aligned}
\end{aligned} \tag{69}$$

where the CIT2 (binary classical irreversible thermodynamics [1,34]) bracket stands for

$$\begin{aligned}
\{F,G\}^{(\text{CIT-2})}(\rho_+,\rho_-,\mathbf{m},s) &= \int \mathrm{d}\mathbf{r}\, \rho_+ \left(\partial_i F_{\rho_+} G_{m_i} - \partial_i G_{\rho_+} F_{m_i} \right) \\
&+ \int \mathrm{d}\mathbf{r}\, \rho_- \left(\partial_i F_{\rho_-} G_{m_i} - \partial_i G_{\rho_-} F_{m_i} \right) \\
&+ \int \mathrm{d}\mathbf{r}\, m_i \left(\partial_j F_{m_i} G_{m_j} - \partial_j G_{m_i} F_{m_j} \right) \\
&+ \int \mathrm{d}\mathbf{r}\, s \left(\partial_i F_s G_{m_i} - \partial_i G_s F_{m_i} \right),
\end{aligned} \tag{70}$$

cf. bracket (A3).

This system is additionally required to satisfy the Gauß laws for electric and magnetic charge, respectively. We have

$$\partial_i D_i = q e_0 \left(\frac{\rho_+}{m_+} - \frac{\rho_-}{m_-} \right) \qquad \text{and} \qquad \partial_i B_i = 0 \,, \tag{71}$$

where the right-hand side of Equation (71)$_{\text{left}}$ is the free charge density.

Total density $\rho = \rho_+ + \rho_-$ and the free charge density can be used for the description instead of ρ_+ and ρ_-. Such transformation allows for the projection to the state variables without free charge density (i.e., where free charge density is relaxed) by letting the functionals depend only on $(\rho, \mathbf{m}, s, \mathbf{D}, \mathbf{B})$. Consequently, bracket (69) transforms into

$$\begin{aligned} \{F,G\}^{(\text{EMHD})}(\rho,\mathbf{m},s,\mathbf{D},\mathbf{B}) &= \{F,G\}^{(\text{FM})}(\rho,\mathbf{m},s) + \{F,G\}^{(\text{EM})}(\mathbf{D},\mathbf{B}) \\ &\quad + \{F,G\}^{(\text{SP})}(\mathbf{D},\mathbf{m}) + \{F,G\}^{(\text{SP})}(\mathbf{B},\mathbf{m}) \,, \end{aligned} \tag{72}$$

and it is equipped with the updated constraint on the displacement field (given by the relaxed value of free charge density, typically zero) and magnetic field. Bracket (72) describes reversible evolution of electroneutral continuum coupled with the Maxwell equations.

Although the continuum described by bracket (72) is electroneutral, it can conduct electric current. This can be seen as a dissipation of the displacement field as suggested in [35]. Let us define dissipation potential

$$\Xi(\mathbf{D}^*) = \int \mathrm{d}\mathbf{r} \frac{\sigma}{2} (\mathbf{D}^*)^2 = \int \mathrm{d}\mathbf{r} \frac{\sigma}{2} \left(\frac{\mathbf{D}^\dagger}{s^\dagger} \right)^2 \,. \tag{73}$$

The reversible evolution generated by (72) and the irreversible evolution due to (73) give together

$$\frac{\partial \rho}{\partial t} = -\partial_k (\rho m_k^\dagger), \tag{74a}$$

$$\begin{aligned} \frac{\partial m_i}{\partial t} &= -\partial_j (m_i m_j^\dagger) - \rho \partial_i \rho^\dagger - m_j \partial_i m_j^\dagger - s \partial_i s^\dagger - D_j \partial_i D_j^\dagger - B_j \partial_i B_j^\dagger \\ &\quad + \partial_j (D_j D_i^\dagger + B_j B_i^\dagger), \end{aligned} \tag{74b}$$

$$\frac{\partial s}{\partial t} = -\partial_k \left(s m_k^\dagger \right) + \frac{\sigma}{(s^\dagger)^2} (\mathbf{D}^\dagger)^2, \tag{74c}$$

$$\frac{\partial D_i}{\partial t} = \varepsilon_{ijk} \partial_j B_k^\dagger - \partial_j \left(D_i m_j^\dagger - m_i^\dagger D_j \right) - m_i^\dagger \partial_j D_j - \frac{\sigma}{s^\dagger} D_i^\dagger, \tag{74d}$$

$$\frac{\partial B_i}{\partial t} = -\varepsilon_{ijk} \partial_j D_k^\dagger - \partial_j \left(B_i m_j^\dagger - m_i^\dagger B_j \right) - m_i^\dagger \partial_j B_j. \tag{74e}$$

The conjugate displacement field $\mathbf{D}^\dagger$ is interpreted as electric intensity $\mathbf{E}$, and the irreversible (last) term in Equation (74d) then tells that the electric current is $\mathbf{J} = \frac{\sigma}{s^\dagger} \mathbf{E}$. Dissipation in the $\mathbf{D}$ field can be thus seen as Ohm's law (Alternatively, Ohm's law can be derived from the relaxation of matter in the presence of the electric field, see [14].).

4.4.2. DynMaxEnt to the Displacement Field—Passage to MHD

Let us apply the DynMaxEnt reduction to the displacement field in Equations (73) so that we approach the magnetohydrodynamics (MHD). The reversible part of the MHD equations can be obtained easily by projection to variables $(\rho, \mathbf{m}, s, \mathbf{B})$ as in [14], but we wish to also obtain the irreversible part of the equations.

Assuming energy quadratic in $\mathbf{D}$, the MaxEnt value is $\tilde{\mathbf{D}} = 0$, which erases all terms containing the displacement field (but not $\mathbf{D}^\dagger$) from the equations. Except for the evolution of entropy, $\mathbf{D}^\dagger$ only remains in Equation (74d), which can be solved and gives

$$\tilde{D_i}^\dagger = \frac{s^\dagger}{\sigma}\varepsilon_{ijk}\partial_j B_k^\dagger\,. \tag{75}$$

Introducing the *curl* of Equation (75) into Equation (74d) yields a dissipative evolution equation for the magnetic field. The complete set of equations after this reduction reads

$$\frac{\partial \rho}{\partial t} = -\partial_k(\rho m_k^\dagger), \tag{76a}$$

$$\frac{\partial m_i}{\partial t} = -\partial_j(m_i m_j^\dagger) - \rho\partial_i\rho^\dagger - m_j\partial_i m_j^\dagger - s\partial_i s^\dagger - B_j\partial_i B_j^\dagger + \partial_j(B_j B_i^\dagger), \tag{76b}$$

$$\frac{\partial s}{\partial t} = -\partial_k\left(s m_k^\dagger\right) + \frac{1}{\sigma}(\nabla\times\mathbf{B}^\dagger)^2, \tag{76c}$$

$$\frac{\partial B_i}{\partial t} = -\partial_j\left(B_i m_j^\dagger - m_i^\dagger B_j\right) - m_i^\dagger\partial_j B_j - \varepsilon_{ijk}\partial_j\left(\frac{s^\dagger}{\sigma}\varepsilon_{klm}\partial_l B_m^\dagger\right), \tag{76d}$$

which is compatible with [36]. The first terms on the right-hand side of Equation (76d) can be further simplified for constant $\sigma/s^\dagger$, provided that the contribution of the magnetic field to the energy is $\frac{\mathbf{B}^2}{\mu_0}$. We can then write

$$\frac{\partial \mathbf{B}}{\partial t} = \frac{s^\dagger}{\mu_0\sigma}\Delta\mathbf{B} - \nabla\times\left(\mathbf{B}\times\mathbf{m}^\dagger\right)\,, \tag{77}$$

where $\partial_i B_i = 0$ was finally used. Keeping in mind that $\mathbf{m}^\dagger = \mathbf{v}$, Equation (77) is the advection–diffusion equation for the magnetic field, *cf.* ([37] Equation 2.15) or [38]. The coefficient $\frac{s^\dagger}{\mu_0\sigma}$ is referred to as the magnetic diffusivity.

In summary, after the relaxation of free charge density, one gets the electroneutral continuum coupled with Maxwell equations. Further dissipation in the displacement field then leads by the DynMaxEnt reduction to the MHD equations including magnetic diffusivity.

5. Contact Geometry

Contact geometry seems to be the so far most general geometric formulation of non-equilibrium thermodynamics. It started with works of Hermann [11] in equilibrium thermodynamics and continued to non-equilibrium thermodynamics, e.g., [12,15,39–41] and many others. Here, we adopt a recent version of contact-geometric formulation of GENERIC from [14].

6. Contact GENERIC

We begin by introducing a space

$$\mathbb{M}^{(cont)} = \mathbf{M}\times\mathbf{M}^*\times\mathbf{N}_{eq}^*\times\mathbf{N}_{eq}\times\mathbb{R} \tag{78}$$

with coordinates (x, x^*, y^*, y, ϕ). The space $\mathbf{M}$ with elements x is the state space, the space $\mathbf{M}^*$ with elements x^* is its dual. Similarly, $\mathbf{N}_{eq}$ with elements y is the state space on the equilibrium level, $\mathbf{N}_{eq}^*$ with elements y^* is its dual. We recall that $y = (E, N)$ and $y^* = (E^*, N^*)$, where $E^* = \frac{1}{T}$ and $N^* = -\frac{\mu}{T}$. We moreover introduce the fundamental thermodynamic relation $S = S(x), y = y(x)$ represented in $\mathbf{M}\times\mathbf{N}_{eq}\times\mathbb{R}$ by the **Gibbs manifold** $\mathcal{M}^{(G)}$ that is the image of the mapping

$$x \hookrightarrow (x, y(x), S(x)). \tag{79}$$

Corresponding to the fundamental thermodynamic relation is the thermodynamic potential $\Phi(x,y^*) = -S(x) + \langle y^*, y(x)\rangle$, where $\langle,\rangle$ denotes the inner product.

The Gibbs manifold $\mathcal{M}^{(G)}$ can be now extended to the **Gibbs–Legendre manifold** $\mathcal{M}^{(GL)}$ (in the shorthand notation *GL manifold*) that is the image of the mapping

$$(x,y^*) \hookrightarrow (x, \Phi_x(x,y^*), y^*, \Phi_{y^*}(x,y^*), \Phi(x,y^*)) \tag{80}$$

in $\mathbb{M}^{(cont)}$.

The thermodynamics in $\mathbf{M}$ is completely expressed in the GL manifold $\mathcal{M}^{(GL)}$. Note that $[\mathcal{M}^{(GL)}]_{y^*=0}$ (i.e., the image of the mapping

$$(x,0) \hookrightarrow (x, -S_x(x), 0, y(x), -S(x)) \tag{81}$$

in the space $\mathbf{M}\times\mathbf{M}^*\times\mathbf{N}_{eq}\times\mathbb{R}$) is an extension of the Gibbs manifold $\mathcal{M}^{(G)}$ by including the conjugate variable x^*. Moreover, the manifold $[\mathcal{M}^{(GL)}]_{x^*=S_x=0}$ displays the states $x_{eq}(y^*)$ that represent in $\mathbf{M}$ the equilibrium states and also the fundamental thermodynamic relation $S^*(y^*), y(y^*)$ in $\mathbf{N}_{eq}$ implied by the fundamental thermodynamic relation $S(x), y(x)$ in $\mathbf{M}$. Indeed, $[\mathcal{M}^{(GL)}]_{x^*=0}$ is the image of the mapping

$$(x,y^*) \hookrightarrow (x_{eq}(y^*), 0, y^*, y(x_{eq}(y^*)), S^*(y^*)). \tag{82}$$

Let us turn to the time evolution in $\mathbb{M}^{(cont)}$. We begin by introducing in $\mathbb{M}^{(cont)}$ a bracket

$$\begin{aligned}
\{A,B\}^{(cont)} &= (\langle A_x, B_{x^*}\rangle - \langle B_x, A_{x^*}\rangle) \\
&\quad -(\langle A_y, B_{y^*}\rangle - \langle B_y, A_{y^*}\rangle) \\
&\quad -(\langle x^*, A_{x^*}\rangle B_\phi - \langle x^*, B_{x^*}\rangle A_\phi) \\
&\quad +(AB_\phi - BA_\phi) \\
&\quad +(\langle A_y, y\rangle B_\phi - \langle B_y, y\rangle A_\phi),
\end{aligned} \tag{83}$$

where A and B are sufficiently regular functions $\mathbb{M}^{(cont)} \to \mathbb{R}$. This bracket consists of two contact brackets (95) of paper [41]. With such bracket, we introduce the time evolution in $\mathbb{M}^{(cont)}$ by an equation

$$\dot{A} = \{A, H^{(cont)}\}^{(cont)} - AH^{(cont)}_\phi \tag{84}$$

that is required to hold for all A. The function $H^{(cont)} : \mathbb{M}^{(cont)} \to \mathbb{R}$, called a contact Hamiltonian, will be specified below. The last term on the right-hand side corresponds to the non-conservation of the phase-space volume [40]. Written explicitly, the time evolution equations (84) take the form

$$\dot{x} = H^{(cont)}_{x^*}, \tag{85a}$$
$$\dot{x^*} = -H^{(cont)}_x - x^* H^{(cont)}_\phi, \tag{85b}$$
$$\dot{y^*} = H^{(cont)}_y, \tag{85c}$$
$$\dot{y} = -H^{(cont)}_{y^*} + yH^{(cont)}_\phi, \tag{85d}$$
$$\dot{\phi} = -H^{(cont)} + \langle x^*, H^{(cont)}_{x^*}\rangle - \langle H^{(cont)}_y, y\rangle. \tag{85e}$$

These are the evolution equations in $\mathbb{M}$.

Next, we specify the contact Hamiltonian $H^{(cont)}$

$$H^{(cont)}(x, x^*, y^*, y, \phi) = -S^{(cont)}(x, x^*, y^*) + \frac{1}{E^*}E^{(cont)}(x, x^*, y^*), \tag{86}$$

where

$$\begin{aligned} S^{(cont)}(x, x^*, y^*) &= \Xi(x, x^*, y^*) - [\Xi(x, x^*, y^*)]_{x^*=\Phi_x}, \\ E^{(cont)}(x, x^*, y^*) &= \langle x^*, L\Phi_x \rangle. \end{aligned} \tag{87}$$

Ξ is the dissipation potential entering GENERIC and L is the Poisson bivector also entering GENERIC. Both Ξ and L are degenerate in the sense

$$\begin{aligned} &\langle x^*, LS_x \rangle = \langle x^*, LN_x \rangle = 0, \quad \forall x^*, \\ &\langle E_x, \Xi_{x^*} \rangle = \langle N_x, \Xi_{x^*} \rangle = 0, \quad \forall x^*, \\ &\langle x^*, [\Xi_{x^*}]_{x^*=E_x} \rangle = \langle x^*, [\Xi_{x^*}]_{x^*=M_x} \rangle = 0, \quad \forall x^*. \end{aligned} \tag{88}$$

We note in particular that the contact Hamiltonian (86) is independent of y and ϕ.
With (86), the time evolution Equations (85a) become

$$\dot{x} = \frac{1}{E^*} L\Phi_x - \Xi_{x^*}, \tag{89a}$$

$$\begin{aligned} \dot{x^*} &= \Phi_{xx}\left(\frac{1}{E^*} Lx^* - [\Xi_{x^*}]_{x^*=\Phi_x}\right) \\ &\quad - \frac{1}{E^*}\langle x^*, L_x\Phi_x \rangle + \Xi_x - [\Xi_x]_{x^*=\Phi_x}, \end{aligned} \tag{89b}$$

$$\dot{\phi} = -\langle x^*, \Xi_{x^*} + \Xi - [\Xi]_{x^*=\Phi_x}, \tag{89c}$$

$$\dot{y^*} = 0, \tag{89d}$$

$$\dot{y} = \Xi_{y^*} - \Xi_{y^*}|_{x^*=\Phi_x}. \tag{89e}$$

If we now evaluate (89a) on the GL manifold $\mathcal{M}^{(GL)}$ (note that $[H^{(cont)}]_{\mathcal{M}^{(GL)}} = 0$), we arrive at

$$\dot{x} = \frac{1}{E^*} L\Phi_x - \Xi_{x^*}|_{(x^*=\Phi_x, y=\Phi_{y^*})}, \tag{90a}$$

$$\dot{x^*} = \Phi_{xx}\left(\frac{1}{E^*} L\Phi_x - [\Xi_{x^*}]_{(x^*=\Phi_x, y=\Phi_{y^*})}\right), \tag{90b}$$

$$\dot{\phi} = -\langle x^*, \Xi_{x^*} \rangle|_{(x^*=\Phi_x, y=\Phi_{y^*})}, \tag{90c}$$

$$\dot{y^*} = 0, \tag{90d}$$

$$\dot{y} = 0, \tag{90e}$$

which are the GENERIC evolution equations. See [14] for more details.

6.1. Relation to DynMaxEnt

Consider state variables $\mathbf{x} = (\mathbf{r}, \mathbf{p})$ as in the Section 3.3 on the damped particle (disregarding entropy for simplicity). The Poisson bivector is then canonical, $\mathbf{L} = \begin{pmatrix} 0 & 1 \\ -1 & 0 \end{pmatrix}$, and the dissipation potential is quadratic in conjugate momentum, $\Xi = \frac{1}{2\tau}(\mathbf{p}^*)^2$. This conjugate momentum, according to Equation (89b), approaches the value where GENERIC evolution equations hold, Equation (11), and eventually reaches the value given by the derivative of thermodynamic potential.

Now, assume that state variable $\mathbf{p}$ evolves faster to the corresponding equilibrium (zero) than both $\mathbf{r}$ and conjugate variables. The GENERIC evolution equations then become Equations (11a) and (15). The conjugate variable $\mathbf{p}^*$ approaches the value where the GENERIC equations are valid, which means that it approaches solutions to Equation (15) as in the DynMaxEnt procedure. Conjugate variables approach the Gibbs–Legendre manifold (80). Contact geometry provides motivation and geometric meaning to the Dynamic MaxEnt reduction.

7. Conclusions

In this paper, we have presented a method for reduction of detailed dynamics to less detailed dynamics called Dynamic MaxEnt. The key feature of the method is that conjugate variables are promoted to independent variables and as such they can relax to a quasi-equilibrium in a different way than state variables. While relaxation of the state variables generates the entropy on the lower level of description, relaxation of conjugate variables ensures that the vector field on the higher level becomes tangent to the quasi-equilibrium manifold.

First, in Section 2, the usual MaxEnt is recalled, which gives state variables on the higher (detailed) level as functions of state variables on the lower (less detailed) level. The DynMaxEnt method is then presented in Section 3 including the infinite chain of higher order DynMaxEnt corrections, and it is compared to asymptotic expansions in Section 3.3.3. Then, the method is used on the reduction of dynamics of complex fluids equipped with conformation tensor and Reynolds stress to the Navier–Stokes equations, reduction of hyperbolic heat conduction to the Fourier law, where we again compare the result to the formal asymptotic methods, and reduction of electromagnetohydrodynamics to magnetohydrodynamics. Finally, motivation for the DynMaxEnt method by contact geometry is shown in Section 5.

In summary, this paper contains a relatively straightforward method for reduction from dynamics on a detailed level of description to dynamics on a less detailed level of description.

Author Contributions: M.G. stands behind the main ideas for DynMaxEnt, V.K. and M.P. formulated the energetic DynMaxEnt and wrote most of the text. P.V. formulated the application of DynMaxEnt on electromagnetic field.

Funding: This work was supported by the Czech Science Foundation, project No. 17-15498Y, and by Charles University Research program No. UNCE/SCI/023. This research has been supported partially by the Natural Sciences and Engineering Research Council of Canada, Grants 3100319 and 3100735.

Acknowledgments: We are grateful to Petr Pelech and Ilya Peshkov for discussing the DynMaxEnt method.

Conflicts of Interest: The authors declare no conflict of interest.

Abbreviations

The following abbreviations are used in this manuscript:

MaxEnt	Maximum Entropy Principle
DynMaxEnt	Dynamic Maximum Entropy Principle
GENERIC	General Equation for Non-Equilibrium Reversible-Irreversible Coupling
FM	Fluid Mechanics
MHD	Magnetohydrodynamics
CIT	Classical Irreversible Thermodynamics

Appendix A.

Appendix A.1. Correction of Upper Entropy ${}^{\uparrow}S$

Appendix A.1.1. General Case

Let us now discuss the possibility to correct the higher level entropy instead of the infinite chain presented above. As a sequence of correction will be produced, we introduce a more detailed notation. Static MaxEnt starts with ${}^{\uparrow}S(\mathbf{x})$, which we shall now denote as ${}^{\uparrow}S_0$. Static MaxEnt provides ${}^{\downarrow}S_0(\mathbf{y})$ and $\tilde{\mathbf{x}}_0^{ME}(\mathbf{y})$ and the reduction of the upper evolution equations to the lower MaxEnt manifold yields $\tilde{\mathbf{x}}_0^*(\mathbf{y})$ (where we rewrote the lower conjugate variables in terms of direct ones $\mathbf{y}^* = \partial_{\mathbf{y}}{}^{\downarrow}S(\mathbf{y})$).

As generally $\tilde{\mathbf{x}}_0^{ME}(\mathbf{y})$ and $\tilde{\mathbf{x}}_0^*(\mathbf{y})$ are independent and hence likely are not conjugate to each other via ${}^{\uparrow}S$ evaluated at the lower MaxEnt manifold, we correct the upper entropy so that they are conjugate variables. Let us denote the conjugate counterpart to $\tilde{\mathbf{x}}_0^*(\mathbf{y})$ via ${}^{\uparrow}S_0^*$ as $\tilde{\mathbf{x}}_0^{evo}(\mathbf{y}) \neq \tilde{\mathbf{x}}_0^{ME}(\mathbf{y})$. Hence, we find ${}^{\uparrow}S_1^*$ (or equivalently ${}^{\uparrow}S_1$ via Legendre transformation) such that

$$\partial_{\mathbf{x}^*} {}^{\uparrow}S_1^*|_{\mathbf{x}^*=\tilde{\mathbf{x}}_0^*(\mathbf{y})} = \tilde{\mathbf{x}}_0^{ME}(\mathbf{y}),$$

which may be rewritten as

$$\partial_{\mathbf{x}^*} \left({}^{\uparrow}S_1^* - {}^{\uparrow}S_0^* \right) \Big|_{\mathbf{x}^*=\tilde{\mathbf{x}}_0^*(\mathbf{y})} = \tilde{\mathbf{x}}_0^{ME}(\mathbf{y}) - \tilde{\mathbf{x}}_0^{evo}(\mathbf{y}). \tag{A1}$$

It might be difficult in practice to find such a correction to the upper entropy in general. However, we provide a worked out example below.

The change in the upper entropy ${}^{\uparrow}S_1$ entails a change in static MaxEnt value and in everything that follows: $\tilde{\mathbf{x}}_1^{ME}(\mathbf{y})$, $\tilde{\mathbf{x}}_0^*(\mathbf{y})$, ${}^{\downarrow}S_1(\mathbf{y}) = {}^{\uparrow}S_1(\tilde{\mathbf{x}}_1^{ME}(\mathbf{y}))$, $\tilde{\mathbf{x}}_1^{evo}(\mathbf{y})$. Hence, a sequence of correction is produced and if they are "small" they may provide a converging sequence.

Appendix A.1.2. The Correction of the Upper Energy for the Damped Particle

Let us illustrate the outlined difficulty of the correction of the upper energy on the simple example of a damped particle. This method corrects upper energy so that the direct and conjugate variables are indeed conjugate. The natural choice

$${}^{\uparrow}E_0 = \frac{(\mathbf{p} + \mathbf{p}_0^{evo})^2}{2m} + V(\mathbf{r}) + \varepsilon(s) = \frac{(\mathbf{p} - m\frac{\tau}{\zeta}V_{\mathbf{r}}(\mathbf{r}))^2}{2m} + V(\mathbf{r}) + \varepsilon(s) \tag{A2}$$

entails

$$\mathbf{p}^{\dagger} = \partial_{\mathbf{p}} {}^{\uparrow}E_0 = \frac{1}{m}(\mathbf{p} + \mathbf{p}_0^{evo})$$

and hence indeed the conjugate value to $\mathbf{p} = 0$ is $\mathbf{p}^{\dagger} = \frac{1}{m}\mathbf{p}_0^{evo}$. Similarly,

$$\mathbf{r}^{\dagger} = \partial_{\mathbf{r}} {}^{\uparrow}E_1 = \frac{1}{m}(\mathbf{p} - m\frac{\tau}{\zeta}V_{\mathbf{r}})(-m\frac{\tau}{\zeta}V_{\mathbf{rr}}) + V_{\mathbf{r}}.$$

Static MaxEnt of ${}^{\uparrow}E_1$ gives (minimum energy for given $\mathbf{r}, s$)

$$\mathbf{p}_1^{ME} = m\frac{\tau}{\zeta}V_{\mathbf{r}}$$

with a conjugate value $\mathbf{p}^{\dagger} = 0$ and also $\mathbf{r}^{\dagger} = V_{\mathbf{r}}$. Note that lower energy is the same as in the previous step ${}^{\uparrow}E_1|_{\mathbf{p}_1^{ME}} = {}^{\uparrow}E_0|_{\mathbf{p}_0^{ME}}$. Finally, the evolution equation yields dependent relations

$$\partial_t \mathbf{p}_1^{ME} = m\frac{\tau}{\zeta}V_{\mathbf{rr}}\partial_t \mathbf{r} = m\frac{\tau}{\zeta}V_{\mathbf{rr}}\mathbf{p}_1^{\dagger} = -\mathbf{r}^{\dagger} - \frac{\zeta}{\tau}\mathbf{p}_1^{\dagger},$$

requiring that

$$\mathbf{p}_1^{\dagger} = -\frac{\tau}{\zeta}\mathbf{r}^{\dagger}\frac{1}{1 + m\frac{\tau^2}{\zeta^2}V_{\mathbf{rr}}} \approx \mathbf{p}_0^{\dagger} - m\frac{\tau^2}{\zeta^2}V_{\mathbf{rr}}\mathbf{p}_0^{\dagger}.$$

Note that this correction method seems to be working well, cf. (25). Namely, both correction methods of dynamic MaxEnt yield an asymptotic type series solution for small τ and, although it does not match the formal asymptotic expansion solution, some similarities can be seen.

However, a second inspection of the proposed upper energy (A2) reveals that energy is no longer an even function with respect to time reversal. One can show that, under the assumption of energy being an analytic function of state variables, the requirement that the conjugate value to $\mathbf{p}^{ME}$ is non-zero requires a presence of a linear term of $\mathbf{p}$ in the corrected energy ${}^{\uparrow}E_1$. In turn, energy cannot be even with respect to time reversal when $\mathbf{p}$ is odd. Additionally, note that a natural term appearing in the correction is of the form $(\mathbf{p} - \mathbf{p}_0^{ME} + \mathbf{p}_0^{evo})^2$, thus again failing to satisfy the requirement of being even with respect to time reversal once there is a change of parity during the transition (as it is here: the odd parity variable $\mathbf{p}$ evolves in such a way that it is enslaved to $\mathbf{r}^\dagger$ on the lower level, which is a variable with even parity).

Appendix B. Fluid Mechanics

The reversible part of fluid mechanics, where the state variables are density, momentum density and entropy density (per volume), $(\rho, \mathbf{m}, s)$, is generated by the Poisson bracket of classical hydrodynamics (see, e.g., [42,43]),

$$\begin{aligned} \{A, B\} = & \int \mathbf{dr}\, \rho \left(\partial_i A_\rho B_{m_i} - \partial_i B_\rho A_{m_i}\right) \\ & + \int \mathbf{dr}\, m_i \left(\partial_j A_{m_i} B_{m_j} - \partial_j B_{m_i} A_{m_j}\right) \\ & + \int \mathbf{dr}\, s \left(\partial_i A_s B_{m_i} - \partial_i B_s A_{m_i}\right). \end{aligned} \tag{A3}$$

Supplied with energy, e.g.,

$$E = \int \mathbf{dr}\, \frac{\mathbf{m}^2}{2\rho} + \varepsilon(\rho, s), \tag{A4}$$

the reversible evolution of an arbitrary functional of the hydrodynamic variables $A(\rho, \mathbf{m}, s)$ is

$$\dot{A} = \{A, E\}. \tag{A5}$$

By rewriting the time-derivative of the functional as

$$\dot{A} = \int \mathbf{dr}\, A_\rho \partial_t \rho + A_{m_i} \partial_t m_i + A_s \partial_t s, \tag{A6}$$

and comparing with Equation (A5), one can read the reversible part of evolution equations for the hydrodynamic fields,

$$\partial_t \rho = -\partial_i (\rho E_{m_i}) = -\partial_i m_i, \tag{A7a}$$

$$\partial_t m_i = -\partial_j \left(m_i E_{m_j}\right) - \rho \partial_i E_\rho - m_j \partial_i E_{m_j} - s \partial_i E_s = -\partial_j \left(\frac{m_i m_j}{\rho}\right) - \partial_i p, \tag{A7b}$$

$$\partial_t s = -\partial_i (s E_{m_i}) = -\partial_i \left(\frac{s m_i}{\rho}\right), \tag{A7c}$$

where $p = -\varepsilon(\rho, s) + \rho \varepsilon_\rho + s \varepsilon_s$ is the pressure. The reversible evolution of hydrodynamic fields with energy (A4) is of course the Euler equations.

References

1. De Groot, S.R.; Mazur, P. *Non-Equilibrium Thermodynamics*; Dover Publications: New York, NY, USA, 1984.
2. Struchtrup, H. *Macroscopic Transport Equations for Rarefied Gas Flows*; Springer: Berlin, Germany, 2005.
3. Zwanzig, R. *Nonequilibrium Statistical Mechanics*; Oxford University Press: New York, NY, USA, 2001.
4. Öttinger, H. *Beyond Equilibrium Thermodynamics*; Wiley: New York, NY, USA, 2005.
5. Gorban, A.N.; Karlin, I.V.; Öttinger, H.C.; Tatarinova, L.L. Ehrenfest's argument extended to a formalism of nonequilibrium thermodynamics. *Phys. Rev. E* **2001**, *63*, 066124. [CrossRef] [PubMed]
6. Karlin, I.V.; Tatarinova, L.L.; Gorban, A.N.; Öttinger, H.C. Irreversibility in the short memory approximation. *Phys. A Stat. Mech. Appl.* **2003**, *327*, 399–424. [CrossRef]
7. Gorban, A.; Karlin, I. *Invariant Manifolds for Physical and Chemical Kinetics*; Lecture Notes in Physics; Springer: Berlin, Germany, 2005.
8. Pavelka, M.; Klika, V.; Grmela, M. Thermodynamic explanation of Landau damping by reduction to hydrodynamics. *Entropy* **2018**, *20*, 457. [CrossRef]

9. Jaynes, E.T. *Delaware Seminar in the Foundation of Physics*; Bunge, M., Ed.; Springer: New York, NY, USA, 1967; chapter Foundations of probability theory and statistical mechanics.
10. Cimmelli, V.; Jou, D.; Ruggeri, T.; Ván, P. Entropy principle and recent results in non-equilibrium theories. *Entropy* **2014**, *16*, 1756–1807. [CrossRef]
11. Hermann, R. *Geometry, Physics and Systems*; Marcel Dekker: New York, NY, USA, 1984.
12. Grmela, M. Contact Geometry of Mesoscopic Thermodynamics and Dynamics. *Entropy* **2014**, *16*, 1652–1686. doi:10.3390/e16031652. [CrossRef]
13. Grmela, M. Geometry of Multiscale Nonequilibrium Thermodynamics. *Entropy* **2015**, *17*, 5938–5964. [CrossRef]
14. Pavelka, M.; Klika, V.; Grmela, M. *Multiscale Thermo-Dynamics*; de Gruyter: Berlin, Germany, 2018.
15. Grmela, M. Role of thermodynamics in multiscale physics. *Comput. Math. Appl.* **2013**, *65*, 1457–1470. doi:10.1016/j.camwa.2012.11.019. [CrossRef]
16. Grmela, M.; Klika, V.; Pavelka, M. Reductions and extensions in mesoscopic dynamics. *Phys. Rev. E* **2015**, *92*. [CrossRef]
17. Beris, A.; Edwards, B. *Thermodynamics of Flowing Systems*; Oxford University Press: Oxford, UK, 1994.
18. Dzyaloshinskii, I.E.; Volovick, G.E. Poisson brackets in condense matter physics. *Ann. Phys.* **1980**, *125*, 67–97. [CrossRef]
19. Peshkov, I.; Pavelka, M.; Romenski, E.; Grmela, M. Continuum Mechanics and Thermodynamics in the Hamilton and the Godunov-type Formulations. *Contin. Mech. Thermodyn.* **2018**, *30*, 1343–1378. [CrossRef]
20. Jizba, P.; Korbel, J. Maximum Entropy Principle in Statistical Inference: Case for Non-Shannonian Entropies. *Phys. Rev. Lett.* **2019**, *122*, 120601. doi:10.1103/PhysRevLett.122.120601. [CrossRef] [PubMed]
21. Grmela, M.; Pavelka, M.; Klika, V.; Cao, B.Y.; Bendian, N. Entropy and Entropy Production in Multiscale Dynamics. *J. Non-Equilibrium Thermodyn.* **2019**, *44*. [CrossRef]
22. Chapman, S.; Cowling, T.; Burnett, D.; Cercignani, C. *The Mathematical Theory of Non-uniform Gases: An Account of the Kinetic Theory of Viscosity, Thermal Conduction and Diffusion in Gases*; Cambridge Mathematical Library; Cambridge University Press: Cambridge, UK, 1990.
23. Grmela, M.; Öttinger, H.C. Dynamics and thermodynamics of complex fluids. I. Development of a general formalism. *Phys. Rev. E* **1997**, *56*, 6620–6632. doi:10.1103/PhysRevE.56.6620. [CrossRef]
24. Öttinger, H.C.; Grmela, M. Dynamics and thermodynamics of complex fluids. II. Illustrations of a general formalism. *Phys. Rev. E* **1997**, *56*, 6633–6655. doi:10.1103/PhysRevE.56.6633. [CrossRef]
25. Beretta, G.P. Steepest entropy ascent model for far-nonequilibrium thermodynamics: Unified implementation of the maximum entropy production principle. *Phys. Rev. E* **2014**, *90*, 042113. doi:10.1103/PhysRevE.90.042113. [CrossRef] [PubMed]
26. Montefusco, A.; Consonni, F.; Beretta, G.P. Essential equivalence of the general equation for the nonequilibrium reversible-irreversible coupling (GENERIC) and steepest-entropy-ascent models of dissipation for nonequilibrium thermodynamics. *Phys. Rev. E* **2015**, *91*, 042138. doi:10.1103/PhysRevE.91.042138. [CrossRef] [PubMed]
27. Callen, H. *Thermodynamics: An Introduction to the Physical Theories of Equilibrium Thermostatics and Irreversible Thermodynamics*; Wiley: New York, NY, USA, 1960.
28. Pavelka, M.; Klika, V.; Grmela, M. Time reversal in nonequilibrium thermodynamics. *Phys. Rev. E* **2014**, *90*, 062131. [CrossRef] [PubMed]
29. Bird, R.B.; Hassager, O.; Armstrong, R.C.; Curtiss, C.F. *Dynamics of Polymeric Fluids*; Wiley: New York, NY, USA, 1987; Volume 2,.
30. Pavelka, M.; Klika, V.; Esen, O.; Grmela, M. A hierarchy of Poisson brackets in non-equilibrium thermodynamics. *Phys. D Nonlinear Phenom.* **2016**, *335*, 54–69. [CrossRef]
31. Müller, I.; Ruggeri, T. *Rational Extended Thermodynamics*; Springer Tracts in Natural Philosophy; Springer: Berlin, Germany, 1998.
32. Grmela, M.; Lebon, G.; Dubois, C. Multiscale thermodynamics and mechanics of heat. *Phys. Rev. E* **2011**, *83*. [CrossRef]
33. Dumbser, M.; Peshkov, I.; Romenski, E.; Zanotti, O. High order ADER schemes for a unified first order hyperbolic formulation of continuum mechanics: Viscous heat-conducting fluids and elastic solids. *J. Comput. Phys.* **2016**, *314*, 824–862. [CrossRef]

34. Jou, D.; Casas-Vázquez, J.; Lebon, G. *Extended Irreversible Thermodynamics*, 4th ed.; Springer: New York, NY, USA, 2010.
35. Dumbser, M.; Peshkov, I.; Romenski, E.; Zanotti, O. High order ADER schemes for a unified first order hyperbolic formulation of Newtonian continuum mechanics coupled with electro-dynamics. *J. Comput. Phys.* **2017**, *348*, 298–342. doi:10.1016/j.jcp.2017.07.020. [CrossRef]
36. Godunov, S. Symmetric form of the magnetohydrodynamic equation. *Chislennye Metody Mekh. Sploshnoi Sredy* **1972**, *3*, 26–34.
37. Biskamp, D. *Magnetohydrodynamic Turbulence*; Cambridge University Press: Cambridge, UK, 2003.
38. Landau, L.; Bell, J.; Kearsley, J.; Pitaevskii, L.; Lifshitz, E.; Sykes, J. *Electrodynamics of Continuous Media*; Course of Theoretical Physics; Elsevier Science: Oxford, United Kingdom, 1984.
39. Favache, A.; Dochain, D.; Maschke, B. An entropy-based formulation of irreversible processes based on contact structures. *Chem. Eng. Sci.* **2010**, *65*, 5204–5216. [CrossRef]
40. Bravetti, A.; Cruz, H.; Tapias, D. Contact Hamiltonian Mechanics. *Ann. Phys.* **2017**, *376*, 17–39. [CrossRef]
41. Esen, O.; Gümral, H. Geometry of Plasma Dynamics II: Lie Algebra of Hamiltonian Vector Fields. *J. Geom. Mech.* **2012**, *4*, 239–269. [CrossRef]
42. Arnold, V. Sur la géometrie différentielle des groupes de Lie de dimension infini et ses applications dans l'hydrodynamique des fluides parfaits. *Annales de l'institut Fourier* **1966**, *16*, 319–361. [CrossRef]
43. Grmela, M. Particle and Bracket Formulations of Kinetic Equations. *Contemp. Math.* **1984**, *28*, 125–132.

entropy

MDPI

Article

A Fourth Order Entropy Stable Scheme for Hyperbolic Conservation Laws

Xiaohan Cheng

School of Science, Chang'an University, Xi'an 710064, China; xhcheng@chd.edu.cn

Received: 7 April 2019; Accepted: 17 May 2019; Published: 19 May 2019

Abstract: This paper develops a fourth order entropy stable scheme to approximate the entropy solution of one-dimensional hyperbolic conservation laws. The scheme is constructed by employing a high order entropy conservative flux of order four in conjunction with a suitable numerical diffusion operator that based on a fourth order non-oscillatory reconstruction which satisfies the sign property. The constructed scheme possesses two features: (1) it achieves fourth order accuracy in the smooth area while keeping high resolution with sharp discontinuity transitions in the nonsmooth area; (2) it is entropy stable. Some typical numerical experiments are performed to illustrate the capability of the new entropy stable scheme.

Keywords: conservation laws; entropy stable; entropy conservative; non-oscillatory reconstruction; sign property

1. Introduction

During the past few decades, abundant numerical methods for solving hyperbolic conservation laws have been designed; one can consult the review papers [1,2] and the references therein. Among the various methods, high order schemes, such as total variation diminishing (TVD) schemes, weighted essentially non-oscillatory (WENO) schemes and discontinuous Galerkin (DG) schemes, have achieved great success. However, it seems that there are few entropy stability results for high order numerical schemes for hyperbolic conservation laws, especially for the nonlinear hyperbolic conservation laws. In view of the above discussion, we limit our research on high order entropy stable methods for solving hyperbolic conservation laws.

In accordance with the idea of Tadmor, entropy schemes are often constructed by utilizing entropy conservative flux in conjunction with suitable numerical diffusion [3]. For example, physical viscosity was discretized and used as numerical diffusion in [4]. Roe-type numerical diffusion was selected for various systems like Euler equations, shallow water equations and ideal magnetohydrodynamic equations [5–7]. Based on the limiter mechanism, Liu et al. constructed a family of entropy consistent schemes with high resolution [8]. Recently, Dubey discussed the amount of suitable diffusion for the sake of devising non-oscillatory entropy stable schemes in the TVD sense [9]. To obtain high order entropy stable schemes, Fjordholm et al. firstly proved that ENO reconstruction satisfies a sign property and presented entropy stable schemes based on ENO reconstruction of arbitrary order accuracy [10,11]. To overcome the drawbacks of ENO reconstruction, we presented a third order reconstruction which is non-oscillatory and satisfies the sign property to construct a third order entropy stable scheme [12]. WENO reconstruction was modified to satisfy the sign property and also used to construct an entropy stable scheme in [13,14], although they are limited to third order accuracy.

In this paper, we are aiming at presenting a new entropy stable scheme of fourth order accuracy to solve hyperbolic conservation laws in one dimension. First, we employ a fourth order entropy conservative flux which is a linear combination of two-point entropy conservative fluxes. Then, we present a non-oscillatory reconstruction of fourth order accuracy which possesses the sign property to obtain a fourth order accurate numerical diffusion operator. By adding this numerical diffusion operator to the entropy conservative flux, the resulting flux is entropy stable.

The remainder of this paper is given as follows. Section 2 describes the procedure for building our fourth order entropy scheme. After that, we present some typical numerical experiments to show the effectiveness of the newly developed scheme. Finally, concluding remarks are given in Section 4.

2. Numerical Method

Consider the scalar conservation law

$$\frac{\partial}{\partial t}u + \frac{\partial}{\partial x}f(u) = 0. \tag{1}$$

The weak solutions for Equation (1) are not unique and we are interested in the so-called entropy solution, which satisfies the entropy condition

$$\frac{\partial}{\partial t}\eta(u) + \frac{\partial}{\partial x}q(u) \leq 0. \tag{2}$$

Here, the entropy function $\eta(u)$ is convex and the entropy flux function $q(u)$ satisfies $\frac{\partial q}{\partial u} = v\frac{\partial f}{\partial u}$ with the entropy variable $v = \frac{\partial \eta}{\partial u}$. To solve Equation (1) with the conservative difference method, we have the semi-discrete scheme

$$\frac{du_i}{dt} = -\frac{f_{i+1/2} - f_{i-1/2}}{\Delta x}, \tag{3}$$

where u_i represents the point valve at the node x_i on a uniform Cartesian mesh with the mesh size $x_{i+1} - x_i = \Delta x$. The scheme (3) is said to be entropy stable if it satisfies a discrete version of the entropy condition (2), namely,

$$\frac{\partial}{\partial t}\eta(u_i) + \frac{q_{i+1/2} - q_{i-1/2}}{\Delta x} \leq 0; \tag{4}$$

the scheme is said to be entropy conservative if it satisfies the discrete entropy equality

$$\frac{\partial}{\partial t}\eta(u_i) + \frac{q_{i+1/2} - q_{i-1/2}}{\Delta x} = 0. \tag{5}$$

In this work, we utilize the familiar Runge–Kutta scheme of order four to solve the ordinary Equation (3). Now, we focus on how to build the entropy stable numerical flux $f_{i+1/2}$.

First, the numerical flux is split into an entropy conservative part and a numerical diffusion part

$$f_{i+1/2} = f^{EC}_{i+1/2} - \frac{1}{2}\delta_{i+1/2}\left(v^+_{i+1/2} - v^-_{i+1/2}\right). \tag{6}$$

Here, $f^{EC}_{i+1/2}$ is a fourth order entropy conservative flux [15] expressed as

$$f^{EC}_{i+1/2} = \frac{4}{3}\tilde{f}\left(u_i, u_{i+1}\right) - \frac{1}{6}\left(\tilde{f}\left(u_{i-1}, u_{i+1}\right) - \tilde{f}\left(u_i, u_{i+2}\right)\right) \tag{7}$$

with $\tilde{f}(\alpha, \beta)$ being the second order entropy conservative flux defined by Tadmor [3]. Generally, $\delta_{i+1/2}$ in the numerical diffusion part is chosen to be $|f'(u_{i+1/2})|$. If the reconstructed values $v^{\pm}_{i+1/2}$ at the interfaces from the entropy variable v_i satisfy

$$sign(v^+_{i+1/2} - v^-_{i+1/2}) = sign(v_{i+1} - v_i), \tag{8}$$

the numerical flux (6) achieves entropy stability. Property (8) in which the jump of the reconstructed point values at each cell interface has the same sign as the jump of the underlying point values across that interface is called the sign property. We present the fourth order reconstruction satisfying the sign property as follows to obtain $v^{\pm}_{i+1/2}$.

Consider a polynomial reconstruction of the form

$$p_i(x) = v_i + d_i\left(\frac{x-x_i}{\Delta x}\right) + \left(\frac{v_{i-1}-2v_i+v_{i+1}}{2}\right)\left(\frac{x-x_i}{\Delta x}\right)^2 + \left(\frac{-v_{i-1}+v_{i+1}-2d_i}{2}\right)\left(\frac{x-x_i}{\Delta x}\right)^3 \quad (9)$$

with d_i being a slope function. For convenience, we introduce the following notation

$$\begin{aligned}
&ds_i = \frac{2}{3}v_{i+1} - \frac{2}{3}v_{i-1} - \frac{1}{12}v_{i+2} + \frac{1}{12}v_{i-2},\\
&WC_i = v_{i+1} - v_{i-1}, \quad WR_i = v_{i+1} - v_i, \quad WC2_i = v_{i+2} - v_{i-2},\\
&ds1_i = 0, \quad ds2_i = \frac{1}{2}\left(WC_i - 8WR_i\right), \quad ds3_i = \frac{1}{2}\left(8WR_i - 7WC_i\right),\\
&S_i = sign(WC_i),\\
&C_1 = \frac{\sqrt{3}}{6}, \quad C_2 = \frac{6}{12+\sqrt{3}},
\end{aligned} \quad (10)$$

and define the slope d_i in the following way:

1. If $S_i = 0$, then $d_i = 0$.
2. If $S_i \neq 0$ and $(2S_i \cdot WC_i \geq S_i \cdot WC2_i)$, then $d_i = ds_i$.
3. If $S_i \neq 0$ and $(2S_i \cdot WC_i < S_i \cdot WC2_i)$, then the following hold:

    (a) If $v_i = \frac{v_{i+1}+v_{i-1}}{2}$, we define

    $$d_i = \begin{cases} \max(ds1_i, ds_i), & \text{if} \quad S_i > 0,\\ \min(ds1_i, ds_i), & \text{if} \quad S_i < 0. \end{cases}$$

    (b) If $v_i \neq \frac{v_{i+1}+v_{i-1}}{2}$, then the following hold:

    i. If $\left|WR_i - \frac{1}{2}WC_i\right| \geq \frac{1}{8}\left|WC2_i - 2WC_i\right|$, then

    $$d_i = \begin{cases} \max(ds2_i, ds3, ds_i), & \text{if} \quad S_i > 0,\\ \min(ds2_i, ds3, ds_i), & \text{if} \quad S_i < 0. \end{cases}$$

    ii. If $\left|WR_i - \frac{1}{2}WC_i\right| < \frac{1}{8}\left|WC2_i - 2WC_i\right|$, then

    $$d_i = \begin{cases} \frac{WC_i}{2} - S_i \cdot C1 \cdot \left|2WR_i - WC_i\right|, & \text{if} \quad \left|\frac{WR_i}{WC_i} - \frac{1}{2}\right| \leq C2,\\ \frac{WC_i}{2}, & \text{if} \quad \left|\frac{WR_i}{WC_i} - \frac{1}{2}\right| > C2. \end{cases}$$

Theorem 1. *With this definition of the slope, the polynomial reconstruction (9) fulfills the shape preserving property, namely,*

- *$p_i(x)$ is monotone in $[x_{i-1/2}, x_{i+1/2}]$ iff the point values $\{v_{i-1}, v_i, v_{i+1}\}$ are;*
- *$p_i(x)$ generates an extremum in the interior of $[x_{i-1/2}, x_{i+1/2}]$ iff v_i is an extremum value.*

The proof of this theorem can be found in [16]. According to this property, the polynomial $p_i(x)$ does not create new extrema in the interior of $[x_{i-1/2}, x_{i+1/2}]$. In other words, the polynomial $p_i(x)$ may create new extrema at the interfaces $\{x_{i\pm1/2}\}$. To keep away from such spurious extrema, we can employ a similar strategy as in [17]. Let us modify the polynomial reconstruction to be the following form:

$$\varphi_i(x) = (1-\theta_i)v_i + \theta_i p_i(x), \quad 0 < \theta_i < 1. \tag{11}$$

The limiter θ_i is determined by

$$\theta_i = \begin{cases} \min\left\{ \frac{M_{i+1/2}-v_i}{M_i-v_i}, \frac{m_{i-1/2}-v_i}{m_i-v_i}, 1 \right\}, & \text{if} \quad v_{i-1} < v_i < v_{i+1}, \\ \min\left\{ \frac{M_{i-1/2}-v_i}{M_i-v_i}, \frac{m_{i+1/2}-v_i}{m_i-v_i}, 1 \right\}, & \text{if} \quad v_{i-1} > v_i > v_{i+1}, \\ 1, & \text{otherwise}, \end{cases} \tag{12}$$

with

$$M_i = \max_{x\in[x_{i-1/2},x_{i+1/2}]} p_i(x), \quad m_i = \min_{x\in[x_{i-1/2},x_{i+1/2}]} p_i(x),$$

and

$$\begin{cases} M_{i\pm1/2} = \max\left\{ \frac{1}{2}(v_i + v_{i\pm1}), p_{i\pm1}(x_{i\pm1/2}) \right\}, \\ m_{i\pm1/2} = \min\left\{ \frac{1}{2}(v_i + v_{i\pm1}), p_{i\pm1}(x_{i\pm1/2}) \right\}. \end{cases}$$

Theorem 2. *The polynomial reconstruction (11) is fourth order accurate and fulfills the sign property (8).*

Theorem 3. *With the definitions of the reconstructed values $v^+_{i+1/2} = \varphi_{i+1}(x_{i+1/2})$ and $v^-_{i+1/2} = \varphi_i(x_{i+1/2})$, the numerical flux (6) is entropy stable and fourth order accurate.*

Remark 1. *The proofs for Theorems 2 and 3 can be carried out very similarly as in [12,17]. We omit the simple but trivial procedure here.*

Remark 2. *For hyperbolic systems, the reconstruction procedure should be implemented in the local characteristic directions for the purpose of achieving entropy stability. The detailed steps can be found in our previous paper [12].*

3. Numerical Examples

In this section, we illustrate the effectiveness of the presented scheme which is abbreviated by ES4 by means of three typical examples. Numerical results include the convergence order and the capacity of dealing with discontinuous problems.

Example 1. *Consider the linear advection equation $u_t + u_x = 0$ on the domain $[-1, 1]$ with two initial data $u(x, 0) = sin(\pi x)$ and $u(x, 0) = sin^4(\pi x)$. For a comparison, a third order entropy stable scheme (ES3) [12] is also implemented for this example. The numerical errors (L^1 error and L^∞ error) and convergence orders are displayed in Tables 1 and 2. We can observe that the fourth order convergence of the proposed scheme is confirmed and ES4 performs better than ES3.*

Table 1. The numerical errors and convergence orders for $u_t + u_x = 0$ with $u(x,0) = sin(\pi x)$ at $t = 8$.

Method	N	L^1 Error	L^1 Order	L^∞ Error	L^∞ Order
ES3	40	7.8941×10^{-3}	2.9838	6.1563×10^{-3}	2.9528
	80	9.8686×10^{-4}	2.9999	7.7371×10^{-4}	2.9922
	160	1.2332×10^{-4}	3.0004	9.6812×10^{-5}	2.9985
	320	1.5413×10^{-5}	3.0002	1.2104×10^{-5}	2.9997
	640	1.9266×10^{-6}	3.0000	1.5131×10^{-6}	2.9999
ES4	40	7.2962×10^{-4}		5.5350×10^{-4}	
	80	4.4746×10^{-5}	4.0273	3.4513×10^{-5}	4.0034
	160	2.7650×10^{-6}	4.0164	2.1523×10^{-6}	4.0032
	320	1.7178×10^{-7}	4.0086	1.3430×10^{-7}	4.0023
	640	1.0702×10^{-8}	4.0046	8.3862×10^{-9}	4.0013

Table 2. The numerical errors and convergence orders for $u_t + u_x = 0$ with $u(x,0) = sin^4(\pi x)$ at $t = 1$.

Method	N	L^1 Error	L^1 Order	L^∞ Error	L^∞ Order
ES3	80	3.8419×10^{-3}		3.7835×10^{-3}	
	160	4.9986×10^{-4}	2.9422	5.8676×10^{-4}	2.6889
	320	6.7841×10^{-5}	2.8813	8.6901×10^{-5}	2.7553
	640	1.0357×10^{-5}	2.7115	1.5669×10^{-5}	2.4715
	1280	1.4533×10^{-6}	2.5625	4.9399×10^{-6}	1.6654
ES4	80	8.1572×10^{-4}		1.2001×10^{-3}	
	160	5.9041×10^{-5}	3.7883	1.4743×10^{-4}	3.0249
	320	4.9006×10^{-6}	3.5907	2.7023×10^{-5}	1.3202
	640	1.6184×10^{-7}	4.9203	1.4716×10^{-7}	7.5207
	1280	1.0013×10^{-8}	4.0146	8.6289×10^{-9}	4.0921

Example 2. *Consider the Burgers equation*

$$u_t + (u^2/2)_x = 0 \tag{13}$$

subjected to the initial data

$$u(x,0) = \begin{cases} 1, & \text{for } |x| \le 1/3, \\ -1, & \text{for } 1/3 < |x| \le 1. \end{cases}$$

For this problem, we can deduce the analytical solution that evolves a rarefaction fan and a stationary shock on the left-hand and right-hand side, respectively. Figure 1 presents the numerical result at time $t = 0.3$ on a mesh of 100 grids. Our scheme resolves the shock wave and the rarefaction wave very well.

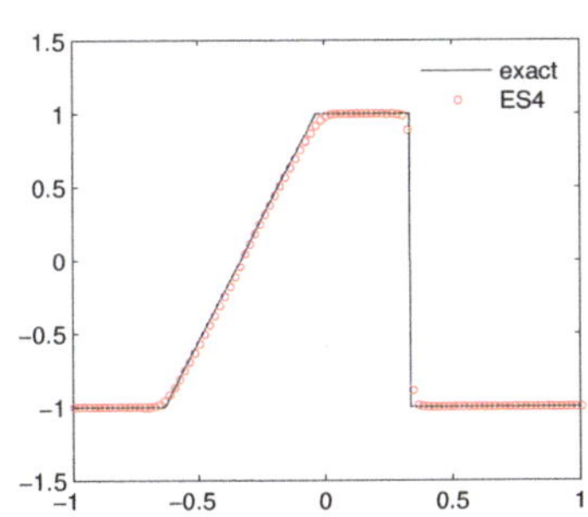

Figure 1. The numerical result for Burgers equation.

Example 3. *Consider the Euler equations from aerodynamics*

$$\frac{\partial}{\partial t}\begin{pmatrix}\rho \\ \rho\mu \\ E\end{pmatrix} + \frac{\partial}{\partial x}\begin{pmatrix}\rho\mu \\ \rho\mu^2 + p \\ \mu(E+p)\end{pmatrix} = 0 \tag{14}$$

with ρ, μ, p and E being the density, velocity, pressure and total energy, respectively. For an idea gas, the total energy E is given by the relation

$$E = \frac{p}{\gamma - 1} + \frac{1}{2}\rho\mu^2 \tag{15}$$

with the specific heats ratio $\gamma = 1.4$. Three Riemann problems are tested by the presented scheme.

Case 1: Sod's shock tube problem. The initial data is given as

$$(\rho, \mu, p) = \begin{cases} (1, 0, 1), & \text{for } x < 0, \\ (0.125, 0, 0.1), & \text{for } x > 0. \end{cases}$$

The numerical simulation is carried out on a mesh of 200 grids on $[-0.5, 0.5]$ up to time $t = 0.16$. The computed density is plotted in Figure 2. We can see that the ES4 scheme performs well by capturing the shock, the contact discontinuity and the rarefaction wave accurately.

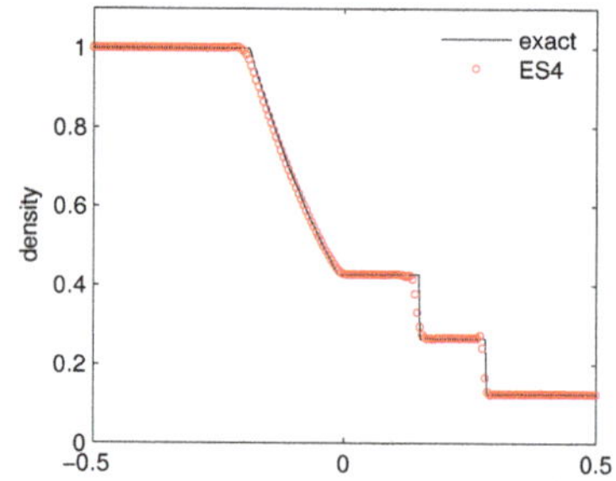

Figure 2. The density for Sod's shock tube problem.

Case 2: Toro's 123 problem. The initial data is given as

$$(\rho, \mu, p) = \begin{cases} (1, -2, 0.4), & \text{for } x < 0, \\ (1, 2, 0.4), & \text{for } x > 0. \end{cases}$$

The difficulty for simulating this problem lies in the fact that the pressure between the evolved rarefactions is very small (near vacuum) and may bring about the blow-ups of the code if the numerical method is not robust. The numerical simulation is carried out on a mesh of 200 grids on $[-0.5, 0.5]$ up to time $t = 0.1$. Figure 3 displays the computed density. It can be observed that the computed result by ES4 compares well with the reference solution.

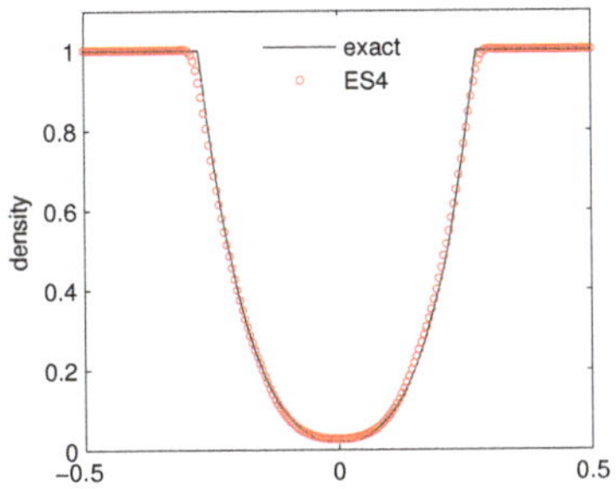

Figure 3. The density for Toro's 123 problem.

Case 3: Shu–Osher problem. The initial data is given as

$$(\rho, \mu, p) = \begin{cases} (3.857, 2.629, 10.333), & \text{for } x < -4, \\ (1 + 0.2\sin(5x), 0, 1), & \text{for } x > -4. \end{cases}$$

This problem, also called the shock density-wave interaction problem, describes a moving Mach 3 shock interacting with sine waves in density. The numerical simulation is carried out on a mesh of 500 grids on $[-5, 5]$ up to time $t = 1.8$. We present the results of density in Figure 4. It can be seen clearly that the ES4 scheme produces accurate results and captures the sine wave well.

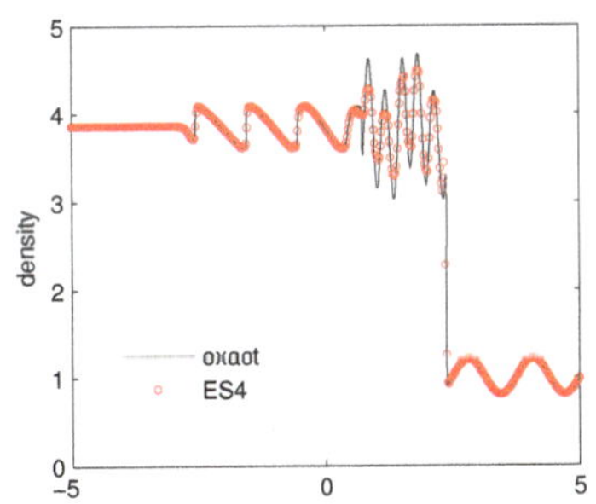

Figure 4. The density for the Shu–Osher problem.

4. Conclusions

This paper presents a fourth order entropy stable scheme for solving one-dimensional hyperbolic conservation laws. Along the lines of [10,12], our scheme is also obtained by utilizing entropy conservative flux in conjunction with suitable numerical diffusion. We first select the existing fourth order entropy conservative scheme based on the combination of the two-point entropy conservative flux. The main novelty lies in the construction of numerical diffusion by presenting a fourth order non-oscillatory reconstruction possessing the sign property. Compared to other high order schemes, the main advantage of our scheme is the entropy stability. Some numerical results are displayed to show the accuracy and shock capturing capacity of our scheme. Ongoing work involves generalizing the idea of this paper to multidimensional cases and other hyperbolic systems such as shallow water equations and magnetohydrodynamic equations.

Funding: This research is supported by the National Natural Science Foundation of China (Grant No. 11601037) and the Natural Science Foundation of Shaanxi Province (Grant No. 2018JQ1027).

Conflicts of Interest: The author declares no conflict of interest.

References

1. Tadmor, E. A review of numerical methods for nonlinear partial differential equations. *Bull. Am. Math. Soc.* **2012**, *49*, 507–554. [CrossRef]
2. Shu, C. High order WENO and DG methods for time-dependent convection-dominated PDEs. *J. Comput. Phys.* **2016**, *316*, 598–613. [CrossRef]
3. Tadmor, E. Entropy stability theory for difference approximations of nonlinear conservation laws and related time-dependent problems. *Acta Numer.* **2003**, *12*, 451–512. [CrossRef]
4. Tadmor, E.; Zhong, W.G. Entropy stable approximations of Navier-Stokes equations with no artificial numerical viscosity. *J. Hyperbolic Differ. Equ.* **2006**, *3*, 529–559. [CrossRef]
5. Ismail, F.; Roe, P.L. Affordable, entropy-consistent Euler flux functions II: Entropy production at shocks. *J. Comput. Phys.* **2009**, *228*, 5410–5436. [CrossRef]
6. Fjordholm, U.S.; Mishra, S.; Tadmor, E. Well-balanced and energy stable schemes for the shallow water equations with discontinuous topography. *J. Comput. Phys.* **2011**, *230*, 5587–5609. [CrossRef]
7. Chandrashekar, P.; Klingenberg, C. Entropy stable finite volume scheme for ideal compressible MHD on 2-D Cartesian meshes. *SIAM J. Numer. Anal.* **2016**, *54*, 1313–1340. [CrossRef]
8. Liu, Y.; Feng, J.; Ren, J. High Resolution, Entropy-Consistent Scheme Using Flux Limiter for Hyperbolic Systems of Conservation Laws. *J. Sci. Comput.* **2015**, *64*, 914–937. [CrossRef]
9. Dubey, R.K.; Biswas, B. Suitable diffusion for constructing non-oscillatory entropy stable schemes. *J. Comput. Phys.* **2018**, *372*, 912–930. [CrossRef]
10. Fjordholm, U.S.; Mishra, S.; Tadmor, E. Arbitrarily high-order accurate entropy stable essentially nonoscillatory schemes for systems of conservation laws. *SIAM J. Numer. Anal.* **2012**, *50*, 544–573. [CrossRef]
11. Fjordholm, U.S.; Mishra, S.; Tadmor, E. ENO reconstruction and ENO interpolation are stable. *Found. Comput. Math.* **2013**, *13*, 139–159. [CrossRef]
12. Cheng, X.; Nie, Y. A third order entropy stable scheme for hyperbolic conservation laws. *J. Hyperbolic Differ. Equ.* **2016**, *13*, 129–145. [CrossRef]
13. Fjordholm, U.S.; Ray, D. A Sign Preserving WENO Reconstruction Method. *J. Sci. Comput.* **2016**, *68*, 42–63. [CrossRef]
14. Biswas, B.; Dubey, R.K. Low dissipative entropy stable schemes using third order WENO and TVD reconstructions. *Adv. Comput. Math.* **2018**, *44*, 1153–1181. [CrossRef]
15. Lefloch, P.G.; Mercier, J.M.; Rohde, C. Fully discrete, entropy conservative schemes of arbitrary order. *SIAM J. Numer. Anal.* **2002**, *40*, 1968–1992. [CrossRef]
16. Balaguer, A.; Conde, C. Fourth-order nonoscillatory upwind and central schemes for hyperbolic conservation laws. *SIAM J. Numer. Anal.* **2005**, *43*, 455–473. [CrossRef]
17. Liu, X.D.; Osher, S. Nonoscillatory high order accurate self-similar maximum principle satisfying shock capturing schemes I. *SIAM J. Numer. Anal.* **1996**, *33*, 760–779. [CrossRef]

entropy

MDPI

Article

Spin Isoenergetic Process and the Lindblad Equation

Congjie Ou [1], Yuho Yokoi [2] and Sumiyoshi Abe [1,2,3,4,*]

1 Physics Division, College of Information Science and Engineering, Huaqiao University, Xiamen 361021, China; jcou@hqu.edu.cn
2 Department of Physical Engineering, Mie University, Mie 514-8507, Japan; yuho_451@yahoo.co.jp
3 Institute of Physics, Kazan Federal University, 420008 Kazan, Russia
4 ESIEA, 9 Rue Vesale, 75005 Paris, France
* Correspondence: suabe@sf6.so-net.ne.jp

Received: 21 March 2019; Accepted: 6 May 2019; Published: 17 May 2019

Abstract: A general comment is made on the existence of various baths in quantum thermodynamics, and a brief explanation is presented about the concept of weak invariants. Then, the isoenergetic process is studied for a spin in a magnetic field that slowly varies in time. In the Markovian approximation, the corresponding Lindbladian operators are constructed without recourse to detailed information about the coupling of the subsystem with the environment called the energy bath. The entropy production rate under the resulting Lindblad equation is shown to be positive. The leading-order expressions of the power output and work done along the isoenergetic process are obtained.

Keywords: quantum thermodynamics of spin; weak invariants; isoenergetic process; Lindblad equation

1. Introduction

Besides its importance for nanoscience, nanotechnology and quantum engineering in general, quantum thermodynamics has a particular status in contemporary physics. It sheds fresh light on both classical and quantum theories. For instance, the quantum-mechanical violation of the law of equipartition of energy seems to require careful reexaminations of even the isothermal process of the ideal gas. It is also the case for the connection between the adiabatic and isoentropic processes. Classical mechanics is described by a set of dynamical variables, whereas quantum mechanics contains not only dynamical variables but also the Hilbert space. Accordingly, quantum mechanics may lead to novel concepts that have no counterparts in classical thermodynamics. The dephasing bath [1] and energy bath [2,3] can be thought of as typical such examples. Therefore, it is of significance to elucidate the implications of such baths to thermodynamics.

In the present paper, we develop a discussion about the isoenergetic process associated with the energy bath within the framework of finite-time quantum thermodynamics. We employ a single Pauli spin in a time-dependent magnetic field and describe its nonequilibrium subdynamics based on the Lindblad equation [4,5], which is known to be unique in the Markovian approximation. It is shown how the Lindbladian operators can be determined without detailed information about the interaction between the subsystem and the energy bath. The resulting subdynamics is seen to be unital [6] and accordingly has a non-negative entropy production rate. The power output and work done are evaluated in the leading order.

The paper is organized as follows. In Section 2, a succinct explanation is presented about the concept of weak invariants, which is directly connected to the isoenergetic process. In Section 3, the Lindbladian operators are determined for the Pauli spin in a time-dependent magnetic field, and the entropy production rate under the Lindblad equation thus obtained is discussed. Then, based on the result in Section 3, finite-time thermodynamics of the power output and work in the leading order is studied in Section 4. Section 5 is devoted to concluding remarks.

2. Weak Invariant and Isoenergetic Process

The concept of weak invariants has wide universality. Let us consider a master equation

$$i\hbar \frac{\partial \rho}{\partial t} = \pounds(\rho) \tag{1}$$

for the density matrix ρ describing the state of a quantum subsystem, where $\pounds$ is a certain linear superoperator. Henceforth, $\hbar$ is set equal to unity for the sake of simplicity. Then, a weak invariant $I = I(t)$ associated with this master equation is defined as a solution of the following equation [7]:

$$i\frac{\partial I}{\partial t} + \pounds^{*}(I) = 0. \tag{2}$$

In this equation, $\pounds^{*}$ stands for the adjoint of $\pounds$ defined by tr $(Q\,\pounds(R)) = \mathrm{tr}(\pounds^{*}(Q)\,R)$, provided that $Q\,\pounds(R)$ and therefore also $\pounds^{*}(Q)\,R]$ should be trace-class. Then, it follows from Equations (1) and (2) that the expectation value of I is conserved:

$$\frac{d\langle I\rangle}{dt} = 0 \tag{3}$$

with the notation $\langle Q\rangle \equiv \mathrm{tr}(Q\rho)$, although the spectrum of I is time-dependent, in general.

Our purpose is to clarify the implication of the energy bath to quantum thermodynamics. For it, what to be contemplated is the isoenergetic processes, along which the internal energy of the subsystem is kept constant through energy transfer between the subsystem and the energy bath. A point is that the energy transfer that may be realized not in the form of heat but rather in the dynamical manner [8,9].

The isoenergetic processes have been discussed for a "three-stroke" engine [3,10], in which however no explicit time evolution of the subsystem has been considered. In view of finite-time quantum thermodynamics, a density matrix evolves in time according to a master equation. Here, let us assume Markovianity of the subdynamics. In this case, the superoperator in Equation (1) has the Lindblad form [4,5]:

$$\pounds(\rho) = [H(t),\, \rho] - \frac{i}{2}\sum_i a_i\left(L_i^{\dagger} L_i\, \rho + \rho\, L_i^{\dagger} L_i - 2L_i\rho L_i^{\dagger}\right), \tag{4}$$

where $H(t)$ is the time-dependent Hamiltonian and a_i's are nonnegative c-number coefficients. Both the coefficients and the Lindbladian operators L_i's may also depend on time, explicitly.

The weak invariant relevant to the isoenergetic process is the time-dependent Hamiltonian itself. Thus, the internal energy

$$U = \mathrm{tr}(H(t)\,\rho) \tag{5}$$

is required to be conserved under time evolution generated by the Lindblad equation. Such a condition is fulfilled if the Hamiltonian obeys the following equation:

$$\frac{\partial H(t)}{\partial t} - \frac{1}{2}\sum_i a_i\left(L_i^{\dagger} L_i\, H(t) + H(t)\, L_i^{\dagger} L_i - 2L_i^{\dagger}\, H(t)\, L_i\right) = 0, \tag{6}$$

which comes from Equation (2) with Equation (4).

In general, it is a nontrivial task to determine the Lindbladian operators in Equations (4) and (6), since it needs detailed knowledge of how the subsystem interacts with the environment. However, Equation (6) tends to make it possible to determine them without such knowledge [11].

Closing this section, we make some comments on the concept of weak invariants. Firstly, it has recently been discovered [12] that there exists a connection between weak invariants and the action principle for corresponding master equations. Secondly, such quantities clearly have their classical analogs. For instance, a weak invariant associated with the classical Fokker-Planck equation is discussed in Reference [13]. Thirdly, it is worth mentioning that the Lindblad equation with a time-dependent Hamiltonian can describe the dynamics toward an "instantaneous attractor" in the nonadiabatic regime [14], inside which isoenergeticity is realized.

3. Weak Invariant of Spin in Time-Dependent Magnetic Field and Lindbladian Operators

In recent years, quantum thermodynamics of a two-level system has been discussed in the literature [15,16]. Here, we consider a single spin in a time-dependent magnetic field $\mathbf{B}(t)$. The Hamiltonian reads

$$H(t) = \mathbf{B}(t) \cdot \sigma \tag{7}$$

with σ being the Pauli-matrix vector. The constant involving the gyromagnetic ratio is set equal to unity. In the thermodynamic context, variation of the magnetic field should be slow. That is, the time scale of the variation is much longer than those of relaxation and quantum dynamics.

From the linearity of Equation (6) with respect to the Hamiltonian and the su(2) Lie algebra of the spin, it is natural to examine the following Lindbladian operators:

$$L_i = \sigma_i \; (i = 1,\, 2,\, 3). \tag{8}$$

These are Hermitian, and accordingly the subdynamics is unital [6]. Substituting Equation (8) into Equation (6) and using linear independence of the Pauli matrices, we have

$$\dot{\mathbf{B}}(t) = -2\,A\,\mathbf{B}(t) + 2c\,\mathbf{B}(t), \tag{9}$$

where the overdot denotes differentiation with respect to time, and A and c are given by

$$A = \begin{pmatrix} a_1 & 0 & 0 \\ 0 & a_2 & 0 \\ 0 & 0 & a_3 \end{pmatrix}, \tag{10}$$

$$c = \operatorname{tr} A = a_1 + a_2 + a_3, \tag{11}$$

respectively. From Equation (9), we see that

$$\mathbf{B}(t) \cdot \dot{\mathbf{B}}(t) = 2(a_2 + a_3)\, B_1^2(t) + 2(a_3 + a_1)\, B_2^2(t) + 2(a_1 + a_2)\, B_3^2(t), \tag{12}$$

which is positive since a_i's are nonnegative and not all of them can be zero. Therefore, the magnitude $B(t) = |\mathbf{B}(t)|$ has to monotonically increase in time. In addition, from Equation (9), we find the coefficients to be given by

$$a_1 = \frac{1}{4}\left(-\frac{\dot{B}_1}{B_1} + \frac{\dot{B}_2}{B_2} + \frac{\dot{B}_3}{B_3}\right),\; a_2 = \frac{1}{4}\left(\frac{\dot{B}_1}{B_1} - \frac{\dot{B}_2}{B_2} + \frac{\dot{B}_3}{B_3}\right),\; a_3 = \frac{1}{4}\left(\frac{\dot{B}_1}{B_1} + \frac{\dot{B}_2}{B_2} - \frac{\dot{B}_3}{B_3}\right). \tag{13}$$

Thus, without detailed information about the interaction between the subsystem and the environment, the explicit form of the Lindblad equation is now fully determined as follows:

$$i\frac{\partial \rho}{\partial t} = [H(t),\, \rho] - \frac{i}{2}\sum_{i=1}^{3} a_i[\sigma_i,\, [\sigma_i,\, \rho]]. \tag{14}$$

We note that the second term on the right-hand side, termed the dissipator, is small and is of the order $\dot{B}_i(t)$'s. Equation (14) belongs to a class of finite-level systems in contact with a singular reservoir consisting of particles with the vanishing correlation time [17]. On the other hand, what is peculiar here is highlighted in Equation (13) that purely comes from isoenergeticity, without recourse to the detailed property of the energy bath.

Hermiticity of the Lindbladian operators in Equation (8), or equivalently the fact that the subdynamics is unital, can have a significant implication for the isoenergetic process. As shown in Reference [18] (see, also Reference [11] and a discussion generalized to the Rényi entropy in Reference [19]), time evolution of the von Neumann entropy

$$S\,[\rho] = -\mathrm{tr}\,(\rho \ln \rho) \tag{15}$$

under the Lindblad equation in its general form in Equation (1) with Equation (4) satisfies

$$\frac{d\,S}{d\,t} = \sum_i a_i \Gamma_i, \tag{16}$$

$$\Gamma_i \geq \left\langle \left[L_i^{\dagger},\, L_i \right] \right\rangle, \tag{17}$$

where the Boltzmann constant is set equal to unity. Since the Lindbladian operators in the present case are Hermitian, the subdynamics tends to produce the entropy in time,

$$\frac{d\,S}{d\,t} \geq 0, \tag{18}$$

as desired.

4. Temporally-Local Equilibrium State, Power Output and Work along Isoenergetic Process

A nonequilibrium thermodynamic system with a slowly-varying Hamiltonian is dominantly described by a locally-equilibrium state, in which the thermodynamic variables also vary slowly. In the present case, what is relevant is the temporally-local equilibrium state given by

$$\rho^{(0)} = \frac{1}{Z\,(t)} \exp\,(-\beta(t) H(t)), \tag{19}$$

where $Z(t)$ is the partition function

$$Z(t) = \mathrm{tr}\ \exp(-\beta(t)\, H(t)). \tag{20}$$

$\beta(t)$ is the time-dependent inverse temperature that slowly varies in time [see Equation (26) below].

For the Hamiltonian in Equation (7), the explicit expression of Equation (19) is the familiar one

$$\rho^{(0)} = \frac{1}{2}\{I - (\mathbf{n}(t)\cdot\sigma)\tanh(\beta(t)\; B(t))\}, \tag{21}$$

where I is the 2×2 unit matrix and $\mathbf{n}(t)$ is a unit vector defined by $\mathbf{n}(t) = \mathbf{B}(t)/B(t)$.

The full density matrix may be expanded around the state in Equation (21) as follows:

$$\rho = \rho^{(0)} + \rho^{(1)} + \cdots, \tag{22}$$

where the expansion should be performed in terms of the elements of $\dot{\mathbf{B}}(t)$ and its higher-order derivatives. It is natural to assume that all of the correction terms are traceless. Substituting Equation (22) into Equation (14), the first-order correction is found to satisfy

$$\left[H(t),\, \rho^{(1)}\right] = i\,\frac{\partial\,\rho^{(0)}}{\partial\,t} + \frac{i}{2}\sum_{i=1}^{3} a_i \left[\sigma_i,\, \left[\sigma_i,\, \rho^{(0)}\right]\right], \tag{23}$$

for instance.

In accordance with Equation (22), the internal energy is also expanded as follows:

$$U = U^{(0)} + U^{(1)} + \cdots. \tag{24}$$

The isoenergeticity condition should be satisfied in each order. For the leading-order term

$$U^{(0)} = \mathrm{tr}\Big(H(t)\,\rho^{\,(0)}\Big) = -B(t)\,\tanh(\beta(t)\,B(t)), \tag{25}$$

we find that the isoenergeticity condition, $dU^{(0)}/d\,t = 0$, in the leading order gives rise to

$$\dot{B}(t)\,[\sinh(2\beta(t)\,B(t)) + 2\beta(t)\,B(t)] = -2B^{\,2}(t)\,\dot{\beta}(t). \tag{26}$$

Since $\dot{B}(t)$ is positive due to Equation (12) resulting from the Lindblad equation, $\dot{\beta}(t)$ is necessarily negative, implying that the temperature monotonically increases in time.

Now, let us discuss the power output defined by

$$P(t) = -\mathrm{tr}\left(\dot{H}(t)\,\rho\right). \tag{27}$$

The leading-order contribution comes from the temporally-local equilibrium state and is calculated to be

$$P(t) = -\,\dot{\mathbf{B}}(t)\cdot \mathrm{tr}\left(\sigma\,\rho^{(0)}\right) = \dot{\mathbf{B}}(t)\cdot \mathbf{n}(t)\,\tanh(\beta(t)\,B(t)). \tag{28}$$

An interesting point is that, similarly to the case of the time-dependent harmonic oscillator [20], this quantity can be expressed in terms of the internal energy as follows:

$$P(t) = -\frac{\dot{B}(t)}{B(t)}\,U^{\,(0)}. \tag{29}$$

From this expression, the work done during the time interval $t_{\,i} \le t \le t_f$ along the isoenergetic process is given, in the leading order, by

$$W = \int_{t_i}^{t_f} dt\; P(t) = -\,U^{\,(0)}(t_i) \int_{t_i}^{t_f} dt\, \frac{\dot{B}(t)}{B(t)} = B(t_i)\tanh(\beta(t_i)\,B(t_i))\;\ln\!\left[\frac{B(t_f)}{B(t_i)}\right], \tag{30}$$

where the initial value is used for the conserved internal energy.

5. Concluding Remarks

Toward clarifications of the physical properties of exotic baths present in quantum thermodynamics but absent in classical thermodynamics, we have focused our attention on the isoenergetic process that is connected with the energy bath. For this purpose, we have studied a single spin in a magnetic field slowly varying in time based on the Lindblad equation. We have shown how the isoenergeticity condition can determine the Lindbladian operators without recourse to detailed knowledge of the interaction between the subsystem and the energy bath. We have developed a discussion about finite-time thermodynamics of such a system and evaluated the power output and the work in the leading order.

The result given in Equation (30) implies that the work is determined only by the initial and final values of the variables without depending on paths of the magnetic field in the parameter **B**-space. This would be a common feature of the isoenergetic processes in the leading order.

In the present work, we have treated a single Pauli spin. As known, by virtue of the structure of spin algebra, any density matrix of a multispin system can be expanded in terms of the spin matrices, their tensor products as well as the unit matrix. Therefore, the temporally-local equilibrium state in Equation (21) can be generalized to the multispin case [21].

Here, we have considered only the energy bath, which is nothing but one of the exotic baths in quantum thermodynamics. Existence of various baths indicates that there may be ensemble-dependent dynamics. In this point, it is worth mentioning that such dynamics are also suggested in nanothermodynamics of classical small systems, in which fluctuations can be very large [22,23]. Much is yet to be clarified about the quantum-classical correspondence in thermodynamics.

Author Contributions: S.A. has provided the idea of the study, performed the calculations and written the manuscript. C.O. and Y.Y. have checked the calculations, made the critical comments and contributed to the improvement of the manuscript. All authors have read and approved the final manuscript.

Funding: The authors would like to thank the support by a grant from the National Natural Science Foundation of China (No. 11775084). The work of S.A. has also been supported in part by the programs of Fujian Province, China, and of Competitive Growth of Kazan Federal University from the Ministry of Education and Science, Russian Federation.

Acknowledgments: This work has been completed while S.A. has stayed at the Wigner Research Centre for Physics with the support of the Distinguished Guest Fellowship of the Hungarian Academy of Sciences. He would like to express his sincere thanks to the Wigner Research Centre for Physics for the warm hospitality extended to him.

Conflicts of Interest: The authors declare no conflict of interest.

References

1. Giusteri, G.G.; Recrosi, F.; Schaller, G.; Celardo, G.L. Interplay of different environments in open quantum systems: Breakdown of the additive approximation. *Phys. Rev. E* **2017**, *96*, 012113. [CrossRef]
2. Wang, J.; He, J.; He, X. Performance analysis of a two-state quantum heat engine working with a single-mode radiation field in a cavity. *Phys. Rev. E* **2011**, *84*, 041127. [CrossRef]
3. Liu, S.; Ou, C. Maximum power output of quantum heat engine with energy bath. *Entropy* **2016**, *18*, 205. [CrossRef]
4. Lindblad, G. On the generators of quantum dynamical semigroups. *Commun. Math. Phys.* **1976**, *48*, 119–130. [CrossRef]
5. Gorini, V.; Kossakowski, A.; Sudarshan, E.C.G. Completely positive dynamical semigroups of *N*-level systems. *J. Math. Phys.* **1976**, *17*, 821–825. [CrossRef]
6. Bhatia, R. *Matrix Analysis*; Springer: New York, NY, USA, 1997.
7. Abe, S. Weak invariants of time-dependent quantum dissipative systems. *Phys. Rev. A* **2016**, *94*, 032116. [CrossRef]
8. Gorman, D.J.; Hemmerling, B.; Megidish, E.; Moeller, S.A.; Schindler, P.; Sarovar, M.; Haeffner, H. Engineering vibrationally assisted energy transfer in a trapped-ion quantum simulator. *Phys. Rev. X* **2018**, *8*, 011038. [CrossRef]
9. Henao, I.; Serra, R.M. Role of quantum coherence in the thermodynamics of energy transfer. *Phys. Rev. E* **2018**, *97*, 062105. [CrossRef]
10. Ou, C.; Abe, S. Exotic properties and optimal control of quantum heat engine. *EPL* **2016**, *113*, 40009. [CrossRef]
11. Ou, C.; Chamberlin, R.V.; Abe, S. Lindbladian operators, von Neumann entropy and energy conservation in time-dependent quantum open systems. *Physica A* **2017**, *466*, 450–454. [CrossRef]
12. Abe, S.; Ou, C. Action principle and weak invariants. *Results Phys.* **2019**. [CrossRef]
13. Abe, S. Invariants of Fokker-Planck equations. *Eur. Phys. J. Special Topics* **2017**, *226*, 529–532. [CrossRef]
14. Dann, R.; Levy, A.; Kosloff, R. Time-dependent Markovian quantum master equation. *Phys. Rev. A* **2018**, *98*, 052129. [CrossRef]
15. Kieu, T.D. The second law, Maxwell's demon, and work derivable from quantum heat engines. *Phys. Rev. Lett.* **2004**, *93*, 140403. [CrossRef]
16. Peterson, J.P.S.; Batalhão, T.B.; Herrera, M.; Souza, A.M.; Sarthour, R.S.; Oliveira, I.S.; Serra, R.M. Experimental characterization of a spin quantum heat engine. *arXiv* **2018**, arXiv:1803.06021.

17. Gorini, V.; Kossakowski, A. *N*-level system in contact with a singular reservoir. *J. Math. Phys.* **1976**, *17*, 1298–1305. [CrossRef]
18. Benatti, F.; Narnhofer, H. Entropy behavior under completely positive maps. *Lett. Math. Phys.* **1988**, *15*, 325–334. [CrossRef]
19. Abe, S. Time evolution of Rényi entropy under the Lindblad equation. *Phys. Rev. E* **2016**, *94*, 022106. [CrossRef] [PubMed]
20. Ou, C.; Abe, S. Weak invariants, temporally local equilibria, and isoenergetic processes described by the Lindblad equation. *EPL* **2019**, *125*, 60004. [CrossRef]
21. Kosloff, R.; Feldmann, T. Optimal performance of reciprocating demagnetization quantum refrigerators. *Phys. Rev. E* **2010**, *82*, 011134. [CrossRef]
22. Hill, T.L.; Chamberlin, R.V. Fluctuations in energy in completely open small systems. *Nano Lett.* **2002**, *2*, 609–613. [CrossRef]
23. Chamberlin, R.V. The big world of nanothermodynamics. *Entropy* **2015**, *17*, 52–73. [CrossRef]